Diabetes

Editor

S. SETHU K. REDDY

ENDOCRINOLOGY AND METABOLISM CLINICS OF NORTH AMERICA

www.endo.theclinics.com

Consulting Editors
ANAT BEN-SHLOMO
MARIA FLESERIU

December 2016 • Volume 45 • Number 4

ELSEVIER

1600 John F. Kennedy Boulevard ● Suite 1800 ● Philadelphia, Pennsylvania, 19103-2899

http://www.theclinics.com

ENDOCRINOLOGY AND METABOLISM CLINICS OF NORTH AMERICA Volume 45, Number 4
December 2016 ISSN 0889-8529, ISBN 13: 978-0-323-47738-3

Editor: Lauren Boyle
Developmental Editor: Meredith Clinton

Endocrinology and Metabolism Clinics of North America (ISSN 0889-8529) is published quarterly by Elsevier Inc., 360 Park Avenue South, New York, NY 10010-1710. Months of issue are March, June, September, and December. Periodicals postage paid at New York, NY and additional mailing offices. Subscription prices are USD 330.00 per year for US individuals, USD 636.00 per year for US institutions, USD 100.00 per year for US students and residents, USD 415.00 per year for Canadian individuals, USD 787.00 per year for Canadian institutions, USD 480.00 per year for international individuals, USD 787.00 per year for international institutions, and USD 245.00 per year for international and Canadian and foreign students/residents. To receive student/resident rate, orders must be accompanied by name of affiliated institution, date of term, and the signature of program/residency coordinator on institution letterhead. Orders will be billed at individual rate until proof of status is received. Foreign air speed delivery is included in all *Clinics* subscription prices. All prices are subject to change without notice. **POSTMASTER:** Send address changes to *Endocrinology and Metabolism Clinics of North America*, Elsevier Health Sciences Division, Subscription Customer Service, 3251 Riverport Lane, Maryland Heights, MO 63043. **Customer Service: Telephone: 1-800-654-2452** (U.S. and Canada); **1-314-447-8871** (outside U.S. and Canada). **Fax: 1-314-447-8029. E-mail: journalscustomerservice-usa@elsevier.com (for print support); journalsonlinesupport-usa@elsevier.com (for online support)**.

Reprints. For copies of 100 or more, of articles in this publication, please contact the Commercial Rights Department, Elsevier Inc., 360 Park Avenue South, New York, NY 10010-1710; phone: +1-212-633-3874; fax: +1-212-633-3820; E-mail: reprints@elsevier.com.

Endocrinology and Metabolism Clinics of North America is covered in *MEDLINE/PubMed (Index Medicus), EMBASE/Excerpta Medica, Current Contents/Clinical Medicine, Current Contents/Life Sciences, Science Citation Index, ISI/BIOMED, BIOSIS,* and *Chemical Abstracts.*

Contributors

CONSULTING EDITORS

ANAT BEN-SHLOMO, MD
Pituitary Center, Division of Endocrinology Diabetes, and Metabolism, Cedars Sinai Medical Center, Los Angeles, California

MARIA FLESERIU, MD, FACE
Division of Endocrinology, Diabetes, & Clinical Nutrition, Departments of Medicine and Neurological Surgery, Northwest Pituitary Center, Oregon Health and Science University, Portland, Oregon

EDITOR

S. SETHU K. REDDY, MD, MBA, FRCPC, FACP, MACE
Senior Consultant, Endocrinology, Diabetes & Metabolism, Cleveland Clinic, Cleveland, Ohio

AUTHORS

HUSSAIN ALQURAINI, MD
Fellow, Division of Metabolism, Endocrinology and Diabetes, Department of Internal Medicine, University of Michigan, Ann Arbor, Michigan

SIDRA AZIM, MD
Department of Endocrinology, Diabetes, and Metabolism, Cleveland Clinic, Cleveland, Ohio

MOHD-YUSOF BARAKATUN-NISAK, PhD
Joslin Diabetes Center, Harvard Medical School, Boston, Massachusetts; Department of Nutrition and Dietetics, Faculty of Medicine and Health Sciences, Universiti Putra Malaysia, Serdang, Selangor, Malaysia

RICHARD S. BEASER, MD
Associate Professor of Medicine, Harvard Medical School; Senior Staff Physician and Chair, Continuing Medical Education Committee, Joslin Diabetes Center, Boston, Massachusetts

FERNANDO BRIL, MD
Assistant Scientist, Division of Endocrinology, Diabetes and Metabolism, Department of Medicine, University of Florida College of Medicine, Gainesville, Florida

KENNETH CUSI, MD, FACP, FACE
Professor of Medicine; Chief, Division of Endocrinology, Diabetes and Metabolism, Department of Medicine, University of Florida College of Medicine; Division of Endocrinology, Diabetes, and Metabolism, Malcom Randall Veterans Affairs Medical Center, Gainesville, Florida

ANDJELA DRINCIC, MD, FACP
Associate Professor of Medicine, Medical Director of Diabetes Center, Nebraska Medicine, Diabetes Center, Omaha, Nebraska

CATHERINE M. EDWARDS, MD
Associate Professor of Medicine, Division of Endocrinology, Diabetes and Metabolism, Department of Medicine, University of Florida College of Medicine, Gainesville, Florida

HERMES FLOREZ, MD, PhD
Miami Veterans Affairs Medical Center, University of Miami Miller School of Medicine, Miami, Florida

ROBERT GABBAY, MD, PhD
Chief Medical Officer and Senior Vice President; Associate Professor of Medicine, Joslin Diabetes Center, Lipid Clinic, Adult Diabetes, Boston, Massachusetts

ABHIMANYU GARG, MD
Professor, Division of Nutrition and Metabolic Diseases, Department of Internal Medicine, Center for Human Nutrition, University of Texas Southwestern Medical Center, Dallas, Texas

JUAN P. GONZÁLEZ-RIVAS, MD
The Andes Clinic of Cardio-Metabolic Studies, Timotes, Venezuela

DEBORAH GREENWOOD, PhD, RN, CDE, FAADE
Diabetes Program Director, Sutter Health Integrated Diabetes Education Network, Clinical Performance Improvement Consultant & Research Scientist, Quality and Clinical Effectiveness Team, Office of Patient Experience, Sutter Health, Sacramento, California

OSAMA HAMDY, MD, PhD, FACE
Department of Endocrinology, Joslin Diabetes Center, Harvard Medical School, Boston, Massachusetts

BETUL HATIPOGLU, MD
Clinical Associate Professor of Medicine, Endocrinology and Metabolism Institute, Cleveland Clinic, Cleveland, Ohio

IRAM HUSSAIN, MD
Assistant Professor, Division of Endocrinology, Department of Internal Medicine, University of Texas Southwestern Medical Center, Dallas, Texas

SANGEETA R. KASHYAP, MD
Department of Endocrinology, Diabetes, and Metabolism, Cleveland Clinic, Cleveland, Ohio

NATASHA B. KHAZAI, MD
Joslin Diabetes Center, Boston, Massachusetts

DAVID C. KLONOFF, MD, FACP, FRCP (Edin)
Fellow AIMBE; Medical Director, Diabetes Research Institute, Mills-Peninsula Health Services, San Mateo, California

MARK MacEACHERN, MLIS
Informationist, Taubman Health Sciences Library, University of Michigan, Ann Arbor, Michigan

JEFFREY I. MECHANICK, MD
Division of Endocrinology, Diabetes, and Bone Disease, Icahn School of Medicine at Mount Sinai, New York, New York

JOANNA MITRI, MD, MS
Research Associate, Joslin Diabetes Center, Lipid Clinic, Adult Diabetes, Boston, Massachusetts

KARA MIZOKAMI-STOUT, MD
Fellow, Division of Metabolism, Endocrinology and Diabetes, Department of Internal Medicine, University of Michigan, Ann Arbor, Michigan

RAMFIS NIETO-MARTÍNEZ, MD, MSc
Department of Physiology, School of Medicine, Universidad Centro-Occidental "Lisandro Alvarado" and Cardiometabolic Unit, Barquisimeto, Venezuela; Department of Physiology, School of Medicine, University of Panamá, Panama City, Panamá

PRIYA PRAHALAD, MD, PhD
Clinical Instructor, Division of Endocrinology and Diabetes, Pediatrics, Stanford University, Stanford, California

S. SETHU K. REDDY, MD, MBA, FRCPC, FACP, MACE
Senior Consultant, Endocrinology, Diabetes & Metabolism, Cleveland Clinic, Cleveland, Ohio

ALISSA R. SEGAL, PharmD, CDE, CDTC, FCCP
Associate Professor of Pharmacy Practice, Department of Pharmacy Practice, MCPHS University; Clinical Pharmacist, Joslin Diabetes Center, Boston, Massachusetts

MENG H. TAN, MD
Professor of Internal Medicine, Division of Metabolism, Endocrinology and Diabetes, Department of Internal Medicine, University of Michigan, Ann Arbor, Michigan

ELENA TOSCHI, MD
Joslin Diabetes Center, Adult Section, Boston, Massachusetts

TEJASWI VOOTLA, MD
Research Associate, Joslin Diabetes Center, Boston, Massachusetts

HOWARD WOLPERT, MD
Joslin Diabetes Center, Adult Section, Boston, Massachusetts

Contents

Prediabetes, defined by blood glucose levels between normal and diabetic levels, is increasing rapidly worldwide. This abnormal physiologic state reflects the rapidly changing access to high-calorie food and decreasing levels of physical activity occurring worldwide, with resultant obesity and metabolic consequences. This is particularly marked in developing countries. Prediabetes poses several threats; there is increased risk of developing type 2 diabetes mellitus (T2DM), and there are risks inherent to the prediabetes state, including microvascular and macrovascular disease. Studies have helped to elucidate the underlying pathophysiology of prediabetes and to establish the potential for treating prediabetes and preventing T2DM.

Nonalcoholic fatty liver disease (NAFLD) is increasingly common in patients with type 2 diabetes mellitus (T2DM), with an estimated prevalence of 60% to 80%. The relationship of NAFLD and T2DM is complex, with each condition negatively affecting the other. Although NAFLD is associated with more metabolic and cardiovascular complications and worse hyperglycemia, T2DM accelerates the progression of liver disease in NAFLD. Despite the high prevalence and serious clinical implications, NAFLD is usually overlooked in clinical practice. This article focuses on understanding the relationship between NAFLD and T2DM, to provide better care for these complex patients.

Lipodystrophies are heterogeneous disorders characterized by varying degrees of body fat loss and predisposition to insulin resistance and its metabolic complications. They are subclassified depending on degree of fat loss and whether the disorder is genetic or acquired. The two most common genetic varieties include congenital generalized lipodystrophy and familial partial lipodystrophy; the two most common acquired varieties include acquired generalized lipodystrophy and acquired partial lipodystrophy. Highly active antiretroviral therapy–induced lipodystrophy in patients infected with human immunodeficiency virus and drug-induced localized lipodystrophy are common subtypes. The metabolic abnormalities associated with lipodystrophy include insulin resistance, hypertriglyceridemia, and hepatic steatosis. Management focuses on preventing and treating metabolic complications.

Medical nutrition therapy (MNT) is a key component of diabetes management. The importance of balancing macronutrients, reducing carbohydrate load, lowering glycemic index, and implementing an overall healthy dietary pattern are emerging as better approaches for MNT in diabetes. Recent research points to improved glycemic control, reduction in body weight, and improvement in many cardiovascular risk factors when these approaches are provided by registered dietitians or health care providers. This review article discusses the current evidence about the role of sensible nutrition in diabetes management. Specific eating plans for weight reduction and for patients with type 1 diabetes are also discussed.

Metformin is the recommended first-line oral glucose-lowering drug initiated to control hyperglycemia in type 2 diabetes mellitus. It acts in the liver, small intestines, and skeletal muscles with its major effect on decreasing hepatic gluconeogenesis. It is safe, inexpensive, and weight neutral and can be associated with weight loss. It can reduce microvascular complication risk and its use is associated with a lower cardiovascular mortality compared with sulfonylurea therapy. It is also used to delay the onset of type 2 diabetes mellitus, in treating gestational diabetes, and in women with polycystic ovary syndrome.

Newer insulin products have advanced the evolution of insulin replacement options to more accurately mimic natural insulin action. There are new, modified, and concentrated insulins; administration devices calibrated for both increased concentrations and administration accuracy to improve adherence and safety; and inhaled insulin. There are new combinations of longer-acting basal insulin and rapid-acting insulin or glucagon like protein-1 receptor agonists. Existing insulin replacement designs and methods can be updated using these tools to improve efficacy and safety. Individualized decisions to use them should be based on patient physiologic needs, self-care ability, comorbidities, and cost considerations.

In hospitalized patients, both hyperglycemia and hypoglycemia have been associated with poor outcomes. During the inpatient period, hyperglycemia has been associated with increased risk of infection, cardiovascular events, and mortality. It is also associated with longer length of hospital stay. Hypoglycemia has also been associated with an increased risk of mortality. Therefore, current evidence supports avoidance of both conditions among hospitalized patients whether they are admitted to critical care units or noncritical care units.

A consensus conference of the American Association of Clinical Endocrinologists and American College of Endocrinology held in February 2016 advocated expanding the use of continuous glucose monitoring (CGM) in the management of diabetes. Based on the data described in this paper, CGM use is shown to improve glucose control and reduce hypoglycemic events, and therefore has the potential to reduce the risk of acute and chronic complications of diabetes. Likely, all of the above would not only improve the quality of life and life expectancy of people with diabetes, but would also have a positive impact on health-related cost.

Diabetes mellitus and obesity are closely interrelated and pose a major burden on health care in terms of morbidity and mortality. Weight loss has favorable metabolic benefits for glycemic control and improvement of metabolic syndrome. Bariatric surgery (BS) is the most effective treatment for weight loss with durable results as compared to lifestyle modification. BS procedures have been associated with significant reduction in abdominal obesity, metabolic syndrome components, and glycemic control requiring fewer medications. Long-term risks of surgery include nutritional deficiencies, osteoporosis, bone fractures, and hyperinsulinemic hypoglycemia, which need to be carefully balanced with metabolic benefits for individual patients.

Even though type 2 diabetes rates plateaued, type 1 diabetes continues to increase. Pancreas transplantation is a treatment modality for patients who suffer hypoglycemic unawareness or complications from diabetes. Islet cell transplantation success rates have improved with modification and advances in isolation, transplantation, and new immunosuppression regimens. The new cell sources as well as delivery ways are explored and being tested in human trials.

A chronic and progressive illness, diabetes requires early diagnosis, effective coordination of care, and self-management to stem its progression. Population health management strategies hold promise to improve outcomes by focusing on reducing the frequency of acute and chronic complications of chronic disease, lowering the cost per service through an integrated care delivery team approach, and promoting patient engagement. This will ultimately result in a better patient experience. The chronic care model targets fragmentation of our health care delivery system and provides a framework for effective care of diabetes and other chronic diseases.

This article reviews mobile medical applications that are commercially available in the United States or European Union (EU) and are (1) associated with published data of clinical outcomes in the peer-reviewed literature during the past 5 years, (2) cleared by the Food and Drug Administration (FDA) in the United States, or (3) a recipient of a Conformité Européenne (CE) mark by the EU. Many of these applications have been shown to positively affect outcomes in the short term, but long-term studies are needed. Until more data are available, consumers and professionals can consider guidance based on FDA/CE status.

Type-2 diabetes (T2D) needs to be prevented and treated effectively to reduce its burden and consequences. White papers, such as evidence-based clinical practice guidelines (CPG) and their more portable versions, clinical practice algorithms and clinical checklists, may improve clinical decision-making and diabetes outcomes. However, CPG are underused and poorly validated. Protocols that translate and implement these CPG are needed. This review presents the global dimension of T2D, details the importance of white papers in the transculturalization process, compares relevant international CPG, analyzes cultural variables, and summarizes translation strategies that can improve care. Specific protocols and algorithmic tools are provided.

Type 2 diabetes is an expensive public health problem threatening society at many levels. Despite many advances in classification of diabetes, we're still in early stages of developing an etio-pathologic ontology of diabetes.

Recognizing the various biologic and social determinants of disease outcomes, precision medicine applies to medical interventions as well as psychosocial measures, nutrition, and exercise that may also affect individuals differently. Using this highly personalized approach, one hopes to achieve cost-effective care. The striking evolution in generating "Big Data," Biomarker Fingerprints, and the Internet of Things will force all clinicians to be familiar with the terminology and understand the clinical relevance.

ENDOCRINOLOGY AND METABOLISM CLINICS OF NORTH AMERICA

ISSUE OF RELATED INTEREST

Pediatric Clinics, August 2015 (Vol. 62, Issue 4)
Pediatric Endocrinology and Obesity
Denis Daneman and Mark R. Palmert, *Editors*
http://www.pediatric.theclinics.com/

VISIT THE CLINICS ONLINE!
Access your subscription at:
www.theclinics.com

Foreword

Diabetes Mellitus

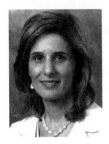 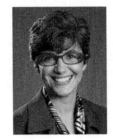

Anat Ben-Shlomo, MD   Maria Fleseriu, MD, FACE
Consulting Editors

Diabetes mellitus (DM) has become a global and costly health problem. In 2015, an estimated 5.5% of the world population had type 2 DM, and the prevalence of type 1 DM in children was reported to increase. Yet, hundreds of billions of dollars have been invested in DM research over the years; the American Diabetes Association alone has invested a staggering sum of $735 million in more than 4500 diabetes research projects since it launched its research programs 64 years ago. This discrepancy between investment and results should make us consider what we have learned about the disease and what changes we need to make in our approach to reverse the upward trend in disease prevalence.

In this issue on Diabetes Mellitus in *Endocrinology and Metabolism Clinics of North America*, our guest editor, Dr Sethu K. Reddy, an internationally recognized authority on DM, has gathered an outstanding group of expert researchers and clinicians to summarize key topics in the field, review current knowledge, and discuss future challenges and new developments; with an aim toward improving prevention, detection, and management of DM. This issue is suitable for all medical professionals involved in the DM field and who interact with diabetic patients.

The issue sheds light on important comorbidities associated with DM, including nonalcoholic fatty liver disease, which is increasingly common in patients with type 2 DM, and lipodystrophies that cause insulin resistance and DM.

Treatment modalities emphasized in this issue include medical nutrition therapy to reduce weight and improve glycemic control, and pharmaceutical compounds such as metformin and insulin in the outpatient and inpatient settings. Surgical interventions are also discussed. Bariatric surgery has been shown to lead to significant improvement in glycemic control and metabolic syndrome components through weight loss. Pancreas and islet cell transplantation can be considered for patients whose type 1 DM cannot be controlled by other modalities; in the near future, human progenitor stem cells may be used to prevent the need for immunosuppressive drugs in these patients.

Endocrinol Metab Clin N Am 45 (2016) xiii–xiv
http://dx.doi.org/10.1016/j.ecl.2016.09.002
0889-8529/16/© 2016 Published by Elsevier Inc.

This issue also provides a more general overview of DM, considering new epidemiological, technological, and individualized approaches to control DM and prediabetes. It is clear today that, beyond the known risk factors associated with some ethnicities and genetic profiles, the dominant drivers of the observed increased prevalence are excess body fat and lifestyle. A globalized approach with transcultural protocols are required to adequately address this issue, and the discussions in this issue focus on the significant changes in disease prevalence between countries and across cultures. Such discussions are critical, as determining goals for population health management in DM will lead to reduced cost and improved quality of care.

Technological developments fast-forward us into the realm of precision medicine in DM. The many mobile medical applications ("apps") available allow the diabetic patient to share glucose pattern analysis with health care providers and to guide more individualized treatment. New devices are also poised to improve DM control: The closed-loop "artificial pancreas" system combining automated continuous glucose monitoring and insulin delivery with minimal patient intervention is under intense study. Yet, new technologies create new challenges along with opportunities. Evidence-based guidance for selecting the most appropriate app and health care system infrastructure to handle big data generated by these modalities is sorely needed and is discussed.

The issue concludes with this emphasis on the future, as we move toward a personalized approach for individual patients with DM. Integrating our current knowledge of the disease, therapeutic approaches, and technologies may provide better results in disease treatment and prevention.

We hope that you, our readers, will find the Diabetes Mellitus issue in *Endocrinology and Metabolism Clinics of North America* helpful in the management of your diabetic patients and prepare you for the upcoming changes that will lead us toward DM personalized medicine. We thank Dr Sethu K. Reddy for guest-editing this stimulating and timely issue, the authors for their work on these topics, and the Elsevier editorial staff for their assistance.

Anat Ben-Shlomo, MD
Pituitary Center
Division of Endocrinology, Diabetes, & Metabolism
Cedars Sinai Medical Center
8700 Beverly Boulevard
Los Angeles, CA 90048, USA

Maria Fleseriu, MD, FACE
Northwest Pituitary Center
Division of Endocrinology, Diabetes
& Clinical Nutrition
Departments of Medicine and Neurological Surgery
Oregon Health & Science University
3138 SW Sam Jackson Park Road
Portland, OR 97239, USA

E-mail addresses:
benshlomoa@cshs.org (A. Ben-Shlomo)
fleseriu@ohsu.edu (M. Fleseriu)

Preface

Rushing to Wholistic Diabetes Care

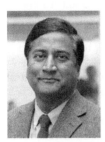

S. Sethu K. Reddy, MD, MBA,
FRCPC, FACP, MACE
Editor

Diabetes continues to be a challenge to all aspects of our society. In both direct and indirect costs, diabetes has a disproportionate amount attributed to it. It is in everyone's interest to support improved diabetes management.

Though the onslaught of diabetes has been compared to a tsunami, in truth, unlike a tsunami lasting for a day, the diabetes waves are likely to go on for decades. For the practitioner, the diagnosis is only the first step. Earlier diagnosis and advances in treatment are necessary to prevent the long-term complications of diabetes. We're also learning more about the natural history of diabetes, the genetic risk factors, and nutritional factors so that we may be able to develop preventive approaches.

We must not forget that diabetes is not just a gluco-centric disorder but a metabolic disorder. To stress this point, nonalcoholic steatohepatitis (NASH) is proving to be as prevalent in our society as type 2 diabetes. The hope is that earlier recognition and treatment of NASH will also ameliorate the tsunami of diabetes. The fascinating conditions of lipodystrophies also give us valuable insights into the link between fat metabolism and glucose regulation.

Nutrition therapy of diabetes is an evolving concept, with periodic fine-tuning based on the latest research. Nutrition remains the cornerstone of diabetes management.

Metformin has been available before many of our colleagues were born and has come to be regarded as the foundational therapy for type 2 diabetes. It behooves us all to reflect on the history of metformin and its clinical utility.

Insulin has been around for almost a hundred years, and there continues to be "tweaking" of the insulin molecule and its formulations to make it more practical and predictable.

With all of the new treatments available for type 2 diabetes, some wonder if we need any more therapies. Clearly, there are still unmet needs, and the Holy Grail for diabetes

Endocrinol Metab Clin N Am 45 (2016) xv–xvi
http://dx.doi.org/10.1016/j.ecl.2016.09.001
0889-8529/16/© 2016 Elsevier Inc. All rights reserved.

endo.theclinics.com

therapy is an agent that can prevent the β-cell burnout and dramatically change the natural history of type 2 diabetes.

A particular new area of specialization has been hospital medicine. Years ago, an often-heard complaint was that future doctors received most of their training in hospitals and were not prepared for ambulatory medicine. Today, the area of inpatient medicine is one of the fastest-growing specialties, and diabetes is one of the most prevalent background conditions ($\geq$20%) for those admitted to hospital. It's important for all of us who take care of diabetes to play our role in inpatient safety and in improving outcomes for those hospitalized with diabetes.

Continuous glucose monitoring is increasingly becoming accepted as a standard of care for those with type 1 diabetes and for some with type 2 diabetes. Continuous glucose monitoring and sharing the data on the "cloud" is rapidly becoming the standard for close monitoring of diabetes, from a safety perspective as well as in helping improve glucose control.

What about the future? Bariatric surgery may become a standard for early type 2 diabetes, and the field of islet cell transplantation will lay the groundwork for stem cell utilization in diabetes. Unlike our typical cadence of quarterly physician-patient visits, telemedicine and companion technology promise to keep the patient connected to family, friends, and/or members of the health care team.

For the number of patients with diabetes, there are not enough practitioners to look after all on an individual basis. In the United States, we're also moving from a fee-for-service model to a value-based model, which will also necessitate changes in how we manage our patients. We have to rely on new means of health care delivery, thinking about population health management as well as leveraging digital solutions. Clinicians are slowly becoming engaged in population health, which will require a change in management style, focusing on population outcomes instead of just individual results. These approaches are complementary in that both allow for reaching a greater number of patients more efficiently.

We're slowly coming to realize that the management of diabetes requires more than technical intervention of attempting to normalize the "numbers": HbA1c, blood pressure, and cholesterol levels. We need to pay attention to the patient as a whole, especially the patient's sociocultural background. In an increasingly diverse patient population, adapting one's approach to the patient's cultural background will lead to greater adherence and improved outcomes. Part of personalized medicine in the future will depend not only on biochemical testing but also on the individual's sociocultural environment.

I would like to thank all the contributing authors for their diligent and scholarly reviews of these important aspects of diabetes in 2016 and for sharing their wisdom. I hope you will enjoy their perspectives and incorporate some of the information into your practice.

I would also like to thank the editors and management of Elsevier, Meredith Clinton and Jessica McCool, for their support and patience.

S. Sethu K. Reddy, MD, MBA, FRCPC, FACP, MACE
Endocrinology, Diabetes, & Metabolism
F20, Cleveland Clinic
9500 Euclid Avenue
Cleveland, OH 44195, USA

E-mail address:
Sethu.k.reddy@gmail.com

Prediabetes
A Worldwide Epidemic

Catherine M. Edwards, MD[a],*, Kenneth Cusi, MD[a,b]

KEYWORDS

- Prediabetes • Impaired glucose tolerance • Impaired fasting glucose
- Type 2 diabetes • Metabolic syndrome • β-Cell • Insulin resistance

KEY POINTS

- Prediabetes is increasing markedly in incidence and prevalence, particularly in Africa and Asia.
- The central reason for this epidemic is increased calorie-dense food and decreased physical activity.
- Prediabetes carries significant risk for both macrovascular and microvascular disease.
- Prospective studies have demonstrated the potential to prevent or delay the onset of type 2 diabetes mellitus in patients with prediabetes with lifestyle changes and pharmacologic therapy.

DEFINITION AND THE DIAGNOSIS OF PREDIABETES

Prediabetes is the state between normal and diabetes; its definition has evolved over time and still varies depending on the defining institution (**Table 1**). It generally reflects the presence of either, or both, impaired fasting glucose (IFG) and impaired glucose tolerance (IGT).[1,2] The American Diabetes Association (ADA) also includes the A1c as a diagnostic criterion. Various terms have been used to refer to this metabolic state, in addition to prediabetes, IFG, and IGT; intermediate hyperglycemia is preferred by the World Health Organization (WHO), and an expert committee convened by the ADA has suggested high-risk state of developing diabetes. The reproducibility of

Disclosure Statements: C.M. Edwards has nothing to disclose; K. Cusi has received research support from Janssen (28431755DIA1054) and Novartis (LCQ908A2226) and served as a consultant for (in alphabetical order) Janssen, Lilly, Pfizer, and Tobira Therapeutics, Inc.
[a] Division of Endocrinology, Diabetes and Metabolism, Department of Medicine, University of Florida College of Medicine, 1600 Southwest Archer Road, Gainesville, FL 32610, USA;
[b] Division of Endocrinology, Diabetes and Metabolism, Malcom Randall Veterans Affairs Medical Center, 1601 South West Archer Road, Gainesville, FL 32608, USA
* Corresponding author. Division of Endocrinology, Diabetes and Metabolism, Department of Medicine, University of Florida College of Medicine, 1600 Southwest Archer Road, Room H-2, Gainesville, FL 32610.
E-mail address: catherine.edwards@medicine.ufl.edu

Table 1
Diagnostic criteria for prediabetes

Institution/Year of Publication	Venous Plasma Glucose
WHO, 2006	IFG: 110–125 mg/dL (6.1–6.9 mmol/L) IGT: 140–200 mg/dL (7.8–11.0 mmol/L) 2 h after a 75 g oral glucose challenge
ADA, 2016	IFG: 100–125 mg/dL (5.5–6.9 mmol/L) IGT: 140–200 mg/dL (7.8–11.0 mmol/L) 2 h after a 75 g oral glucose challenge A1c: 5.7% to 6.4%

the definition of prediabetes (50%) is less than that of diabetes (>70%).[3] The variations in defining threshold glucose levels and this low reproducibility of the tests themselves result in variability in populations of patients defined as having prediabetes in clinical studies.

Prediabetes is clearly the major risk factor for the future development of type 2 diabetes mellitus (T2DM). In addition, other risk factors, like family history of T2DM, or a personal history of gestational diabetes, polycystic ovary syndrome (PCOS), nonalcoholic fatty liver disease (NAFLD), obesity, or metabolic syndrome (MS), can markedly increase the risk of developing T2DM. Various biomarkers have been examined and risk scores developed in an effort to improve the ability to predict the progression of prediabetes to T2DM, but these have not yet achieved frequent clinical use.[4] In addition, there are important ethnic differences in the risk of developing diabetes, perhaps necessitating different algorithms depending on ethnicity.[5]

EPIDEMIOLOGY

The incidence and prevalence of prediabetes is increasing in both developed and developing countries. The Centers for Disease Control and Prevention (CDC) estimated that 37% of adults in the United States over the age of 20, and 51% of those over 65, had prediabetes in the period 2009 to 2012, as determined by fasting glucose or A1c.[6] The International Diabetes Federation (IDF) estimated the worldwide prevalence of IGT at 280 million in 2011 with projections of 398 million by 2030.[7] Emphasizing the risk of progression of prediabetes to diabetes, the recent 2016 WHO Global Report on Diabetes[8] reports that in 2014, 422 million adults had diabetes. This increase has been particularly marked in African and Asian countries.[8]

The chronicity of the disease and the high cost of care make these predictions an issue of great concern, and necessitate estimates of the financial burden for future policy making and planning. A review by Lam and LeRoith in 2012[9] summarized evidence that rapid urbanization has altered diet, with increased intake of vegetable fat and increased glycemic load and index. The rapid changes in urbanization and diet in developing countries have thus likely resulted in an accelerated increase in average body mass index (BMI) and prediabetes. Lam and LeRoith[9] also stress that genetic differences in different populations may play an important role in the global prediabetes and diabetes epidemic.

PATHOGENESIS OF PREDIABETES

Both resistance to the action of insulin and impaired β-cell function are present during even early stages of prediabetes and are required for most of the hyperglycemia seen in prediabetes. Insulin resistance (IR) appears to be the earliest abnormality, although there is marked heterogeneity between individuals and populations in studies that investigate the course of pathogenicity of prediabetes. This is not surprising; genome-wide sequencing studies (GWAS) have revealed at least 60 genes that confer risk for the development of type 2 diabetes, most of these related to β-cell biology.[10,11] The Whitehall study looked at the time course of physiologic changes during the development of diabetes in British subjects[12] and found evidence of IR and of early intermittent hyperglycemia about 13 years before the diagnosis of diabetes. Blood glucose remained close to normal, presumably due to compensatory mechanisms to allow for increased insulin production by pancreatic beta cells, until their failure 2 to 6 years before the diagnosis at a time where more sustained hyperglycemia developed, which also correlated with worsening IR. A steeper decline in pancreatic β-cell function seemed to follow a few years later, now with frank hyperglycemia, at this point resulting in the clinical diagnosis of diabetes.

But what precisely causes an elevation in plasma glucose levels, either in the fasting or fed state? Basu and colleagues[13] used euglycemic hyperinsulinemic clamp studies to investigate the pathophysiology of IFG and IGT. Their data showed that isolated IFG (with normal postmeal blood glucose [BG]) was associated with increased gluconeogenesis, but no evidence of hepatic IR (ie, glycogenolysis was normally suppressed). In contrast, subjects with combined IFG/IGT had a combination of increased gluconeogenesis, lack of suppression of glycogenolysis by insulin, and impaired glucose disposal with extrahepatic IR. Whether isolated IFG reflects an earlier stage in progressive loss of glucose metabolic control compared with more advanced disease in patients with isolated IGT or combined IFG and IGT, or whether there are different pathogenic mechanisms at play when postprandial hyperglycemia develops, remains unclear, and different groups have found discordant results.[14]

Another perspective to help dissect out the pathogenesis of prediabetes is the biology of the pancreatic β-cell itself, including an understanding of normal β-cell life span, pancreatic β-cell mass, and responses to stress. In normal individuals, β-cell mass peaks in the first decade, plateaus during adolescence, and declines in later years. There is wide variability in beta mass between individuals, irrespective of age or BMI, with overlapping mass between normoglycemic and hyperglycemic individuals.[15] It is thought that β-cells have a variety of responses to different stressors, probably differing according to genetic background and to the details of the stressor and physiology at that time. In general, the β-cell likely develops a compensatory response that allows for ongoing or increased insulin production and secretion, for a time, but at a cost. With ongoing stress, any of a variety of pathologic pathways can be taken by the β-cell, leading to permanent dysfunction and eventual death.[15] Research is ongoing in the area of noninvasive techniques to measure or estimate β-cell mass; this will be a critical element in the goal of early detection of those individuals at highest risk of developing prediabetes and diabetes.

Much attention has been devoted to understanding the effects of obesity-related stressors on the β-cell. A prominent hypothesis is that of β-cell lipotoxicity,[16] leading to cell apoptosis, not only impairing insulin secretion, but also affecting other key tissues involved in the regulation of glucose metabolism, such as skeletal muscle or the liver.[17] In a setting of chronic excessive energy supply, adipose tissue is maximally utilized, and fats accumulate in other tissues that would not normally store fats. Lipids are redirected in this setting, into nonoxidative metabolic pathways, with resultant accumulation of toxic metabolites. There is substantial evidence in vivo[16] and in people[18] on the role of β-cell lipotoxicity in the development of T2DM. For instance, in healthy individuals with normal glucose tolerance who are genetically predisposed to T2DM (ie, having both parents with T2DM), a sustained (48–72 h) physiologic increase in plasma free fatty acid (FFA) concentration impairs insulin secretion in response to mixed meals and to intravenous glucose stimulation, suggesting that in subjects at high risk of developing T2DM, β-cell lipotoxicity may play an important role in the progression from normal glucose tolerance to overt hyperglycemia.[19] As proof of concept, when in these individuals plasma FFA levels are lowered for 7 days with the administration of acipimox (a nicotinic acid derivative and potent inhibitor of triglyceride lipolysis in adipose tissue), insulin secretion improves.[20] The role of hyperglycemia is also important in the prediabetic state to alter β-cell function and precipitate clinical diabetes, so that the combined effects of glucose and lipotoxicity results in the activation of inflammatory pathways that lead eventually to severe β-cell dysfunction and cell apoptosis.[21] Components of the inflammatory pathways that participate in this process include C-reactive protein (CRP), interleukin (IL)-6, IL-2 and IL2RA.[22] Local islet inflammation can also be triggered when islet amyloid polypeptide (IAPP) accumulates, due to parallel increases in synthesis along with insulin. High levels of IAPP lead to IL-1β recruitment of macrophages and eventual apoptosis.[15]

The compensatory action of the β-cell to increase insulin production in the face of IR may itself trigger destructive pathways for the β-cell. Endoplasmic reticulum (ER) stress occurs in this setting, resulting from increased flux of proinsulin through the rough ER. There is an increase in misfolded proinsulin, potentially exceeding the capacity of the β-cell to handle this load and leading to β-cell failure and death. In some monogenic forms of diabetes, this may be an important cause of stress leading to apoptosis, although the role of this pathway in most cases of T2DM remains unclear.[23]

Additional pathogenic mechanisms may include disruption of the architecture of the islets of Langerhans. This is often seen histopathologically, and the consequences are being investigated. Cell–cell communication may be impaired in this setting, with resultant abnormalities in insulin secretion. Beta cell incretin signaling may be impaired in disrupted islets, with consequent hyperglucagonemia.[15]

THE RELATIONSHIP BETWEEN METABOLIC SYNDROME, INSULIN RESISTANCE, AND PREDIABETES

MS, IR, and prediabetes are closely related but distinct entities. One of the challenges in investigating these relationships and interpreting the literature is the variability in definitions of these disease states. The NCEP-ATP III (National Cholesterol Education Program-Adult Treatment Panel III) definition has been frequently used (**Table 2**),[24] as

Table 2
ATP III definition of metabolic syndrome (diagnosis made with at least 3 of the 5 criteria)

Risk Factor	Defining Value
Abdominal obesity (waist circumference)	
Men	>102 cm
Women	>88 cm
Triglycerides	$\geq$1.7 mmol/L ($\geq$150 mg/dL)
HDL cholesterol	
Men	<1.04 mmol/L (<40 mg/dL)
Women	<1.30 mmol/L (<50 mg/dL)
Blood pressure	$\geq$130/85 mm Hg
Fasting glucose	$\geq$6.1 mmol/L ($\geq$110 mg/dL)

have the International Diabetes Federation (IDF),[25] the IDF/American Heart Association/National Heart, Lung and Blood Institute criteria,[26] as well as the World Health Organization (WHO) criteria (**Box 1**).[27] The American Association of Clinical Endocrinologists (AACE) proposed a different set of criteria and a different name to denote MS that is more aligned with the underlying pathophysiology of this condition, calling it instead the insulin resistance syndrome (**Table 3**).[28] However, it should be noted that these definitions overlap substantially.[29]

MS is closely linked to IR and is a major, independent risk factor for the development of both microvascular and macrovascular disease. Bianchi and colleagues[30] investigated the relative roles of IR and insulin secretion in varying degrees of glucose intolerance in patients at risk for type 2 diabetes, and found that patients with MS (defined by ATP III criteria) had more IR irrespective of glucose tolerance, while insulin secretion was less related. However, only 59% of patients with IR had MS. They cited potential mechanisms in addition to IR that may account for clustering of the components of MS, including visceral obesity, inflammation, and endothelial dysfunction.[30] Other investigators have shown that MS, IR, and prediabetes/type 2 diabetes are all independent predictors of coronary heart disease.[31]

Many areas of debate remain in this field: ethnic differences in the MS criteria, whether the associated components of metabolic syndrome confer more cardiovascular disease risk than the sum of the individual components, the precise role of insulin resistance in the development of metabolic syndrome and prediabetes, and which of the multitude of risk factors are the best predictors of future prediabetes/diabetes and cardiovascular disease, as well as how the severity of the risk factor components vary over time and impact future outcomes.[32–36] The overall sense that IR is the most fundamental pathogenic mechanism in the development of MS remains a prominent hypothesis in this area of investigation and thought.

Box 1
World Health Organization criteria for metabolic syndrome

Insulin resistance, defined by 1 of the following:

- Type 2 diabetes

- Impaired fasting glucose

- Impaired glucose tolerance

- Glucose uptake less than the lowest quartile for the background population under investigation under hyperinsulinemic, euglycemic conditions

Plus 2 of the following:

- Antihypertensive medication and/or hypertension ($\geq$140 mm Hg systolic or $\geq$90 mm Hg diastolic)

- Plasma triglycerides at least 1.7 mmol/L ($\geq$150 mg/dL)

- Plasma HDL cholesterol less than 0.9 mmol/L (<35 mg/dL) in men or less than 1.0 mmol/L (<40 mg/dL) in women

- BMI greater than 30 kg/m^2 and/or waist to hip ratio greater than 0.9 in men or greater than 0.85 in women

- Urinary albumin excretion rate of at least 20 μg/min or albumin to creatinine at least 3.4 mg/mmol ($\geq$30 mg/g)

Table 3
American Association of Clinical Endocrinologists criteria for diagnosis of insulin resistance syndrome (diagnosis made by clinical judgment rather than number of criteria met)

Risk Factor	Defining Value
Overweight/obesity	BMI $\geq$25 kg/m^2
Plasma triglycerides	$\geq$1.70 mmol/L ($\geq$150 mg/dL)
Plasma HDL-cholesterol	
Men	<1.04 mmol/L (<40 mg/dL)
Women	<1.30 mmol/L (<50 mg/dL)
Blood pressure	$\geq$130/85 mm Hg
2 h postglucose challenge	>7.8 mmol/L (>140 mg/dL)
Fasting plasma glucose	6.1–6.9 mmol/L
Other risk factors	Family history of T2DM, hypertension, or cardiovascular disease Polycystic ovarian syndrome Sedentary lifestyle Advancing age Ethnic groups at high-risk for T2DM or cardiovascular disease

COMPLICATIONS OF PREDIABETES

Prediabetes has been associated with an increased risk for both early microvascular and macrovascular complications. It appears to increase the risk of early forms of nephropathy as demonstrated in the National Health and Nutrition Examination Survey (NHANES) 1999 to 2006 data (**Table 4**).[37] However, as with other epidemiologic links to complications, it has been difficult to associate prediabetes with risk for more advanced disease, including decreased GFR (glomerular filtration rate),[37] and to separate out the contribution that prediabetes makes as opposed to other clustered risk factors associated with metabolic syndrome.[38] There also appears to be an increased risk for autonomic neuropathy[39–41] and early sensorimotor neuropathy.[39] Similarly, the literature suggests an increased risk of early retinopathy.[42,43] Of note, over 7% of participants in the US Diabetes Prevention Program (DPP) had evidence of early retinopathy.[44] Studies have shown variable results in the association of prediabetes with microvascular disease, probably reflecting the variability of testing strategies and their sensitivities.[45]

The data linking prediabetes with macrovascular disease are stronger for coronary disease compared with cerebrovascular disease and other macrovascular disease.[46]

Table 4
Relationship between glycemia and nephropathy

Glycemia	Microalbuminuria, %	Macroalbuminuria, %
Normoglycemia	6	0.6
Impaired fasting glucose	10	1.1
Undiagnosed diabetes	29	3.3
Diagnosed diabetes	29	7.7

Data from Bianchi C, Miccoli R, Bonadonna RC, et al. Metabolic syndrome in subjects at high risk for type 2 diabetes: the genetic, physiopathology and evolution of type 2 diabetes (GENFIEV) study. Nutr Metab Cardiovasc Dis 2011;21:699–705.

Prospective studies do show an association between premeal and postmeal blood glucose, and A1c in patients with prediabetes with risk of cardiovascular disease,[47–49] but again, it is difficult to define the absolute risk in the presence of other clustered risk factors for cardiovascular disease in this patient population.[38]

TREATMENT OF PREDIABETES AND THE PREVENTION OF TYPE 2 DIABETES AND ITS COMPLICATIONS

Multiple prospective randomized controlled trials with intervention during prediabetes have demonstrated the potential for delaying and possibly preventing type 2 diabetes. The DPP[50] demonstrated a 58% decrease in the development of type 2 diabetes with the use of lifestyle changes, supported by frequent visits and counseling, and a 31% decrease with metformin use. The Da Qing IGT and Diabetes Study done in China,[51] the Finnish Diabetes Prevention Study,[52] the ACT NOW study (Actos Now for the Prevention of Diabetes study),[53] and the Diabetes Reduction Assessment With Ramipril and Rosiglitazone Medication (DREAM),[54] have all shown significant benefits of lifestyle changes and/or various pharmacologic agents in preventing or delaying diabetes, in a wide variety of populations.

Perhaps even more intriguing, follow-up studies after these trials[55–59] show that at least some of the benefit of the treatment groups is sustained over time, delaying the progression toward diabetes and its complications long after the intervention has ended, occurring despite attenuation of the effect of therapy on the blood glucose. This important observation suggests that early intervention, perhaps with normalization of the blood glucose, would be optimal with regard to prevention and limiting the high toll of diabetes.[53,60]

A closer look at the types of lifestyle changes is warranted, particularly because the data suggest that lifestyle has achieved the greatest benefits in these studies. Several recent reviews[61–64] have been published that detail the types of dietary changes and physical activity interventions that have been effective in diabetes prevention. The consensus is that a diet rich in whole grains, vegetables, fruit, monounsaturated fat, and low in animal fat, trans fats, and simple sugars is beneficial, along with maintenance of ideal body weight and an active lifestyle. Good specific or regional diets include the Mediterranean diet,[64] and indeed this diet has been associated with a lower risk of diabetes in prospective studies.[65,66] Two of these reviews[61,62] particularly emphasized the challenges and best practice approaches to a broader implementation of lifestyle recommendations in the real world, and in a variety of cultural settings. This is surely among the most daunting and necessary challenges faced by those committed to intervening in the relentless increase in diabetes incidence.

The prevention of the complications of prediabetes and diabetes, with regard to microvascular and macrovascular disease, is a vital aspect of the therapeutic approach to prediabetes. The data are clear that tighter blood glucose control decreases microvascular disease in type 2 diabetes; clearly demonstrating this in prediabetes is more challenging. Prediabetes is associated with an increased risk of microalbuminuria and macroalbuminuria; the risk of these early renal complications increases as hyperglycemia increases, as shown by the NHANES 1999 to 2006 data.[67] Prediabetes is associated with an increased risk of autonomic neuropathy[39,40] and sensorimotor neuropathy.[39] Retinopathy may also occur with an increased incidence in prediabetes.[68] The sum of the data thus suggests that microvascular complications occur in prediabetes, and the data in tight glucose control in diabetes suggest the possibility that normalizing glycemia in prediabetes may be effective in preventing these complications, but clearly more data are needed.

Cardiovascular disease is responsible for up to 80% of the mortality in type 2 diabetes.[69] There is ongoing discussion regarding whether hyperglycemia is a cause of macrovascular disease, and the data directly linking prediabetes to cardiovascular disease are difficult to interpret, largely because it has been impossible to separate out the confounding influences of the metabolic syndrome. This includes obesity, hypertension, and dyslipidemia, as well as a proinflammatory and prothrombotic state. Regardless of how the pathogenic mechanisms are understood, multiple studies have demonstrated cardiovascular mortality in prediabetes close to that in type 2 diabetes,[49,70–72] an aspect that calls for aggressive risk factor management in this population.[73,74]

In light of the data detailed above regarding the potential to delay, and to possibly prevent type 2 diabetes and its complications with lifestyle and pharmacologic intervention, it seems reasonable to take a proactive position regarding intervention in this population. As stated so clearly by many authors,[53,59,60,74] early intervention with lifestyle changes, aggressive treatment of other risk factors for cardiovascular diseases such as hypertension and hyperlipidemia, and, in the highest-risk patients, pharmacologic treatment to prevent diabetes, is the rational approach. The authors agree with this. There are, however, no US Food and Drug Administration (FDA) approved pharmacologic therapies for prediabetes. The current ADA recommendations suggest consideration of metformin in patients with both IFG and IGT, and at least 1 high-risk factor including family history of diabetes, age less than 60, BMI $\geq$35 kg/m^2, hypertriglyceridemia, low high density lipoprotein (HDL), hypertension, and A1c of at least 6.0%.[75] In their practice, the authors urge optimal lifestyle, provide resources for them to try to achieve that, and offer metformin to those patients at higher risk of progression to diabetes. The authors also have discussions with their prediabetes patients regarding pioglitazone therapy, given the data showing both stabilization of ß-cell function and decreased progression to diabetes during treatment with thiazolidinediones.[53,57,76–78] For those patients who show signs of nonalcoholic fatty liver disease (NAFLD), particularly if there is early evidence of fibrosis, the recommendation to start pioglitazone is even stronger, given the data linking this drug to beneficial effects on liver metabolism and histology in this setting.[79–84]

THE FUTURE

Many challenges remain in this field; the epidemiologic and economic data emphasize an urgent need to view the prediabetes epidemic seriously and to institute effective measures for limiting the burden of this disease on future generations. A deeper understanding of the pathogenesis of prediabetes, the metabolic syndrome, diabetes, and complications will help point toward novel targets of pharmacologic intervention. However, whatever the details, the underlying pathogenesis is certainly reflective of the inability of some patients' physiology to adapt to an overabundance of food and a decrease in physical activity. An enormous challenge is thus the prospect of trying to change the lifestyle habits of populations with different cultures and genetic make-ups. Despite considerable research in this field,[55,58,60–63] more needs to be done, and social systems need to become engaged in this task.

Identifying a high-risk population on which to focus the effort to prevent diabetes is another aspect of the challenge in this area. A variety of approaches has been taken in this area that may inform future public heath efforts, including screening with biomarkers,[85–87] clinical screening for the metabolic syndrome, and identifying a particularly high-risk group of patients that continues to have hyperglycemia despite lifestyle intervention.[58]

Most agree that early intervention, whether lifestyle or pharmacologic, will be key in diabetes prevention. Methodology for more accurately measuring β-cell mass and function, in order to identify those with a higher rate of loss and therefore a higher risk of prediabetes and diabetes, would be extremely helpful in this goal. The next step would be an intervention that could halt the process of β-cell loss, or even increase β-cell mass and function; the search continues for these important tools and interventions.

The economic costs of global recognition of prediabetes as a disease, with all the implications thereof, are staggering. However, this must be put into the context of the much higher costs if this urgent need to intervene early in the disease process of the diabetes spectrum is ignored. Later stages of the disease with frank hyperglycemia carry the otherwise almost inevitable consequences of microvascular complications, with a higher personal and economic impact to society.

REFERENCES

1. American Diabetes Association. Classification and diagnosis of diabetes. Diabetes Care 2016;39(Suppl 1):S13–22.
2. World Health Organization. Definition and diagnosis of diabetes mellitus and intermediate hyperglycemia; report of a WHO/IDF consultation. Geneva (Switzerland): World Health Organization; 2006. p. 1–50.
3. Balion CM, Raina PS, Gerstein HC, et al. Reproducibility of impaired glucose tolerance (IGT) and impaired fasting glucose (IFG) classification: a systematic review. Clin Chem Lab Med 2007;45:1180–5.
4. Buijsse B, Simmons RK, Griffin SJ, et al. Risk assessment tools for identifying individuals at risk of developing type 2 diabetes. Epidemiol Rev 2011;33:46–62.
5. Noble D, Mathur R, Dent T, et al. Risk models and scores for type 2 diabetes: systematic review. BMJ 2011;343:d7163.
6. National diabetes statistics report: estimates of diabetes and its burden in the United States. Centers for Disease Control and Prevention national diabetes statistics report. Atlanta (GA): U.S. Department of Health and Human Services; 2014. Available at: https://www.cdc.gov/diabetes/pubs/statsreport14/national-diabetes-report-web.pdf.
7. Aguirre F, Brown A, Cho NH, et al. International Diabetes Federation. IDF Diabetes Atlas, 6th edition. Brussels (Belgium): International Diabetes Federation; 2013.
8. WHO Global report on diabetes. Geneva (Switzerland): World Health Organization; 2016.
9. Lam DW, LeRoith D. The worldwide diabetes epidemic. Curr Opin Endocrinol Diabetes Obes 2012;19:93–6.
10. Voight BF, Scott LJ, Steinthorsdottir V, et al. Twelve type 2 diabetes susceptibility loci identified through large-scale association analysis. Nat Genet 2010;42: 579–89.
11. Pal A, McCarthy MI. The genetics of type 2 diabetes and its clinical relevance. Clin Genet 2013;83:297–306.
12. Tabak AG, Jokela M, Akbaraly TN, et al. Trajectories of glycaemia, insulin sensitivity, and insulin secretion before diagnosis of type 2 diabetes: an analysis from the Whitehall II study. Lancet 2009;373:2215–21.
13. Basu R, Barosa C, Jones J, et al. Pathogenesis of prediabetes: role of the liver in isolated fasting hyperglycemia and combined fasting and postprandial hyperglycemia. J Clin Endocrinol Metab 2013;98:E409–17.

14. Perreault L, Bergman BC, Playdon MC, et al. Impaired fasting glucose with or without impaired glucose tolerance: progressive or parallel states of prediabetes? Am J Physiol Endocrinol Metab 2008;295:E428–35.

15. Halban PA, Polonsky KS, Bowden DW, et al. beta-cell failure in type 2 diabetes: postulated mechanisms and prospects for prevention and treatment. Diabetes Care 2014;37:1751–8.

16. Unger RH. Lipotoxicity in the pathogenesis of obesity-dependent NIDDM. Genetic and clinical implications. Diabetes 1995;44:863–70.

17. Cusi K. Role of obesity and lipotoxicity in the development of nonalcoholic steatohepatitis: pathophysiology and clinical implications. Gastroenterology 2012; 142:711–25.e6.

18. Cusi K. The role of adipose tissue and lipotoxicity in the pathogenesis of type 2 diabetes. Curr Diab Rep 2010;10:306–15.

19. Kashyap S, Belfort R, Gastaldelli A, et al. A sustained increase in plasma free fatty acids impairs insulin secretion in nondiabetic subjects genetically predisposed to develop type 2 diabetes. Diabetes 2003;52:2461–74.

20. Cusi K, Kashyap S, Gastaldelli A, et al. Effects on insulin secretion and insulin action of a 48-h reduction of plasma free fatty acids with acipimox in nondiabetic subjects genetically predisposed to type 2 diabetes. Am J Physiol Endocrinol Metab 2007;292:E1775–81.

21. Poitout V, Amyot J, Semache M, et al. Glucolipotoxicity of the pancreatic beta cell. Biochim Biophys Acta 2010;1801:289–98.

22. Donath MY, Shoelson SE. Type 2 diabetes as an inflammatory disease. Nat Rev Immunol 2011;11:98–107.

23. Sun J, Cui J, He Q, et al. Proinsulin misfolding and endoplasmic reticulum stress during the development and progression of diabetes. Mol Aspects Med 2015;42: 105–18.

24. Expert Panel on Detection, Evaluation, and Treatment of High Blood Cholesterol in Adults. Executive summary of the third report of The National Cholesterol Education Program (NCEP) Expert Panel on Detection, Evaluation, and Treatment of High Blood Cholesterol in Adults (adult treatment panel III). JAMA 2001;285: 2486–97.

25. Alberti KG, Zimmet P, Shaw J, et al. The metabolic syndrome—a new worldwide definition. Lancet 2005;366:1059–62.

26. Alberti KG, Eckel RH, Grundy SM, et al. Harmonizing the metabolic syndrome: a joint interim statement of the International Diabetes Federation Task Force on Epidemiology and Prevention; National Heart, Lung, and Blood Institute; American Heart Association; World Heart Federation; International Atherosclerosis Society; and International Association for the Study of Obesity. Circulation 2009;120: 1640–5.

27. Alberti KG, Zimmet PZ. Definition, diagnosis and classification of diabetes mellitus and its complications. Part 1: diagnosis and classification of diabetes mellitus provisional report of a WHO consultation. Diabet Med 1998;15:539–53.

28. Einhorn D, Reaven GM, Cobin RH, et al. American College of Endocrinology position statement on the insulin resistance syndrome. Endocr Pract 2003;9:237–52.

29. Beilby J. Guidelines review: definition of metabolic syndrome: report of the National Heart, Lung, and Blood Institute/American Heart Association Conference on scientific issues related to definition. Clin Biochem Rev 2004;25:195–8.

30. Bianchi C, Miccoli R, Bonadonna RC, et al. Metabolic syndrome in subjects at high risk for type 2 diabetes: the genetic, physiopathology and evolution of type 2 diabetes (GENFIEV) study. Nutr Metab Cardiovasc Dis 2011;21:699–705.

31. Saely CH, Aczel S, Marte T, et al. The metabolic syndrome, insulin resistance, and cardiovascular risk in diabetic and nondiabetic patients. J Clin Endocrinol Metab 2005;90:5698–703.
32. Kahn R, Buse J, Ferrannini E, et al. The metabolic syndrome: time for a critical appraisal: joint statement from the American Diabetes Association and the European Association for the Study of Diabetes. Diabetes Care 2005;28:2289–304.
33. Eckel RH, Grundy SM, Zimmet PZ. The metabolic syndrome. Lancet 2005; 365(9468):1415–28.
34. Grundy SM. Metabolic syndrome: connecting and reconciling cardiovascular and diabetes worlds. J Am Coll Cardiol 2006;47:1093–100.
35. Gurka MJ, Lilly CL, Oliver MN, et al. An examination of sex and racial/ethnic differences in the metabolic syndrome among adults: a confirmatory factor analysis and a resulting continuous severity score. Metabolism 2014;63:218–25.
36. Vishnu A, Gurka MJ, DeBoer MD. The severity of the metabolic syndrome increases over time within individuals, independent of baseline metabolic syndrome status and medication use: the Atherosclerosis Risk in Communities Study. Atherosclerosis 2015;243:278–85.
37. Plantinga LC, Crews DC, Coresh J, et al. Prevalence of chronic kidney disease in US adults with undiagnosed diabetes or prediabetes. Clin J Am Soc Nephrol 2010;5:673–82.
38. Sarwar N, Gao P, Seshasai SR, et al, Emerging Risk Factor Collaboration. Diabetes mellitus, fasting blood glucose concentration, and risk of vascular disease: a collaborative meta-analysis of 102 prospective studies. Lancet 2010;375: 2215–22.
39. Tesfaye S, Boulton AJ, Dyck PJ, et al. Diabetic neuropathies: update on definitions, diagnostic criteria, estimation of severity, and treatments. Diabetes Care 2010;33:2285–93.
40. Wu JS, Yang YC, Lin TS, et al. Epidemiological evidence of altered cardiac autonomic function in subjects with impaired glucose tolerance but not isolated impaired fasting glucose. J Clin Endocrinol Metab 2007;92:3885–9.
41. Putz Z, Tabak AG, Toth N, et al. Noninvasive evaluation of neural impairment in subjects with impaired glucose tolerance. Diabetes Care 2009;32:181–3.
42. Gabir MM, Hanson RL, Dabelea D, et al. Plasma glucose and prediction of microvascular disease and mortality: evaluation of 1997 American Diabetes Association and 1999 World Health Organization criteria for diagnosis of diabetes. Diabetes Care 2000;23:1113–8.
43. Nguyen TT, Wang JJ, Islam FM, et al. Retinal arteriolar narrowing predicts incidence of diabetes: the Australian Diabetes, Obesity and Lifestyle (AusDiab) Study. Diabetes 2008;57:536–9.
44. Diabetes Prevention Program Research Group. The prevalence of retinopathy in impaired glucose tolerance and recent-onset diabetes in the Diabetes Prevention Program. Diabet Med 2007;24:137–44.
45. Tabak AG, Herder C, Rathmann W, et al. Prediabetes: a high-risk state for diabetes development. Lancet 2012;379:2279–90.
46. Brunner EJ, Shipley MJ, Witte DR, et al. Relation between blood glucose and coronary mortality over 33 years in the Whitehall Study. Diabetes Care 2006;29: 26–31.
47. Barr EL, Zimmet PZ, Welborn TA, et al. Risk of cardiovascular and all-cause mortality in individuals with diabetes mellitus, impaired fasting glucose, and impaired glucose tolerance: the Australian Diabetes, Obesity, and Lifestyle Study (AusDiab). Circulation 2007;116:151–7.

48. Sarwar N, Aspelund T, Eiriksdottir G, et al. Markers of dysglycaemia and risk of coronary heart disease in people without diabetes: Reykjavik prospective study and systematic review. PLoS Med 2010;7:e1000278.

49. Decode Study Group, the European Diabetes Epidemiology Group. Glucose tolerance and cardiovascular mortality: comparison of fasting and 2-hour diagnostic criteria. Arch Intern Med 2001;161:397–405.

50. Knowler WC, Barrett-Connor E, Fowler SE, et al. Reduction in the incidence of type 2 diabetes with lifestyle intervention or metformin. N Engl J Med 2002;346: 393–403.

51. Pan XR, Li GW, Hu YH, et al. Effects of diet and exercise in preventing NIDDM in people with impaired glucose tolerance. The Da Qing IGT and Diabetes Study. Diabetes Care 1997;20:537–44.

52. Tuomilehto J, Lindstrom J, Eriksson JG, et al. Prevention of type 2 diabetes mellitus by changes in lifestyle among subjects with impaired glucose tolerance. N Engl J Med 2001;344:1343–50.

53. DeFronzo RA, Tripathy D, Schwenke DC, et al. Pioglitazone for diabetes prevention in impaired glucose tolerance. N Engl J Med 2011;364:1104–15.

54. Gerstein HC, Yusuf S, Bosch J, et al. Effect of rosiglitazone on the frequency of diabetes in patients with impaired glucose tolerance or impaired fasting glucose: a randomised controlled trial. Lancet 2006;368:1096–105.

55. Lindstrom J, Peltonen M, Eriksson JG, et al. Improved lifestyle and decreased diabetes risk over 13 years: long-term follow-up of the randomised Finnish Diabetes Prevention Study (DPS). Diabetologia 2013;56:284–93.

56. Li G, Zhang P, Wang J, et al. Cardiovascular mortality, all-cause mortality, and diabetes incidence after lifestyle intervention for people with impaired glucose tolerance in the Da Qing Diabetes Prevention Study: a 23-year follow-up study. Lancet Diabetes Endocrinol 2014;2:474–80.

57. Gerstein HC, Mohan V, Avezum A, et al. Long-term effect of rosiglitazone and/or ramipril on the incidence of diabetes. Diabetologia 2011;54:487–95.

58. Perreault L, Pan Q, Mather KJ, et al. Effect of regression from prediabetes to normal glucose regulation on long-term reduction in diabetes risk: results from the Diabetes Prevention Program Outcomes Study. Lancet 2012;379:2243–51.

59. Tripathy D, Schwenke DC, Banerji M, et al. Diabetes incidence and glucose tolerance after termination of pioglitazone therapy: results from ACT NOW. J Clin Endocrinol Metab 2016;101:2056–62.

60. Phillips LS, Ratner RE, Buse JB, et al. We can change the natural history of type 2 diabetes. Diabetes Care 2014;37:2668–76.

61. Schwarz PE, Greaves CJ, Lindstrom J, et al. Nonpharmacological interventions for the prevention of type 2 diabetes mellitus. Nat Rev Endocrinol 2012;8:363–73.

62. Dunkley AJ, Bodicoat DH, Greaves CJ, et al. Diabetes prevention in the real world: effectiveness of pragmatic lifestyle interventions for the prevention of type 2 diabetes and of the impact of adherence to guideline recommendations: a systematic review and meta-analysis. Diabetes Care 2014;37:922–33.

63. Ley SH, Hamdy O, Mohan V, et al. Prevention and management of type 2 diabetes: dietary components and nutritional strategies. Lancet 2014;383: 1999–2007.

64. Salas-Salvado J, Martinez-Gonzalez MA, Bullo M, et al. The role of diet in the prevention of type 2 diabetes. Nutr Metab Cardiovasc Dis 2011;21(Suppl 2):B32–48.

65. Salas-Salvado J, Bullo M, Estruch R, et al. Prevention of diabetes with Mediterranean diets: a subgroup analysis of a randomized trial. Ann Intern Med 2014;160: 1–10.

66. Esposito K, Maiorino MI, Ceriello A, et al. Prevention and control of type 2 diabetes by Mediterranean diet: a systematic review. Diabetes Res Clin Pract 2010;89:97–102.
67. Ogunniyi MO, Croft JB, Greenlund KJ, et al. Racial/ethnic differences in microalbuminuria among adults with prehypertension and hypertension: National Health and Nutrition Examination Survey (NHANES), 1999-2006. Am J Hypertens 2010; 23:859–64.
68. Gong Q, Gregg EW, Wang J, et al. Long-term effects of a randomised trial of a 6-year lifestyle intervention in impaired glucose tolerance on diabetes-related microvascular complications: the China Da Qing Diabetes Prevention Outcome Study. Diabetologia 2011;54:300–7.
69. Morrish NJ, Wang SL, Stevens LK, et al. Mortality and causes of death in the WHO Multinational Study of Vascular Disease in Diabetes. Diabetologia 2001; 44(Suppl 2):S14–21.
70. Tominaga M, Eguchi H, Manaka H, et al. Impaired glucose tolerance is a risk factor for cardiovascular disease, but not impaired fasting glucose. The Funagata Diabetes Study. Diabetes Care 1999;22:920–4.
71. Lawes CM, Parag V, Bennett DA, et al. Blood glucose and risk of cardiovascular disease in the Asia Pacific region. Diabetes Care 2004;27:2836–42.
72. de Vegt F, Dekker JM, Ruhe HG, et al. Hyperglycaemia is associated with all-cause and cardiovascular mortality in the Hoorn population: the Hoorn Study. Diabetologia 1999;42:926–31.
73. DeFronzo RA, Abdul-Ghani M. Assessment and treatment of cardiovascular risk in prediabetes: impaired glucose tolerance and impaired fasting glucose. Am J Cardiol 2011;108:3B–24B.
74. Grundy SM. Pre-diabetes, metabolic syndrome, and cardiovascular risk. J Am Coll Cardiol 2012;59:635–43.
75. Nathan DM, Davidson MB, DeFronzo RA, et al. Impaired fasting glucose and impaired glucose tolerance: implications for care. Diabetes Care 2007;30:753–9.
76. Knowler WC, Hamman RF, Edelstein SL, et al. Prevention of type 2 diabetes with troglitazone in the Diabetes Prevention Program. Diabetes 2005;54:1150–6.
77. Azen SP, Peters RK, Berkowitz K, et al. TRIPOD (TRoglitazone In the Prevention Of Diabetes): a randomized, placebo-controlled trial of troglitazone in women with prior gestational diabetes mellitus. Control Clin Trials 1998;19:217–31.
78. Kahn SE, Haffner SM, Heise MA, et al. Glycemic durability of rosiglitazone, metformin, or glyburide monotherapy. N Engl J Med 2006;355:2427–43.
79. Belfort R, Harrison SA, Brown K, et al. A placebo-controlled trial of pioglitazone in subjects with nonalcoholic steatohepatitis. N Engl J Med 2006;355:2297–307.
80. Cusi K. Treatment of patients with type 2 diabetes and non-alcoholic fatty liver disease: current approaches and future directions. Diabetologia 2016;59: 1112–20.
81. Gastaldelli A, Harrison SA, Belfort-Aguilar R, et al. Importance of changes in adipose tissue insulin resistance to histological response during thiazolidinedione treatment of patients with nonalcoholic steatohepatitis. Hepatology 2009;50: 1087–93.
82. Aithal GP, Thomas JA, Kaye PV, et al. Randomized, placebo-controlled trial of pioglitazone in nondiabetic subjects with nonalcoholic steatohepatitis. Gastroenterology 2008;135:1176–84.
83. Sanyal AJ, Chalasani N, Kowdley KV, et al. Pioglitazone, vitamin E, or placebo for nonalcoholic steatohepatitis. N Engl J Med 2010;362:1675–85.

84. Cusi K, Orsak B, Bril F, et al. Long-term pioglitazone treatment for patients with nonalcoholic steatohepatitis and prediabetes or type 2 diabetes mellitus: a randomized, controlled trial. Ann Intern Med 2016. [Epub ahead of print].

85. Kolberg JA, Jorgensen T, Gerwien RW, et al. Development of a type 2 diabetes risk model from a panel of serum biomarkers from the Inter99 cohort. Diabetes Care 2009;32:1207–12.

86. Watkins SM, Rowe MW, Kolberg JA, et al. Biomarker models as surrogates for the disposition index in the Insulin Resistance Atherosclerosis Study. Diabet Med 2012;29:1399–406.

87. Lyssenko V, Jorgensen T, Gerwien RW, et al. Validation of a multi-marker model for the prediction of incident type 2 diabetes mellitus: combined results of the Inter99 and Botnia studies. Diab Vasc Dis Res 2012;9:59–67.

Nonalcoholic Fatty Liver Disease
The New Complication of Type 2 Diabetes Mellitus

Fernando Bril, MD[a], Kenneth Cusi, MD[a,b],*

KEYWORDS

- Obesity • Nonalcoholic fatty liver disease (NAFLD)
- Nonalcoholic steatohepatitis (NASH) • Thiazolidinediones • Pioglitazone • Diabetes
- Insulin resistance

KEY POINTS

- Nonalcoholic fatty liver disease (NAFLD) is increasingly common in patients with type 2 diabetes mellitus (T2DM).
- NAFLD should be considered as part of a systemic disease, characterized by the accumulation of lipids in tissues where they are usually not stored, causing cellular dysfunction (known as lipotoxicity).
- Although the presence of NAFLD results in worse atherogenic dyslipidemia and more difficult to control hyperglycemia, the presence of T2DM accelerates the progression of liver disease in patients with NAFLD.
- A high level of suspicion is required by health care providers to diagnose NAFLD in patients with T2DM, especially because plasma aminotransferases are not reliable as markers of liver disease in patients with NAFLD.
- Among the different pharmacologic agents tested, pioglitazone has the highest degree of evidence for patients with T2DM and nonalcoholic steatohepatitis, and should be strongly considered in this population.

Disclosure: K. Cusi has received research support from Janssen and Novartis, and served as a consultant for (in alphabetical order) Janssen, Lilly, Pfizer, and Tobira Therapeutics, Inc; F. Bril has nothing to disclose.
[a] Division of Endocrinology, Diabetes and Metabolism, Department of Medicine, University of Florida College of Medicine, 1600 South West Archer Road - Room H2, Gainesville, FL 32610, USA; [b] Division of Endocrinology, Diabetes, and Metabolism, Malcom Randall Veterans Affairs Medical Center, 1601 South West Archer Road, Gainesville, FL 32608, USA
* Corresponding author. Division of Endocrinology, Diabetes and Metabolism, Department of Medicine, University of Florida College of Medicine, 1600 Southwest Archer Road, Room H-2, Gainesville, FL 32610.
E-mail address: Kenneth.Cusi@medicine.ufl.edu

INTRODUCTION

Nonalcoholic fatty liver disease (NAFLD) is defined as the presence of hepatic steatosis (>5% of hepatocytes by histology or >5.6% by nuclear magnetic resonance techniques) in the absence of secondary causes such as alcohol consumption, viral hepatitis, medications (eg, amiodarone, methotrexate, valproate), and autoimmune hepatitis.[1,2] It encompasses a wide range of liver diseases from fairly benign forms such as isolated steatosis (hepatic triglyceride accumulation with minimal or no inflammation) to nonalcoholic steatohepatitis (NASH; steatosis with inflammation and necrosis) and eventually cirrhosis and/or hepatocellular carcinoma (HCC).[1,2] Although NAFLD has been proposed to increase the incidence of new-onset type 2 diabetes mellitus (T2DM),[3] there is also a consensus that the presence of T2DM is a key factor for the progression of NAFLD to its most severe forms, with worse steatohepatitis, relentless fibrosis, and a higher incidence of HCC.[4–6]

However, unlike retinopathy, neuropathy, and nephropathy, NAFLD is currently a largely unrecognized complication of T2DM. Frequently overlooked in clinical practice by both endocrinologists and primary care physicians, NAFLD results in serious metabolic,[7,8] cardiovascular (CV),[9] and hepatic[10,11] consequences to patients with T2DM. Understanding the complicated relationship between NAFLD and T2DM is extremely important, in order to provide better clinical care to these complex patients. Although it may be argued that NAFLD often precedes the development of T2DM,[3] this can also be said about retinopathy,[12] neuropathy,[13,14] and nephropathy,[15] which are also found in insulin-resistant patients with prediabetes but without overt hyperglycemia.

This article focuses on the underlying mechanisms and health risks associated with the development of NASH in patients with T2DM, in the hope that a better understanding of the broad metabolic, hepatic, and CV implications will alert clinicians to be more proactive in the early diagnosis and treatment of these challenging patients.

EPIDEMIOLOGY

As a result of the obesity epidemic, NAFLD has become the most frequent chronic liver disease in the United States, with an estimated prevalence of 34% in the general population (based on screening using liver proton magnetic resonance spectroscopy [^{1}H-MRS]).[16] In the setting of T2DM, the prevalence of NAFLD is at least 2-fold higher, with a range from 57% to 80%, depending on the diagnostic test performed.[17–19]

Most importantly, the presence of T2DM has been associated with a faster progression to NASH and advanced fibrosis,[4,5] supporting the concept that NASH should be considered as a complication of T2DM. In cross-sectional studies involving middle-aged patients with T2DM and NAFLD, Leite and colleagues[20] found that 78% of 92 patients had NASH and ~50% had advanced fibrosis, whereas Fracanzani and colleagues[21] reported that the association of T2DM with NASH and advanced fibrosis was independent of any other risk factors in a larger cohort of 458 patients. In a report in 698 patients with NASH from the Nonalcoholic Steatohepatitis Clinical Research Network (NASH CRN)[22] patients with definite NASH were much more likely to have diabetes and insulin resistance than those with milder liver disease. Among 1069 middle-aged patients with NAFLD, diabetes was associated with an adjusted odds ratio (OR) of 1.76 for NASH (95% confidence interval [CI], 1.1–2.7; $P<.001$) and of 2.57 for fibrosis (95% CI, 1.6–4.1; $P<.0001$).[23] Two recent large population-based studies have confirmed that ~17% of patients with T2DM may have significant fibrosis when assessed by noninvasive imaging tools.[24,25]

Longitudinal studies produced similar conclusions. In a small (n = 103) study with paired biopsies, Adams and colleagues[5] found that, after a mean interval of

3.2 ± 3.0 years, diabetes was independently associated with a much higher rate of fibrosis progression and cirrhosis, in another report being more than 2-fold higher compared with nondiabetics.[26] Pais and colleagues[27] reported that, after a mean follow-up of 3.7 years, two-thirds of patients with isolated steatosis developed NASH and about 40% of these had severe fibrosis. Presence of T2DM at baseline or during follow-up was the most important risk factor for poor prognosis. Other prospective studies have shown that NASH is associated with increased overall and liver-related mortality (**Fig. 1**) and that the presence of T2DM increases the risk of both in these patients.[28–31]

In a similar way, the link between T2DM, cirrhosis, and HCC has long been recognized in the literature.[26] Epidemiologic studies indicate that patients with diabetes have 2-fold to 4-fold higher prevalence rates of cirrhosis and HCC.[6] Whether T2DM, insulin resistance, or another unidentified factor promotes HCC in the end is still under debate. However, NASH seems to be a reasonable intermediary in the association of T2DM and HCC. Although in a meta-analysis by White and colleagues[32] the investigators concluded that the progression from NASH to HCC was almost invariably characterized by the transition to cirrhosis, this has recently been challenged by a large study that included 1500 patients with HCC.[33] This finding reinforces the need for early diagnosis and treatment, in order to delay the progression of liver disease. Moreover, this becomes even more compelling because studies suggest that NASH is the third most common risk factor for HCC in middle-aged individuals, and that they are less likely to undergo HCC surveillance (compared with other classic liver diseases).[34] Taken together, there is an urgent need for early identification of NASH in patients with T2DM.

PATHOPHYSIOLOGY

Nonalcoholic fatty liver disease results from the complex interaction of multiple factors (**Fig. 2**). Hepatic steatosis develops as a consequence of intrahepatic triglyceride accumulation from free fatty acids (FFAs) released from the adipose tissue (lipolysis), FFAs synthesized in the liver from excess carbohydrate (*de novo* lipogenesis) that are then esterified to storage triglycerides for future energy needs, or triglycerides coming from the diet. Of these, FFAs from the adipose tissue are the most important source, and correspond to 60% to 70% of the total lipids reaching the liver.[35,36]

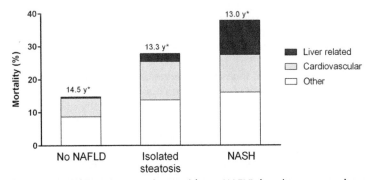

Fig. 1. All-cause mortality among patients without NAFLD by ultrasonography compared with patients with and without NASH by liver biopsy (liver related, cardiovascular, and other). * A weighted mean was performed to calculate time of follow-up. (*Data from* Refs.[10,11,28–31])

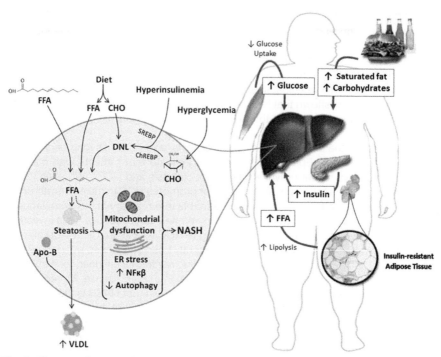

Fig. 2. The contribution of insulin resistance and obesity to the development of hepatic steatosis (see text for details). Apo-B, apolipoprotein B; CHO, carbohydrates; ChREBP, carbo-hydrate-responsive element-binding protein; DNL, de novo lipogenesis; ER, endoplasmic re-ticulum; FFA, free fatty acids; NFkβ, nuclear factor kappa beta; SREBP, sterol regulatory element-binding protein-1c; VLDL, very-low-density lipoprotein.

In the setting of insulin resistance (secondary to obesity, genetic predisposition, or others), lipolysis in the adipose tissue is increased, resulting in an increased release of FFAs into the circulation. This oversecretion of FFAs, in turn, results in lipotoxicity, a term that implies lipid accumulation in tissues that, under normal conditions, do not store large amounts of fat (ie, liver, skeletal muscle, pancreatic beta cell),[36] leading to cellular dysfunction and/or death. Ectopic fat accumulation is associated with hy-perglycemia caused by reduced insulin suppression of hepatic glucose production and altered insulin-stimulated glucose uptake in the skeletal muscle, which in turn pro-duces hyperinsulinemia, a strong promoter of de novo lipogenesis, thus fueling a pos-itive feedback loop (ie, steatosis causes hyperglycemia/hyperinsulinemia, which then worsen steatosis).[37]

Compensatory increases of triglyceride synthesis and very-low-density lipoprotein (VLDL) oversecretion are unable to restore the equilibrium, because they are rapidly exceeded by the high FFA influx.[38] Chronically increased fatty acid oxidation in the mitochondria, unable to fully compensate for the excess FFA flux, leads to a state of mitochondrial dysfunction and accumulation of toxic lipid intermediates.[39] Mito-chondrial dysfunction triggers hepatocyte inflammatory pathways and macrophage (Kupffer cell) recruitment and activation as observed in NASH.[40]

In summary, given the essential role of dysfunctional adipose tissue and lipotoxicity in the development of NAFLD/NASH, the authors think that it would be more appro-priate for the condition to be termed lipotoxic liver disease to more accurately describe its pathophysiology and help focus the target of treatment in clinical practice.

METABOLIC AND CARDIOVASCULAR IMPLICATIONS

In addition to the deleterious consequences on the liver, the presence of NAFLD is associated with a myriad of negative metabolic consequences that ultimately result in increased cardiovascular disease (CVD).[9] Because these metabolic disturbances closely resemble those typical of patients with T2DM, there continues to be considerable debate as to whether the presence of NAFLD in patients with T2DM predisposes them to an even worse metabolic profile. Emerging evidence suggests the coexistence of NAFLD and T2DM as a synergic interaction with unique associated health risks.[7,8,41]

Among these, one of the most extensively assessed is the association between NAFLD and the presence of atherogenic dyslipidemia.[7] In patients with hepatic steatosis, insulin fails to appropriately suppress hepatic VLDL secretion.[38] Increased hepatic VLDL secretion is at the core of the typical atherogenic dyslipidemia of insulin-resistant states leading to high plasma triglyceride levels; low high-density lipoprotein cholesterol levels; and small, dense low-density lipoprotein cholesterol particles.[35] As the authors recently showed, these changes occur in patients with NAFLD, independently of the presence of obesity and/or T2DM.[7,8] Worse liver histology (ie, presence or severity of NASH) was not associated with more atherogenic dyslipidemia.[7] Among the other metabolic consequences of NAFLD, hyperglycemia is of particular concern, because it results in worse diabetes control and the need for more medications to reduce glucose levels. This requirement is probably the result of decreased insulin suppression of hepatic glucose production, as recently shown by our group.[8] In the setting of worse hyperglycemia, and in combination with impaired insulin clearance, these patients frequently show severe hyperinsulinemia.[42]

The common final pathway of all these disturbances is increased CV risk. There is an increasing body of evidence suggesting that the presence of NAFLD is associated with increased CVD.[43] Investigators have addressed this question in a variety of ways, examining the spectrum of vascular disease using different surrogate markers ranging from carotid intima-media thickness[44] to calcium score by computed tomography,[45] but also in a few longitudinal studies.[28–31] Results vary among the different studies, and to date it is still unclear whether NAFLD independently increases CV risk in high-risk patients, such as those with T2DM. Most of the available information comes from studies that have included a small percentage of patients with T2DM and have secondarily performed multivariable analyses including T2DM as a covariate.[46,47] In most reports, the association between NAFLD and CVD persisted even after adjusting for traditional CVD risk factors. The lingering question is whether statistical adjustment for traditional CV variables (eg, obesity, age, hyperglycemia, dyslipidemia) is enough to account for the many confounding factors involved in this relationship. Another caveat is that the diagnosis of NAFLD in most studies has relied on surrogate markers, such as liver aminotransferases or liver ultrasonography, rather than liver ^{1}H-MRS or histology. Many studies are of poor quality because of inadequate controls, short-term follow-up, or few CV events. Only a few longitudinal studies have focused on the association between NAFLD and CVD in patients with T2DM, with conflicting results (**Table 1**). In summary, the metabolic milieu of NAFLD supports the notion of an increased risk for CVD, but the current evidence remains inconclusive for patients with an already increased risk, such as patients with T2DM.

Another important question is whether NAFLD in diabetes worsens microvascular disease. The strongest evidence in this regard comes from studies assessing the association between NAFLD and chronic kidney disease (CKD) and/or proteinuria. In a

Table 1
Longitudinal and cross-sectional studies assessing the association of CV outcomes and/or mortality and nonalcoholic fatty liver disease (NAFLD) in patients with type 2 diabetes mellitus (T2DM)

	Country	n	NAFLD	CV Risk	Outcome
Longitudinal Studies					
Targher et al,[9] 2007	Italy	2103	Ultrasonography	↑	CV events
Adams et al,[10] 2010	United States	337	Biopsy	↔	CV mortality
Dunn et al,[109] 2013	United States	2343	CT	↔	CV mortality
Cross-sectional Studies					
Targher et al,[110] 2006	Italy	245	Biopsy	↑	CIMT
McKimmie et al,[111] 2008	United States	623	CT	↔	CIMT and CACS
Petit et al,[19] 2009	France	101	MRS	↔	CIMT
Khashper et al,[112] 2013	Israel	93	CT	↔	CACS
Kim et al,[44] 2014	Korea	4437	Ultrasonography	↑	CIMT
Idilman et al,[113] 2015	Turkey	273	CT	↔	CACS
Silaghi et al,[114] 2015	Romania	336	Ultrasonography	↔	CIMT
Kwak et al,[115] 2015	Korea	213	Ultrasonography	↔	CACS
Mantovani et al,[116] 2015	Italy	222	Ultrasonography	↑	LV diastolic dysfunction

Abbreviations: CACS, coronary artery calcium score; CIMT, carotid intima-media thickness; CT, computed tomography; LV, left ventricle; MRS, magnetic resonance spectroscopy.

meta-analysis by Musso and colleagues,[48] there was a significant association between NAFLD and kidney disease in both cross-sectional and longitudinal studies. This association was true for different outcomes, such as prevalence (cross sectional) or incidence (longitudinal) of CKD, estimated glomerular filtration rate considered as a continuous variable, or presence of proteinuria. Moreover, the presence of NASH and advanced fibrosis was associated with worse CKD compared with patients with isolated steatosis or those without fibrosis, respectively. The magnitude and direction of effects remained unaffected by diabetes status or other classic risk factors of CKD.

Available information on the association between NAFLD and retinopathy or neuropathy is much more limited. In a study of 2103 patients with T2DM, patients with NAFLD had a higher prevalence of proliferative/laser-treated retinopathy (OR, 1.8 [1.1–3.7]) after adjusting for typical CV risk factors.[49] However, a better understanding of the role of NAFLD, if any, in microvascular complications in T2DM is greatly needed.

DIAGNOSIS

Based on the evidence discussed earlier, diagnosis of NAFLD in patients with T2DM is important in order to detect patients with a potentially higher CV (and microvascular) risk, as well as to identify patients who may benefit from specific treatment modalities (discussed later). However, clinically available diagnostic tools have important limitations for the diagnosis of NAFLD, which probably contributes to the current underdiagnosis of NAFLD.

Although plasma aminotransferases have frequently been trusted as markers of liver disease, 56% of overweight/obese patients with T2DM have a diagnosis of

NAFLD by ^{1}H-MRS despite normal aspartate transaminase (AST) and alanine transaminase (ALT) levels.[50] Moreover, even in patients without diabetes, around one-third of patients with normal ALT levels had NASH or advanced fibrosis, further supporting that ALT is a poor marker of liver disease in NAFLD.[51] Liver ultrasonography, another frequently prescribed test for the diagnosis of NAFLD, has only modest sensitivity and specificity, which are significantly reduced when liver triglyceride content is lower than 12.5%.[52] More recently, the use of vibration-controlled transient elastography and controlled attenuation parameter have allowed liver fat and fibrosis to be quantified in an easy and noninvasive way.[53] However, application of this methodology to NAFLD can be challenging, because worse performance and higher rates of measurement failure have been described in obese individuals.[54] A recent study by Imajo and colleagues[55] suggested that this tool underperformed compared with nuclear magnetic resonance techniques (MRI proton density fat fraction and magnetic resonance elastography). As these magnetic resonance techniques become more accessible and readily available, the authors envision that they will soon become more widely used for the diagnosis of steatosis and fibrosis, relegating the liver biopsy for only particular cases.

In spite of these advances, diagnosis of NASH (ie, presence of inflammation and necrosis in the liver) remains elusive to noninvasive techniques. Different plasma biomarkers and clinical scores have been tested in recent years in order to better diagnose patients with NASH.[56] Cytokeratin-18 fragments, probably among the most promising biomarkers in the past, have been shown to be inadequate as a stand-alone test for the diagnosis of this condition,[57] as have most of the plasma biomarkers individually assessed for the prediction of NASH. Because of the multifactorial nature of this condition, it is to be expected that no single molecule will be able to reasonably detect NAFLD in all scenarios, much less to distinguish isolated steatosis from NASH. Using a combination of different factors, such as AST/ALT, body mass index (BMI), platelets, albumin, presence of diabetes, insulin, and cytokeratin-18, different groups have tried to develop clinical models to use in the clinical setting for the diagnosis of NAFLD.[58–60] Although acceptable to distinguish between opposite extremes of the disease (absence of NAFLD vs NASH with advanced fibrosis), none of these clinical models has proved useful to correctly classify most of the patients in the middle of the disease spectrum (ie, those with mild to moderate fibrosis). Similar approaches have been tried in patients with T2DM, but with comparable results. Bazick and colleagues[61] developed a clinical model to predict the presence of NASH in patients with T2DM using ethnicity, BMI, waist, ALT, AST, albumin, hemoglobin A1c (A1c), homeostatic model assessment–insulin resistance (HOMA-IR), and ferritin. However, 44% of the patients were in the gray zone of the model, and therefore the presence of NASH could not be established. Moreover, the percentage of patients in the gray zone increased to 87% for the prediction of advanced fibrosis, reinforcing the notion that these models may only help to distinguish patients who are healthy (without NASH or fibrosis) from those with advanced liver disease.

Because NAFLD is usually asymptomatic (and with normal ALT/AST levels, as discussed earlier), physicians must have a high degree of clinical suspicion in order to reach a diagnosis of NAFLD or NASH in patients with T2DM. In the last few years, there has been great progress in the development of novel diagnostic tools that are likely to improve the detection threshold for NAFLD. This improvement is likely to result in a significant increase in the number of patients being diagnosed with NAFLD, and will require a more active role among health care providers in the treatment of NAFLD and NASH.

TREATMENT
Diet and Lifestyle Intervention

Lifestyle modification and weight loss should be at the core of the management of NAFLD. However, most studies have had significant shortcomings by being small, uncontrolled, including few patients with diabetes, and by using surrogate end points of liver disease (plasma aminotransferases, liver ultrasonography, or ^{1}H-MRS) and not liver histology to assess treatment success.[62,63] Overall, a large body of literature can be summarized by saying that even a modest weight reduction of 5% to 10% with lifestyle modification markedly reduces intrahepatic triglyceride (IHTG) levels by about 40%.[36] A weight loss of ~10% induced by lifestyle modification improves steatosis, necrosis, and inflammation on liver biopsies of most patients with NASH,[64,65] and this is even more consistent after greater weight loss with bariatric surgery.[63,66] However, improvement in fibrosis by lifestyle changes and/or bariatric surgery is less well established and awaits assessment in long-term studies. In summary, weight loss is essential for the successful management of patients with T2DM and NAFLD.

Insulin Sensitizers in Nonalcoholic Steatohepatitis: Role of Pioglitazone

Restoring insulin action is a major goal of therapy given the central role of adipose tissue insulin resistance and lipotoxicity in the pathogenesis of NASH.[36] In this setting, insulin sensitizers have often been tested for the treatment of NASH. Although early open-label studies with metformin were promising,[67,68] benefits seemed to be more associated with weight loss from the biguanide and not drug specific, with more recent controlled trials being negative in both children[69] and adults.[1,2,70,71]

Patients with T2DM and steatohepatitis have worse adipose tissue and hepatic insulin resistance compared with matched obese controls with only isolated steatosis on liver histology.[8] They also have profound mitochondrial defects associated with insulin resistance and lipotoxicity,[39,40,72–74] with accumulation of toxic lipid metabolites that suggest inadequate disposal of excess fatty acids through the Krebs cycle. Pioglitazone is a thiazolidinedione that targets the transcription factor peroxisome proliferator–activated receptor (PPAR)–gamma and modulates glucose and lipid metabolism,[36,75] preventing excessive rates of adipose tissue lipolysis[76,77] and increasing plasma adiponectin concentration.[78] Histologic response in pioglitazone-treated patients can be predicted by the magnitude of the early increase in plasma adiponectin level.[79] The study by Belfort and colleagues[76] established that patients with prediabetes or T2DM treated with pioglitazone had a marked improvement in hepatic steatosis and necroinflammation, and that steatohepatitis could be resolved within 6 months. Liver fibrosis improved compared with baseline ($P = .002$), but not compared with placebo ($P = .08$). Recently, a 3-year study in 101 patients with NASH, and either prediabetes or T2DM, confirmed its long-term safety and efficacy in this population.[79] Patients with NASH but without diabetes also improve with pioglitazone.[80,81] These results suggest that pioglitazone may modify the natural history of the disease in patients with (or without) T2DM and become the standard of care for treatment of NASH, at least in the future.

Weight gain with pioglitazone treatment may occur from enhanced adipocyte triglyceride storage (typically 2–3 kg gain over 12–18 months), and less often from fluid retention.[82] Congestive heart failure is unusual but may occur in patients with unrecognized diastolic dysfunction.[83] Bone loss may occur in women, and this is one of the main reasons for restricting use to adults only.[84] A 10-year prospective study showed no association between pioglitazone and bladder cancer.[85] In addition, given the increased CV risk of patients with NAFLD, it is of interest that pioglitazone decreases CV events, although long-term studies in this population have not been conducted.[36,75]

Glucagonlike Peptide-1 Receptor Agonists and Dipeptidyl Peptidase-4 Inhibitors

During clinical development it was observed that liraglutide reduced the increased plasma aminotransferase levels in patients with T2DM,[86] but it was not until recently that the glucagonlike peptide-1 receptor agonist (GLP-1RA) class of drugs showed efficacy in a randomized controlled trial (RCT) in patients with NASH, although only one-third had T2DM.[87] In a 48-week study in 52 patients, resolution of NASH occurred in 39% patients treated with GLP-1RA versus 9% treated with placebo (Relative risk, 4.3; 95% CI, 1.0–17.7; $P = .019$; treatment difference ~30%). Liver and adipose tissue insulin sensitivity improved in a subset of patients undergoing in-depth metabolic studies at 3 months.[88] It remains to be established whether the benefit is from changes in specific hepatocyte glucagonlike peptide-1 signaling pathways[89,90] or only secondary to weight loss with improved hepatic insulin action or amelioration of glucotoxicity.[91] Several long-acting (weekly dosing) GLP-1RAs are currently undergoing testing. In contrast, largely negative results have tempered excitement about the treatment of NASH with dipeptidyl peptidase-4 (DPP-4) inhibitors, although there are no controlled studies with liver histology as the primary end point to fully assess their impact on steatohepatitis in humans. A reduction in plasma aminotransferase levels has been reported with sitagliptin,[92] but not in all studies.[93] Another study reported a modest decrease in liver IHTG levels with the DPP-4 inhibitor vildagliptin in patients with T2DM with overall mild steatosis, which correlated with an improvement in hyperglycemia.[94]

Sodium-Glucose Cotransporter 2 Inhibitors

Inhibitors of proximal tubule glucose reabsorption have become widely used agents for the treatment of T2DM[95] and have been reported to decrease plasma aminotransferase levels in RCTs.[96] Its rationale for use in NAFLD is based on the hypothesis that sodium-glucose cotransporter 2 (SGLT2)–induced euglycemia deprives de novo lipogenesis from glucose carbons for FFA synthesis and eventual IHTG accumulation. In addition, in vivo evidence suggests that SGLT2 is an inhibitor of hepatic fibrogenesis.[97] Although ongoing studies are examining the role of SGLT2 inhibitors in patients with NAFLD and T2DM, in pooled data from 6 RCTs of canagliflozin versus placebo or sitagliptin (~3800 patients), a greater reduction in plasma alanine aminotransferase levels was observed with canagliflozin 300 mg versus either comparator.[98] Of note, decreases in plasma aminotransferase levels seemed to be unspecific and closely linked to changes in A1c or body weight.

Other Pharmacologic Treatments Tested in Patients Without Diabetes

Many agents have been tested for the treatment of NASH.[1,36,70,71] However, most have included only small numbers of patients with T2DM, or simply excluded them. Perhaps the best studied has been vitamin E. At a dose of 800 IU/d, the primary histologic outcome was reached in 43% on vitamin E versus 19% on placebo ($P = .001$) in nondiabetic adults with NASH.[81] However, resolution of NASH was of borderline significance (36% vs 21%; $P = .05$ vs placebo), in contrast with the significant effect of pioglitazone on resolution of NASH in the same trial (47% vs 21%; $P = .001$ vs placebo).[81] Vitamin E is not effective compared with placebo in nondiabetic children with NASH.[69] The mechanisms by which vitamin E may ameliorate steatohepatitis remain uncertain, but are thought to be related to amelioration of intracellular oxidative stress. Controversy still surrounds its long-term safety because of the fear of an increased risk of prostate cancer and, to a lesser extent, of CVD. Its safety and efficacy in patients with T2DM, either alone or combined with pioglitazone, is being explored in an RCT that will report results in early 2017 (NCT01002547).

Many agents that reduce lipid levels (eg, statins, fibrates) have been tested in this population to reduce IHTG levels or treat steatohepatitis, but largely without success[99–104] (reviewed in depth by Bril and colleagues[35]). Pentoxifylline, a tumor necrosis factor-alpha agonist and nonselective phosphodiesterase inhibitor, has been studied in 2 small RCTs with either a modest[105] or no[106] histologic improvement. As recently reviewed,[107] several pharmacologic agents are undergoing testing for NASH in phase 2a/2b or early phase 3 trials: obeticholic acid (a farnesoid X receptor agonist), elafibranor (a dual PPARα/PPARδ agonist), cenicriviroc (an inhibitor of ligand binding of chemokine receptor [CCR] 2 and CCR5), as well as drugs primarily targeting fibrosis, such as emricasan (a pancaspase inhibitor); galectin-3 protein inhibitors; or lysyl oxidase–like 2 inhibitors, which prevent collagen cross-linking.

SUMMARY

Rapid changes in the diagnosis and management of NASH are likely to occur in the near future. In contrast with the recent past, there is consensus about the increased risk associated with having diabetes in patients with NASH, and most RCTs now include a large number of patients with T2DM. However, there is a lack of more specific screening and treatment recommendations for such patients. The future will include genetic testing, searching for specific polymorphisms linked with worse prognosis in NASH, combined with novel plasma biomarkers and more accurate liver fibrosis imaging techniques.[108] Because recent studies suggest that liver fibrosis is common in patients with T2DM,[24,25] screening for NASH, and specifically for fibrosis, will become routine and will be done in the same way as is now done for microvascular complications such as retinopathy, neuropathy, and nephropathy.

Early intervention will be important to modify the natural history of the disease. For the first time, there is now a safe and effective long-term treatment (pioglitazone) that seems to halt disease progression in many patients with T2DM and NASH.[79] The authors envision that pioglitazone is likely to be used as first-line therapy in NASH, in the same way as metformin is currently prescribed for the treatment of T2DM. As novel agents become available, combination of several agents to treat NASH will become common practice, and management will be viewed more and more as it currently is for the treatment of diabetes, dyslipidemia, or hypertension. Clinicians are at the dawn of a new era of greater awareness about the impact of NASH to overall health and better treatment options are available. If taken together, this will significantly improve the quality of life of many patients who are currently overlooked and undertreated in clinical practice.

REFERENCES

1. Toplak H, Stauber R, Sourij H. EASL-EASD-EASO clinical practice guidelines for the management of non-alcoholic fatty liver disease: guidelines, clinical reality and health economic aspects. Diabetologia 2016;59:1148–9.

2. Chalasani N, Younossi Z, Lavine JE, et al. The diagnosis and management of non-alcoholic fatty liver disease: practice guideline by the American Gastroenterological Association, American Association for the Study of Liver Diseases, and American College of Gastroenterology. Gastroenterology 2012;142: 1592–609.

3. Ballestri S, Zona S, Targher G, et al. Nonalcoholic fatty liver disease is associ- ated with an almost two-fold increased risk of incident type 2 diabetes and metabolic syndrome. Evidence from a systematic review and meta-analysis. J Gastroenterol Hepatol 2015;31:936–44.

4. Hossain N, Afendy A, Stepanova M, et al. Independent predictors of fibrosis in patients with nonalcoholic fatty liver disease. Clin Gastroenterol Hepatol 2009;7: 1224–9.e1–2.

5. Adams LA, Sanderson S, Lindor KD, et al. The histological course of nonalco- holic fatty liver disease: a longitudinal study of 103 patients with sequential liver biopsies. J Hepatol 2005;42:132–8.

6. Wang C, Wang X, Gong G, et al. Increased risk of hepatocellular carcinoma in patients with diabetes mellitus: a systematic review and meta-analysis of cohort studies. Int J Cancer 2012;130:1639–48.

7. Bril F, Sninsky JJ, Baca AM, et al. Hepatic steatosis and insulin resistance, but not steatohepatitis, promote atherogenic dyslipidemia in NAFLD. J Clin Endocri- nol Metab 2016;101:644–52.

8. Lomonaco R, Bril F, Portillo-Sanchez P, et al. Metabolic impact of nonalcoholic steatohepatitis in obese patients with type 2 diabetes. Diabetes Care 2016; 39:632–8.

9. Targher G, Bertolini L, Rodella S, et al. Nonalcoholic fatty liver disease is inde- pendently associated with an increased incidence of cardiovascular events in type 2 diabetic patients. Diabetes Care 2007;30:2119–21.

10. Adams LA, Harmsen S, St Sauver JL, et al. Nonalcoholic fatty liver disease in- creases risk of death among patients with diabetes: a community-based cohort study. Am J Gastroenterol 2010;105:1567–73.

11. Angulo P, Kleiner DE, Dam-Larsen S, et al. Liver fibrosis, but no other histologic features, is associated with long-term outcomes of patients with nonalcoholic fatty liver disease. Gastroenterology 2015;149:389–97.e10.

12. Nguyen TT, Wang JJ, Wong TY. Retinal vascular changes in pre-diabetes and prehypertension: new findings and their research and clinical implications. Dia- betes Care 2007;30:2708–15.

13. Smith AG, Russell J, Feldman EL, et al. Lifestyle intervention for pre-diabetic neuropathy. Diabetes Care 2006;29:1294–9.

14. Lee CC, Perkins BA, Kayaniyil S, et al. Peripheral neuropathy and nerve dysfunction in individuals at high risk for type 2 diabetes: the PROMISE cohort. Diabetes Care 2015;38:793–800.

15. Melsom T, Schei J, Stefansson VT, et al. Prediabetes and risk of glomerular hy- perfiltration and albuminuria in the general nondiabetic population: a prospec- tive cohort study. Am J Kidney Dis 2016;67(6):841–50.

16. Browning JD, Szczepaniak LS, Dobbins R, et al. Prevalence of hepatic steatosis in an urban population in the United States: impact of ethnicity. Hepatology 2004;40:1387–95.

17. Williamson RM, Price JF, Glancy S, et al. Prevalence of and risk factors for he- patic steatosis and nonalcoholic fatty liver disease in people with type 2 dia- betes: the Edinburgh Type 2 Diabetes Study. Diabetes Care 2011;34:1139–44.

18. Targher G, Bertolini L, Padovani R, et al. Prevalence of nonalcoholic fatty liver disease and its association with cardiovascular disease among type 2 diabetic patients. Diabetes Care 2007;30:1212–8.

19. Petit JM, Guiu B, Terriat B, et al. Nonalcoholic fatty liver is not associated with carotid intima-media thickness in type 2 diabetic patients. J Clin Endocrinol Metab 2009;94:4103–6.

20. Leite NC, Villela-Nogueira CA, Pannain VL, et al. Histopathological stages of nonalcoholic fatty liver disease in type 2 diabetes: prevalences and correlated factors. Liver Int 2011;31:700–6.

21. Fracanzani AL, Valenti L, Bugianesi E, et al. Risk of severe liver disease in nonalcoholic fatty liver disease with normal aminotransferase levels: a role for insulin resistance and diabetes. Hepatology 2008;48:792–8.

22. Neuschwander-Tetri BA, Clark JM, Bass NM, et al. Clinical, laboratory and histological associations in adults with nonalcoholic fatty liver disease. Hepatology 2010;52:913–24.

23. Loomba R, Abraham M, Unalp A, et al. Association between diabetes, family history of diabetes, and risk of nonalcoholic steatohepatitis and fibrosis. Hepatology 2012;56:943–51.

24. Koehler EM, Plompen EP, Schouten JN, et al. Presence of diabetes mellitus and steatosis is associated with liver stiffness in a general population: The Rotterdam study. Hepatology 2016;63:138–47.

25. Kwok R, Choi KC, Wong GL, et al. Screening diabetic patients for non-alcoholic fatty liver disease with controlled attenuation parameter and liver stiffness measurements: a prospective cohort study. Gut 2015;65(8):1359–68.

26. El-Serag HB, Tran T, Everhart JE. Diabetes increases the risk of chronic liver disease and hepatocellular carcinoma. Gastroenterology 2004;126:460–8.

27. Pais R, Charlotte F, Fedchuk L, et al. A systematic review of follow-up biopsies reveals disease progression in patients with non-alcoholic fatty liver. J Hepatol 2013;59:550–6.

28. Ekstedt M, Franzen LE, Mathiesen UL, et al. Long-term follow-up of patients with NAFLD and elevated liver enzymes. Hepatology 2006;44:865–73.

29. Dam-Larsen S, Becker U, Franzmann MB, et al. Final results of a long-term, clinical follow-up in fatty liver patients. Scand J Gastroenterol 2009;44:1236–43.

30. Soderberg C, Stal P, Askling J, et al. Decreased survival of subjects with elevated liver function tests during a 28-year follow-up. Hepatology 2010;51:595–602.

31. Stepanova M, Rafiq N, Makhlouf H, et al. Predictors of all-cause mortality and liver-related mortality in patients with non-alcoholic fatty liver disease (NAFLD). Dig Dis Sci 2013;58:3017–23.

32. White DL, Kanwal F, El-Serag HB. Association between nonalcoholic fatty liver disease and risk for hepatocellular cancer, based on systematic review. Clin Gastroenterol Hepatol 2012;10:1342–59.e2.

33. Mittal S, El-Serag HB, Sada YH, et al. Hepatocellular carcinoma in the absence of cirrhosis in United States veterans is associated with nonalcoholic fatty liver disease. Clin Gastroenterol Hepatol 2016;14:124–31.e1.

34. Mittal S, Sada YH, El-Serag HB, et al. Temporal trends of nonalcoholic fatty liver disease-related hepatocellular carcinoma in the veteran affairs population. Clin Gastroenterol Hepatol 2015;13:594–601.e1.

35. Bril F, Lomonaco R, Cusi K. The challenge of managing dyslipidemia in patients with nonalcoholic fatty liver disease. Clin Lipidol 2012;7:471–81.

36. Cusi K. Role of obesity and lipotoxicity in the development of nonalcoholic steatohepatitis: pathophysiology and clinical implications. Gastroenterology 2012;142:711–25.e6.

37. Neuschwander-Tetri BA. Hepatic lipotoxicity and the pathogenesis of nonalcoholic steatohepatitis: the central role of nontriglyceride fatty acid metabolites. Hepatology 2010;52:774–88.

38. Fabbrini E, Mohammed BS, Magkos F, et al. Alterations in adipose tissue and hepatic lipid kinetics in obese men and women with nonalcoholic fatty liver disease. Gastroenterology 2008;134:424–31.

39. Sunny NE, Parks EJ, Browning JD, et al. Excessive hepatic mitochondrial TCA cycle and gluconeogenesis in humans with nonalcoholic fatty liver disease. Cell Metab 2011;14:804–10.

40. Satapati S, Kucejova B, Duarte JA, et al. Mitochondrial metabolism mediates oxidative stress and inflammation in fatty liver. J Clin Invest 2015;125:4447–62.

41. Hazlehurst JM, Woods C, Marjot T, et al. Non-alcoholic fatty liver disease and diabetes. Metabolism 2016;65(8):1096–108.

42. Bril F, Lomonaco R, Orsak B, et al. Relationship between disease severity, hyperinsulinemia, and impaired insulin clearance in patients with nonalcoholic steatohepatitis. Hepatology 2014;59:2178–87.

43. Armstrong MJ, Adams LA, Canbay A, et al. Extrahepatic complications of nonalcoholic fatty liver disease. Hepatology 2014;59:1174–97.

44. Kim SK, Choi YJ, Huh BW, et al. Nonalcoholic fatty liver disease is associated with increased carotid intima-media thickness only in type 2 diabetic subjects with insulin resistance. J Clin Endocrinol Metab 2014;99:1879–84.

45. Kim D, Choi SY, Park EH, et al. Nonalcoholic fatty liver disease is associated with coronary artery calcification. Hepatology 2012;56:605–13.

46. El Azeem HA, Khalek el SA, El-Akabawy H, et al. Association between nonalcoholic fatty liver disease and the incidence of cardiovascular and renal events. J Saudi Heart Assoc 2013;25:239–46.

47. Lazo M, Hernaez R, Bonekamp S, et al. Non-alcoholic fatty liver disease and mortality among US adults: prospective cohort study. BMJ 2011;343:d6891.

48. Musso G, Gambino R, Tabibian JH, et al. Association of non-alcoholic fatty liver disease with chronic kidney disease: a systematic review and meta-analysis. PLoS Med 2014;11:e1001680.

49. Targher G, Bertolini L, Rodella S, et al. Non-alcoholic fatty liver disease is independently associated with an increased prevalence of chronic kidney disease and proliferative/laser-treated retinopathy in type 2 diabetic patients. Diabetologia 2008;51:444–50.

50. Portillo-Sanchez P, Bril F, Maximos M, et al. High prevalence of nonalcoholic fatty liver disease in patients with type 2 diabetes mellitus and normal plasma aminotransferase levels. J Clin Endocrinol Metab 2015;100:2231–8.

51. Verma S, Jensen D, Hart J, et al. Predictive value of ALT levels for non-alcoholic steatohepatitis (NASH) and advanced fibrosis in non-alcoholic fatty liver disease (NAFLD). Liver Int 2013;33:1398–405.

52. Bril F, Ortiz-Lopez C, Lomonaco R, et al. Clinical value of liver ultrasound for the diagnosis of nonalcoholic fatty liver disease in overweight and obese patients. Liver Int 2015;35:2139–46.

53. Hannah WN, Harrison SA. NAFLD and elastography - incremental advances but work still to be done. Hepatology 2016;63(6):1762–4.

54. Wong VW, Vergniol J, Wong GL, et al. Liver stiffness measurement using XL probe in patients with nonalcoholic fatty liver disease. Am J Gastroenterol 2012;107:1862–71.

55. Imajo K, Kessoku T, Honda Y, et al. Magnetic resonance imaging more accurately classifies steatosis and fibrosis in patients with nonalcoholic fatty liver disease than transient elastography. Gastroenterology 2016;150:626–37.e7.

56. Papagianni M, Sofogianni A, Tziomalos K. Non-invasive methods for the diagnosis of nonalcoholic fatty liver disease. World J Hepatol 2015;7:638–48.

57. Cusi K, Chang Z, Harrison S, et al. Limited value of plasma cytokeratin-18 as a biomarker for NASH and fibrosis in patients with non-alcoholic fatty liver disease. J Hepatol 2014;60:167–74.
58. Ratziu V, Massard J, Charlotte F, et al. Diagnostic value of biochemical markers (FibroTest-FibroSURE) for the prediction of liver fibrosis in patients with non-alcoholic fatty liver disease. BMC Gastroenterol 2006;6:6.
59. Harrison SA, Oliver D, Arnold HL, et al. Development and validation of a simple NAFLD clinical scoring system for identifying patients without advanced disease. Gut 2008;57:1441–7.
60. Angulo P, Bugianesi E, Bjornsson ES, et al. Simple noninvasive systems predict long-term outcomes of patients with nonalcoholic fatty liver disease. Gastroenterology 2013;145:782–9.e4.
61. Bazick J, Donithan M, Neuschwander-Tetri BA, et al. Clinical model for NASH and advanced fibrosis in adult patients with diabetes and NAFLD: guidelines for referral in NAFLD. Diabetes Care 2015;38:1347–55.
62. Marchesini G, Petta S, Dalle Grave R. Diet, weight loss, and liver health in NAFLD: pathophysiology, evidence and practice. Hepatology 2016;63(6):2032–43.
63. Hannah WN, Harrison SA. Effect of weight loss, diet, exercise, and bariatric surgery on nonalcoholic fatty liver disease. Clin Liver Dis 2016;20:339–50.
64. Promrat K, Kleiner DE, Niemeier HM, et al. Randomized controlled trial testing the effects of weight loss on nonalcoholic steatohepatitis. Hepatology 2010;51:121–9.
65. Vilar-Gomez E, Martinez-Perez Y, Calzadilla-Bertot L, et al. Weight loss through lifestyle modification significantly reduces features of nonalcoholic steatohepatitis. Gastroenterology 2015;149:367–78.
66. Moretto M, Kupski C, da Silva VD, et al. Effect of bariatric surgery on liver fibrosis. Obes Surg 2012;22:1044–9.
67. Bugianesi E, Gentilcore E, Manini R, et al. A randomized controlled trial of metformin versus vitamin E or prescriptive diet in nonalcoholic fatty liver disease. Am J Gastroenterol 2005;100:1082–90.
68. Loomba R, Lutchman G, Kleiner DE, et al. Clinical trial: pilot study of metformin for the treatment of non-alcoholic steatohepatitis. Aliment Pharmacol Ther 2009;29:172–82.
69. Lavine JE, Schwimmer JB, Van Natta ML, et al, The Nonalcoholic Steatohepatitis Clinical Research Network. Effect of vitamin E or metformin for treatment of nonalcoholic fatty liver disease in children and adolescents: the TONIC randomized controlled trial. JAMA 2011;305:1659–68.
70. Lomonaco R, Sunny NE, Bril F, et al. Nonalcoholic fatty liver disease: current issues and novel treatment approaches. Drugs 2013;73:1–14.
71. Ahmed A, Wong RJ, Harrison SA. Nonalcoholic fatty liver disease review: diagnosis, treatment and outcomes. Clin Gastroenterol Hepatol 2015;13:2062–70.
72. Sunny NE, Kalavalapalli S, Bril F, et al. Cross-talk between branched-chain amino acids and hepatic mitochondria is compromised in nonalcoholic fatty liver disease. Am J Physiol Endocrinol Metab 2015;309:E311–9.
73. Patterson RE, Kalavalapalli S, Williams CM, et al. Lipotoxicity in steatohepatitis occurs despite an increase in tricarboxylic acid cycle activity. Am J Physiol Endocrinol Metab 2016;310:E484–94.
74. Koliaki C, Szendroedi J, Jelenik T, et al. Adaptation of hepatic mitochondrial function in humans with non-alcoholic fatty liver or steatohepatitis. Cell Metab 2015;21:739–46.

75. Soccio RE, Chen ER, Lazar MA. Thiazolidinediones and the promise of insulin sensitization in type 2 diabetes. Cell Metab 2014;20:573–91.
76. Belfort R, Harrison SA, Brown K, et al. A placebo-controlled trial of pioglitazone in subjects with nonalcoholic steatohepatitis. N Engl J Med 2006;355:2297–307.
77. Lomonaco R, Ortiz-Lopez C, Orsak B, et al. Effect of adipose tissue insulin resistance on metabolic parameters and liver histology in obese patients with nonalcoholic fatty liver disease. Hepatology 2012;55:1389–97.
78. Gastaldelli A, Harrison S, Belfort-Aguiar R, et al. Pioglitazone in the treatment of NASH: the role of adiponectin. Aliment Pharmacol Ther 2010;32:769–75.
79. Cusi K, Orsak B, Bril F, et al. Long-term pioglitazone treatment for patients with nonalcoholic steatohepatitis and prediabetes or type 2 diabetes mellitus: a randomized trial. Ann Intern Med 2016;165(5):305–15.
80. Aithal GP, Thomas JA, Kaye PV, et al. Randomized, placebo-controlled trial of pioglitazone in nondiabetic subjects with nonalcoholic steatohepatitis. Gastroenterology 2008;135:1176–84.
81. Sanyal AJ, Chalasani N, Kowdley KV, et al. Pioglitazone, vitamin E, or placebo for nonalcoholic steatohepatitis. N Engl J Med 2010;362:1675–85.
82. Balas B, Belfort R, Harrison S, et al. Pioglitazone treatment increases whole body fat but not total body water in patients with non-alcoholic steatohepatitis. J Hepatol 2007;47:565–70.
83. VanWagner LB, Wilcox JE, Colangelo LA, et al. Association of nonalcoholic fatty liver disease with subclinical myocardial remodeling and dysfunction: a population-based study. Hepatology 2015;62:773–83.
84. Yau H, Rivera K, Lomonaco R, et al. The future of thiazolidinedione therapy in the management of type 2 diabetes mellitus. Curr Diab Rep 2013;13:329–41.
85. Lewis JD, Habel LA, Quesenberry CP, et al. Pioglitazone use and risk of bladder cancer and other common cancers in persons with diabetes. JAMA 2015;314:265–77.
86. Armstrong MJ, Houlihan DD, Rowe IA, et al. Safety and efficacy of liraglutide in patients with type 2 diabetes with elevated liver enzymes: individual patient data meta-analysis of the LEAD programme. Aliment Pharmacol Ther 2013;37:234–42.
87. Armstrong MJ, Gaunt P, Aithal GP, et al. Liraglutide Safety and Efficacy in Patients with Non-alcoholic Steatohepatitis (LEAN): a multicentre, double-blind, randomised, placebo-controlled phase 2 study. Lancet 2016;387:679–90.
88. Armstrong MJ, Hull D, Guo K, et al. Glucagon-like peptide 1 decreases lipotoxicity in non-alcoholic steatohepatitis. J Hepatol 2016;64:399–408.
89. Gupta NA, Mells J, Dunham RM, et al. Glucagon-like peptide-1 receptor is present on human hepatocytes and has a direct role in decreasing hepatic steatosis in vitro by modulating elements of the insulin signaling pathway. Hepatology 2010;51:1584–92.
90. Svegliati-Baroni G, Saccomanno S, Rychlicki C, et al. Glucagon-like peptide-1 receptor activation stimulates hepatic lipid oxidation and restores hepatic signalling alteration induced by a high-fat diet in nonalcoholic steatohepatitis. Liver Int 2011;31:1285–97.
91. Portillo P, Yavuz S, Bril F, et al. Role of insulin resistance and diabetes in the pathogenesis and treatment of nonalcoholic fatty liver disease. Curr Hepatol Rep 2014;13:159–70.
92. Fukuhara T, Hyogo H, Ochi H, et al. Efficacy and safety of sitagliptin for the treatment of nonalcoholic fatty liver disease with type 2 diabetes mellitus. Hepatogastroenterology 2014;61:323–8.

93. Iwasaki T, Yoneda M, Inamori M, et al. Sitagliptin as a novel treatment agent for non-alcoholic fatty liver disease patients with type 2 diabetes mellitus. Hepato-gastroenterology 2011;58:2103–5.

94. Macauley M, Hollingsworth KG, Smith FE, et al. Effect of vildagliptin on hepatic steatosis. J Clin Endocrinol Metab 2015;100:1578–85.

95. Mudaliar S, Polidori D, Zambrowicz B, et al. Sodium-glucose cotransporter in-hibitors: effects on renal and intestinal glucose transport: from bench to bedside. Diabetes Care 2015;38:2344–53.

96. Lavalle-Gonzalez FJ, Januszewicz A, Davidson J, et al. Efficacy and safety of canagliflozin compared with placebo and sitagliptin in patients with type 2 dia-betes on background metformin monotherapy: a randomised trial. Diabetologia 2013;56:2582–92.

97. Hayashizaki-Someya Y, Kurosaki E, Takasu T, et al. Ipragliflozin, an SGLT2 inhib-itor, exhibits a prophylactic effect on hepatic steatosis and fibrosis induced by choline-deficient l-amino acid-defined diet in rats. Eur J Pharmacol 2015;754: 19–24.

98. Leiter LA, Forst T, Polidori D, et al. Effect of canagliflozin on liver function tests in patients with type 2 diabetes. Diabetes Metab 2016;42:25–32.

99. Athyros VG, Mikhailidis DP, Didangelos TP, et al. Effect of multifactorial treatment on non-alcoholic fatty liver disease in metabolic syndrome: a randomised study. Curr Med Res Opin 2006;22:873–83.

100. Nelson A, Torres DM, Morgan AE, et al. A pilot study using simvastatin in the treatment of nonalcoholic steatohepatitis: a randomized placebo-controlled trial. J Clin Gastroenterol 2009;43:990–4.

101. Fabbrini E, Mohammed BS, Korenblat KM, et al. Effect of fenofibrate and niacin on intrahepatic triglyceride content, very low-density lipoprotein kinetics, and in-sulin action in obese subjects with nonalcoholic fatty liver disease. J Clin Endo-crinol Metab 2010;95:2727–35.

102. Le TA, Chen J, Changchien C, et al. Effect of colesevelam on liver fat quantified by magnetic resonance in nonalcoholic steatohepatitis: a randomized controlled trial. Hepatology 2012;56:922–32.

103. Dasarathy S, Dasarathy J, Khiyami A, et al. Double-blind randomized placebo-controlled clinical trial of omega 3 fatty acids for the treatment of diabetic pa-tients with nonalcoholic steatohepatitis. J Clin Gastroenterol 2015;49:137–44.

104. Loomba R, Sirlin CB, Ang B, et al. Ezetimibe for the treatment of nonalcoholic steatohepatitis: assessment by novel magnetic resonance imaging and mag-netic resonance elastography in a randomized trial (MOZART Trial). Hepatology 2015;61:1239–50.

105. Zein CO, Yerian LM, Gogate P, et al. Pentoxifylline improves nonalcoholic stea-tohepatitis: a randomized placebo-controlled trial. Hepatology 2011;54:1610–9.

106. Van Wagner LB, Koppe SW, Brunt EM, et al. Pentoxifylline for the treatment of non-alcoholic steatohepatitis: a randomized controlled trial. Ann Hepatol 2011; 10:277–86.

107. Cusi K. Treatment of patients with type 2 diabetes and non-alcoholic fatty liver disease: current approaches and future directions. Diabetologia 2016;59: 1112–20.

108. Yki-Järvinen H. Diagnosis of non-alcoholic fatty liver disease (NAFLD). Diabeto-logia 2016;59:1104–11.

109. Dunn MA, Behari J, Rogal SS, et al. Hepatic steatosis in diabetic patients does not predict adverse liver-related or cardiovascular outcomes. Liver Int 2013;33: 1575–82.

110. Targher G, Bertolini L, Padovani R, et al. Non-alcoholic fatty liver disease is associated with carotid artery wall thickness in diet-controlled type 2 diabetic patients. J Endocrinol Invest 2006;29:55–60.
111. McKimmie RL, Daniel KR, Carr JJ, et al. Hepatic steatosis and subclinical cardiovascular disease in a cohort enriched for type 2 diabetes: the diabetes heart study. Am J Gastroenterol 2008;103:3029–35.
112. Khashper A, Gaspar T, Azencot M, et al. Visceral abdominal adipose tissue and coronary atherosclerosis in asymptomatic diabetics. Int J Cardiol 2013;162: 184–8.
113. Idilman IS, Akata D, Hazirolan T, et al. Nonalcoholic fatty liver disease is associated with significant coronary artery disease in type 2 diabetic patients: a computed tomography angiography study 2. J Diabetes 2015;7:279–86.
114. Silaghi CA, Silaghi H, Craciun AE, et al. Age, abdominal obesity, and glycated hemoglobin are associated with carotid atherosclerosis in type 2 diabetes patients with nonalcoholic fatty liver disease. Med Ultrason 2015;17:300–7.
115. Kwak MS, Yim JY, Kim D, et al. Nonalcoholic fatty liver disease is associated with coronary artery calcium score in diabetes patients with higher HbA1c. Diabetol Metab Syndr 2015;7:28.
116. Mantovani A, Pernigo M, Bergamini C, et al. Nonalcoholic fatty liver disease is independently associated with early left ventricular diastolic dysfunction in patients with type 2 diabetes. PLoS One 2015;10:e0135329.

Lipodystrophy Syndromes

Iram Hussain, MD[a], Abhimanyu Garg, MD[b],*

KEYWORDS

- Lipodystrophy • Congenital generalized lipodystrophy
- Familial partial lipodystrophy • Acquired generalized lipodystrophy
- Acquired partial lipodystrophy • Metreleptin

KEY POINTS

- Lipodystrophies are a group of heterogeneous disorders characterized by varying degrees of body fat loss and predisposition to insulin resistance–related metabolic complications.
- They are classified as generalized, partial or localized by extent of fat loss; and genetic and acquired by etiology.
- Highly active antiretroviral therapy–induced lipodystrophy in HIV-infected patients and drug-induced localized lipodystrophy are more prevalent subtypes, followed by genetic and acquired autoimmune lipodystrophies.
- Common metabolic abnormalities and complications include insulin resistance and diabetes mellitus, hypertriglyceridemia, and hepatic steatosis.
- Management options include diet and exercise; conventional antihyperglycemic agents and lipid-lowering therapy; and metreleptin therapy, which is the only drug approved specifically for generalized lipodystrophy.

INTRODUCTION

Lipodystrophies are a group of rare disorders of diverse cause characterized by variable loss of body fat. The loss of body fat may affect nearly the entire body (generalized), only certain body regions (partial), or small areas under the skin (localized). Depending on the severity and extent of body fat loss, patients may be predisposed

Grant Support: This work was supported by the National Institutes of Health grant RO1 DK105448, CTSA grants UL1RR024982 and UL1TR001105, and the Southwest Medical Foundation.
Disclosure Statement: Dr I. Hussain has no disclosures. Dr A. Garg coholds a patent regarding use of leptin for treating human lipoatrophy and the method of determining predisposition to this treatment but receives no financial compensation. He receives research grant support from Aegerion, Pfizer, and Ionis Pharmaceuticals and is a consultant for Aegerion.
[a] Division of Endocrinology, Department of Internal Medicine, UT Southwestern Medical Center, 5323 Harry Hines Boulevard, Dallas, TX 75390-8537, USA; [b] Division of Nutrition and Metabolic Diseases, Department of Internal Medicine, Center for Human Nutrition, UT Southwestern Medical Center, 5323 Harry Hines Boulevard, Dallas, TX 75390-8537, USA
* Corresponding author.
E-mail address: abhimanyu.garg@utsouthwestern.edu

Endocrinol Metab Clin N Am 45 (2016) 783–797
http://dx.doi.org/10.1016/j.ecl.2016.06.012
0889-8529/16/Published by Elsevier Inc.

to metabolic complications associated with insulin resistance.[1,2] These metabolic complications include early onset of diabetes mellitus, hypertriglyceridemia, and hepatic steatosis.[1–3] In some patients, these metabolic complications are challenging to manage and can lead to complications including diabetic nephropathy and retinopathy, acute pancreatitis (from extreme hypertriglyceridemia and chylomicronemia), hepatic cirrhosis, and premature cardiovascular disease. Other common clinical manifestations include polycystic ovarian syndrome (PCOS), acanthosis nigricans as a result of severe insulin resistance, and eruptive xanthomas caused by extreme hypertriglyceridemia.[1–3]

The loss of body fat can result from underlying genetic defects (genetic lipodystrophies including autosomal-recessive or autosomal-dominant subtypes) or from autoimmune mechanisms (acquired lipodystrophies including generalized or partial subtypes) or drugs (eg, highly active antiretroviral therapy [HAART]-induced partial lipodystrophy in human immunodeficiency virus [HIV]-infected patients or localized lipodystrophies from insulin and other injected drugs).[1–3] The localized lipodystrophies and lipodystrophy in HIV-infected patients are the most prevalent subtype of lipodystrophies, whereas the other genetic and acquired lipodystrophies are rare.[2] Localized lipodystrophies do not predispose to metabolic complications because the loss of fat is trivial; however, other partial or generalized lipodystrophies cause variable predisposition to metabolic complications.

The major subtypes of lipodystrophy are described in **Table 1** and shown in **Fig. 1**. However, given the heterogeneity of manifestations, variable patterns of fat loss, and genetic basis that have yet to be identified, all lipodystrophy syndromes cannot be classified into these categories.[4] Regardless of the cause, patients with generalized lipodystrophy have extremely low serum levels of adipocytokines, such as leptin and adiponectin,[5,6] whereas serum leptin and adiponectin levels in those with partial lipodystrophies can range from low to high. Marked hypoleptinemia may induce excessive appetite and can exacerbate metabolic complications of insulin resistance.[3] This article covers the major types of lipodystrophy syndromes.

Table 1
General classification of major lipodystrophy subtypes

Lipodystrophy Subtype	Main Characteristics
Congenital generalized lipodystrophy	Presents with near total loss of body fat at birth or during infancy. Autosomal-recessive inheritance.
Familial partial lipodystrophy	Presents with variable loss of subcutaneous fat from the upper and lower extremities and the truncal region at puberty or later. Autosomal-dominant inheritance.
Acquired generalized lipodystrophy	Characterized by gradual loss of subcutaneous fat from nearly all over the body. Associated with autoimmune diseases.
Acquired partial lipodystrophy	Characterized by gradual loss of fat from the upper body, including head, neck, upper extremities, and truncal region during childhood. Associated with autoantibodies called complement 3 nephritic factor and in ~20% of patients with membranoproliferative glomerulonephritis.
HAART-induced lipodystrophy in HIV patients	Associated with therapy including HIV protease inhibitors or nucleoside analogues.
Localized lipodystrophy	Usually caused by insulin injections or other injectables, such as steroids.

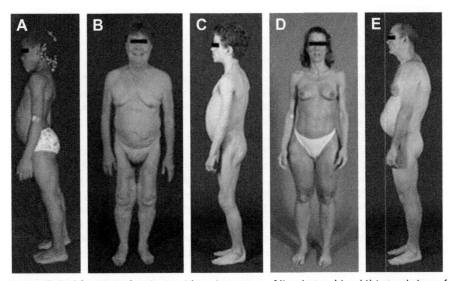

Fig. 1. Clinical features of patients with various types of lipodystrophies. (*A*) Lateral view of an 8-year-old African American girl with congenital generalized lipodystrophy (also known as Berardinelli-Seip congenital lipodystrophy) type 1 caused by homozygous c.377insT (p.Leu126fs*146) mutation in *AGPAT2*. The patient had generalized loss of subcutaneous fat at birth and developed mild acanthosis nigricans in the axillae and neck later during childhood. She had umbilical prominence and acromegaloid features (enlarged mandible, hands, and feet). (*B*) Anterior view of a 65-year-old white woman with familial partial lipodystrophy of the Dunnigan variety caused by heterozygous p.Arg482Gln mutation in *LMNA*. She noticed loss of subcutaneous fat from the limbs at the time of puberty and later lost subcutaneous fat from the anterior truncal region. The breasts were atrophic. She had increased subcutaneous fat deposits in the face, anterior neck, suprapubic and vulvar region, and medial parts of the knees. (*C*) Lateral view of an 8-year-old German boy with acquired generalized lipodystrophy. He started experiencing generalized loss of subcutaneous fat at age 3 with marked acanthosis nigricans in the neck, axillae, and groin. He developed Crohn's disease at age 11 requiring hemicolectomy at age 13. (*D*) Anterior view of a 39-year-old white woman with acquired partial lipodystrophy (Barraquer-Simons syndrome). She noticed marked loss of subcutaneous fat from the face, neck, upper extremities, chest, and abdomen at the age of 12 years but later developed increased subcutaneous fat deposition in the lower extremities. (*E*) Lateral view of a 39-year-old white man infected with HIV with protease inhibitor–containing highly active antiretroviral therapy–induced lipodystrophy. He had marked loss of subcutaneous fat from the face and limbs but had increased subcutaneous fat deposition in the neck region anteriorly and posteriorly showing buffalo hump. Abdomen was protuberant because of excess intra-abdominal fat. He had been on protease inhibitor–containing antiretroviral therapy for more than 7 years. (*[A] From* Simha V, Garg A. Lipodystrophy: lessons in lipid and energy metabolism. Curr Opin Lipidol 2006;17:162–9; with permission; *[B–E]* Garg A. Lipodystrophies: genetic and acquired body fat disorders. J Clin Endocrinol Metab 2011;96:3317; with permission.)

GENETIC LIPODYSTROPHIES

The two main types of genetic lipodystrophies are congenital generalized lipodystrophy (CGL), an autosomal-recessive syndrome (**Tables 2** and **3**), and familial partial lipodystrophy (FPLD), mostly an autosomal-dominant syndrome (**Table 4**). There are other extremely rare types that have been reported in approximately 30 patients or less (**Table 5**). These extremely rare types of genetic lipodystrophies are not discussed further in this article.

Congenital Generalized Lipodystrophy

CGL, or Berardinelli-Seip syndrome, is an autosomal-recessive disorder characterized by generalized lack of adipose tissue either at birth or within the first year of life. Patients have prominent musculature and subcutaneous veins.[1,7,8] Most cases are diagnosed at birth or early in childhood because of the striking fat loss, but a few patients without access to regular medical care may be identified later in life.

Patients with CGL can develop hyperphagia as a result of profound leptin deficiency in early childhood, and may have accelerated linear growth; advanced bone age; and features suggestive of acromegaly, such as enlarged hands, feet, and jaw.[5,6] Severe metabolic complications, along with hepatomegaly and splenomegaly, develop at an early age. Hyperinsulinemia leads to development of widespread acanthosis nigricans, followed by onset of diabetes mellitus during adolescence.[7,8] Diabetes is generally ketosis-resistant. Some patients develop extreme hypertriglyceridemia especially after the onset of insulin-resistant diabetes mellitus and are prone to recurrent attacks of acute pancreatitis.[7,8]

Hepatic steatosis is common and severe, and can progress to steatohepatitis, cirrhosis, and liver failure.[4] Female patients with CGL have additional clinical features including hirsutism, clitoromegaly, irregular menstrual periods, polycystic ovaries, and/or infertility.[1] There are four genetically distinct subtypes of CGL[7–12] and besides common clinical features listed previously, each one has some peculiar clinical features (see **Tables 2** and **3**).

Table 2
Subtypes of CGL

Subtype	Gene	Molecular Basis	Prevalence
CGL1	AGPAT2	AGPAT enzymes play a key role in biosynthesis of triglycerides and phospholipids in various organs. AGPAT isoform 2 is highly expressed in the adipose tissue.	Most common subtype[7,8,10]
CGL2	BSCL2	Seipin, encoded by BSCL2, plays a key role in fusion of small lipid droplets in the adipocytes and in adipocyte differentiation.	Second most common subtype[7–9]
CGL3	CAV1	Caveolin 1 is an integral component of caveolae, which are present on adipocyte membranes. Caveolae translocate fatty acids and other lipids to lipid droplets.	Only one patient reported[11]
CGL4	PTRF	PTRF (also known as cavin-1) is involved in biogenesis of caveolae and regulates expression of caveolins 1 and 3.	About 20 patients reported[12,43,44]

Abbreviations: AGPAT2, 1-acylglycerol-3-phosphate O-acyltransferase 2; BSCL2, Berardinelli-Seip congenital lipodystrophy 2; CAV1, caveolin 1; PTRF, polymerase I and transcript release factor.

Familial Partial Lipodystrophy

FPLD is mostly inherited as an autosomal-dominant disorder and is characterized by subcutaneous fat loss from the upper and lower extremities and variable fat loss from the trunk.[13,14] These patients have normal fat distribution during childhood, followed by onset around late childhood or puberty of progressive and variable subcutaneous

Table 3
Unique clinical features in CGL subtypes

Affected Feature	CGL Type 1 (AGPAT2)	CGL Type 2 (BSCL2)	CGL Type 3 (CAV1)	CGL Type 4 (PTRF)
Body fat loss	Only metabolically active adipose tissue is lost Mechanical adipose tissue preserved	Both metabolically active and mechanical adipose tissues are lost	Absent metabolically active adipose tissue Preserved mechanical and bone marrow adipose tissue	Absent metabolically active adipose tissue Preserved mechanical and bone marrow adipose tissue
Cardiovascular complications	N/A	Cardiomyopathy	N/A	Cardiomyopathy, catecholaminergic polymorphic ventricular tachycardia, prolonged QT, and sudden death
Lytic bone lesions in long bones	Most frequent	Occasional	Not reported	Not reported
Gastrointestinal complications	N/A	N/A	Functional megaesophagus	Congenital pyloric stenosis achalasia
Skeletal muscle	N/A	N/A	N/A	Congenital myopathy Developmental delay Muscle weakness, Percussion-induced myotonia
Other features	N/A	Teratozoospermia in one patient	Short stature, hypocalcemia, vitamin D resistance	Low bone density for age, distal metaphyseal deformation with joint stiffness, atlantoaxial instability Late onset of lipodystrophy in infancy

Abbreviation: N/A, not applicable.

Table 4
Subtypes of FPLD

Subtype	Genetic Mutation	Prevalence
FPLD1 (Kobberling-type)	Molecular basis unknown	Rare[16]
FPLD2 (Dunnigan-type)	Missense mutations in *LMNA*	Most common subtype; more than 500 patients reported[17–19]
FPLD3	Heterozygous mutations in *PPARG*	Second most common subtype; about 30–50 patients reported[20,21]
FPLD4	Heterozygous mutations in *PLIN1*	Reported in three families[22]
FPLD5	Homozygous nonsense mutation in *CIDEC* (autosomal recessive)	One patient reported[23]
FPLD6	Homozygous mutation in *LIPE* (autosomal recessive)	Six patients reported[24,25]
FPLD7	Heterozygous mutation in *ADRA2A*	Reported in one family[27]
AKT2-linked lipodystrophy	Heterozygous mutation in *AKT2*	Reported in one family[26]

Abbreviations: *AKT2*, v-akt murine thymoma viral oncogene homolog 2; *CIDEC*, cell death-inducing DFFA-like effector c; *LIPE*, hormone sensitive lipase; *LMNA*, lamin A/C; *PLIN1*, perilipin 1; *PPARG*, peroxisome proliferator-activated receptor gamma.

fat loss typically from the extremities (causing the musculature to appear prominent), but variably from the anterior abdomen and chest.[13,14] Some patients may have small size of the breasts because of reduced or lack of overlying subcutaneous fat. At the same time, there is often fat accumulation in the face, neck, perineal, and intra-abdominal areas, particularly in women. Excess fat accumulation in the dorsocervical (causing a buffalo-hump), supraclavicular, and submental regions gives these patients a cushingoid appearance and many of these patients may be confused with having Cushing's syndrome. These patients may be clinically hard to detect if the fat loss is subtle, especially in males because many normal men are also quite muscular.[13]

FPLD in women may present with masculinization and menstrual irregularity and metabolic complications. Women with FPLD have a high prevalence of PCOS compared with the 6% to 8% prevalence observed in the general population; however, infertility is not common.[13] This increased prevalence of PCOS and metabolic complications occurs more frequently in those women who have excess fat accumulation in nonlipodystrophic regions.

As compared to patients with generalized lipodystrophies, hepatic steatosis and acanthosis nigricans is less pronounced; however, hypertriglyceridemia is common and severe, with high risk of acute pancreatitis. In addition, these patients may also develop myopathy, cardiomyopathy, and/or conduction system abnormalities.[15] There are several genetically distinct varieties of FPLD[16–26]; however, the clinical differences among these various subtypes have not been clear so far (see **Table 4**).

ACQUIRED LIPODYSTROPHIES
Acquired Generalized Lipodystrophy

Acquired generalized lipodystrophy (AGL), or Lawrence syndrome, is characterized by generalized loss of subcutaneous fat that occurs gradually in individuals who are born

Table 5
Extremely rare genetic lipodystrophy syndromes

Lipodystrophy Type	Gene	Molecular Basis	Clinical Features
MAD type A	*LMNA*	Mutations may disrupt nuclear function resulting in premature cell death in many tissues.	Mandibular and clavicular hypoplasia, acro-osteolysis. Partial lipodystrophy affecting the extremities and trunk.[45,46]
MAD type B	*ZMPSTE24*	Mutations result in accumulation of farnesylated prelamin A that can disrupt nuclear function in several tissues.	Mandibular and clavicular hypoplasia, acro-osteolysis. More generalized loss of fat, premature renal failure, progeroid features.[47]
JMP/CANDLE	*PSMB8*	PSMB8 encodes subunit of immunoproteasomes that degrade abnormal/excess proteins in cells.	Joint contractures, muscle atrophy, microcytic anemia and panniculitis-induced lipodystrophy. Recurrent fevers, annular erythematous skin lesions, violaceous eyelid swelling, partial lipodystrophy.[48,49]
SHORT syndrome	*PIK3R1*	PIK3R1 plays a role in metabolic actions of insulin, mutations associated with insulin resistance.	Variable loss of subcutaneous fat, short stature, hyperextensibility, ocular depression, teething delay.[50]
MDP syndrome	*POLD1*	Critical for DNA replication and repair.	Mandibular hypoplasia, deafness, and progeroid features.[51,52]
Neonatal progeroid syndrome, type A	*FBN1*	Fibrillin 1	Generalized loss of body fat and muscle mass, and progeroid appearance at birth. Marfanoid habitus.[53,54]
Neonatal progeroid syndrome, type B	*CAV1*	Caveolin 1, present on adipocyte membranes, binds fatty acids and translocates them to lipid droplets.	Generalized loss of body fat and muscle mass, and progeroid appearance at birth.[55]
Atypical progeroid syndrome	*LMNA*	Different heterozygous, mostly de novo mutations cause nuclear dysfunction.	Partial or generalized loss of subcutaneous fat, progeroid features.[56]
Hutchinson-Gilford progeria	*LMNA*	Specific de novo mutations induce abnormal splicing and accumulation of truncated farnesylated prelamin A.	Generalized loss of subcutaneous fat, progeroid features.[57]

Abbreviations: CANDLE, chronic atypical neutrophilic dermatosis with lipodystrophy and elevated temperature; *CAV1*, caveolin 1; JMP, joint contractures, muscle atrophy, microcytic anemia and panniculitis-induced lipodystrophy; *LMNA*, lamin A/C; MAD, mandibuloacral dysplasia; MDP, mandibular hypoplasia, deafness, progeroid features; *PIK3R1*, phosphoinositide-3-kinase regulatory subunit 1; *POLD1*, polymerase (DNA) delta 1, catalytic subunit; *PSMB8*, proteasome subunit beta 8; SHORT, short stature, hyperextensibility or inguinal hernia, ocular depression, Rieger anomaly, and teething delay; *ZMPSTE24*, zinc metalloprotease STE24.

with a normal fat distribution. The fat loss typically begins in childhood or adolescence, but can rarely begin after 30 years of age.[28] It can occur over a variable time period, ranging from a few weeks to months or years, and affects all subcutaneous areas of the body especially the face and extremities and may include the palms and soles. Orbital and bone marrow fat depots seem to be preserved, whereas intra-abdominal fat loss is variable. AGL is more frequent in the females than males (3:1).[28] Patients with AGL are predisposed to the same metabolic complications as other patients with lipodystrophies, such as insulin resistance associated with diabetes mellitus and hypertriglyceridemia. Hypoleptinemia is thought to contribute to the metabolic complications. Usually these complications are quite severe. Most of the patients have associated autoimmune diseases, especially juvenile dermatomyositis, or panniculitis (pathologically infiltration of adipose tissue with inflammatory cells of various types resulting in loss of subcutaneous fat) (**Table 6**). In some patients, the underlying mechanism of fat loss is not clear (idiopathic variety). Usually the metabolic complications are less severe in patients with panniculitis-associated AGL compared with the other two subtypes.

Table 6 Classification of AGL		
Subtype	**Prevalence**	**Clinical Features**
Panniculitis-associated AGL	~ 25%	Initial development of panniculitis (subcutaneous inflammatory nodules) followed by localized fat loss when these lesions heal. Ongoing panniculitis later results in generalized loss of subcutaneous fat.[28]
Autoimmune AGL	~ 25%	Gradual generalized fat loss associated with autoimmune diseases, especially juvenile dermatomyositis. Some patients have low levels of serum complement 4.[28,58]
Idiopathic AGL	~ 50%	Gradual generalized subcutaneous fat loss of unclear etiology.[28]

Acquired Partial Lipodystrophy (Barraquer-Simons Syndrome)

Acquired partial lipodystrophy is characterized by gradual loss of subcutaneous fat from the upper body (ie, the face, neck, upper extremities, and upper trunk).[29] Usually the lower abdomen, hips, and lower extremities are spared. In fact, after puberty, patients, especially females, may accumulate excess fat there. Acquired partial lipodystrophy is more frequent in females than males (4:1). It is often associated with autoimmune diseases. Most patients have a circulating autoantibody called complement 3 nephritic factor, and have low circulating levels of serum complement 3.[29] Approximately 20% of these patients develop membranoproliferative glomerulonephritis and some develop end-stage renal disease requiring renal transplantation. Rare patients have drusen on fundus examination. Metabolic complications are not seen as frequently as in other types of lipodystrophy.[29]

Highly Active Antiretroviral Therapy–Induced Lipodystrophy in Patients Infected with Human Immunodeficiency Virus

Lipodystrophy in HIV-infected patients usually occurs after approximately 2 to 4 years of HAART consisting of HIV-1 protease inhibitors or nucleoside reverse transcriptase inhibitors (**Table 7**).[30,31] It is characterized by the loss of subcutaneous fat from the upper and lower extremities and from the face, with increased fat accumulation in the neck, anteriorly and posteriorly, and in the upper trunk and intra-abdominal

Table 7	
Etiology of drug-induced lipodystrophy in HIV-infected patients	
Type/Etiology	**Pathogenesis and Molecular Basis**
PI-induced	PIs inhibit ZMPSTE24, which is important for the correct maturation and processing of prelamin A. Thus, PIs result in accumulation of toxic farnesylated prelamin A.[32] May also cause dysregulation of transcription factors involved in adipogenesis. They may also inhibit glucose transporter 4 expression leading to insulin resistance.
NRTI-induced	NRTIs (especially stavudine and zidovudine) inhibit mitochondrial polymerase-γ and subsequently cause mitochondrial toxicity.[33]

Abbreviations: NRTI, nucleoside reverse transcriptase inhibitor; PI, protease inhibitor; polymerase-γ, polymerase gamma; ZMPSTE24, zinc mellatoproteinase STE24.

region.[30,31] Many protease inhibitors have been shown to inhibit zinc metalloprotease, the key enzyme involved in posttranslation processing of prelamin A to mature lamin A.[32] Thus, protease inhibitor–based HAART may result in accumulation of toxic prelamin A. Nucleoside reverse transcriptase inhibitors may induce lipodystrophy by causing mitochondrial dysfunction.[33]

Localized Lipodystrophies

Localized lipodystrophies are characterized by loss of fat from small areas, either single or multiple. Sometimes it can affect portions of the limbs or large contiguous areas on the trunk. Patients with localized lipodystrophies do not develop any metabolic abnormalities. There are several etiologies of localized lipodystrophies (**Table 8**).[34]

MANAGEMENT

The treatment of lipodystrophy is focused on managing the metabolic abnormalities to prevent complications, and cosmetic appearance. Although there is no cure for lipodystrophy, morbidity and mortality are improved through early intervention. Diet and exercise form an integral part of the treatment plan, although clinical trial data are not available.

A diet with a well-balanced macronutrient composition of about 50% to 60% carbohydrates, 20% to 30% fat, and about 10% to 20% protein is appropriate for most patients. Overfeeding should be avoided, especially in infants and children (despite their lack of weight gain), because this can accelerate hepatic steatosis and worsen diabetes and hyperlipidemia. Energy-restricted diets are more appropriate in adults, because children with growth and developmental needs may otherwise develop deficiencies.

Exercise, in the absence of contraindications, can help improve metabolic parameters, so patients should be encouraged to be physically active. Those who are predisposed to cardiomyopathy, such as patients with CGL4, FPLD2, and progeroid syndromes, should undergo a cardiac evaluation before engaging in an exercise program, and should avoid strenuous exercise. To avoid traumatic injuries, patients with severe hepatosplenomegaly and patients with CGL with lytic lesions in the bones should avoid contact sports.

Strategies to reduce hypertriglyceridemia include medium-chain triglyceride-based formulas in infants,[35] and very-low-fat diets in older individuals. Any fat intake should be in the form of *cis*-monounsaturated fats and long-chain omega-3 fatty acids. In patients who have developed acute pancreatitis secondary to hypertriglyceridemia,

Table 8
Characteristics of different types of localized lipodystrophies

Type	Etiology	Clinical Features
Drug-induced localized lipodystrophy	Insulin therapy (more common before purified/human insulin was available), steroids, and antibiotics. High local production of TNF-α may cause dedifferentiation of adipocytes. Other mechanisms include presence of lipases, repeated trauma and/or autoimmune processes.	More common in patients with high titers of anti-insulin antibodies. May have deposition of IgA and C3 locally. Sometimes responds to local corticosteroids.
Pressure-induced localized lipodystrophy	Trauma and decreased perfusion caused by repeated pressure to the same area over a long period of time.	Fat atrophy localized to the area exposed to repeated pressure. This tends to improve when the pressure is avoided.
Panniculitis-associated localized lipodystrophy	Associated with serum ANA or anti dsDNA antibodies; may also have autoimmune diseases, such as SLE.	Initial development of panniculitis (subcutaneous inflammatory nodules in several areas) followed by localized fat loss when these lesions heal.
Centrifugal lipodystrophy (lipodystrophia centrifugalis abdominalis infantalis)	Cause is unknown and most patients recover spontaneously with no intervention.	More common in Asians. Fat loss spreads in a centrifugal pattern from abdomen and groin area and is associated with peripheral panniculitis. It begins in infancy, stops spreading between the ages of 3 and 8 and then in most cases, resolves by itself.
Idiopathic localized lipodystrophy	Undetermined etiology.	

Abbreviations: ANA, antinuclear antibodies; anti dsDNA Ab, anti-double-stranded deoxyribonucleic acid antibodies; C3, complement 3; SLE, systemic lupus erythematosus; TNF-α, tumor necrosis factor alpha.
Data from Garg A. Lipodystrophies. Am J Med 2000;108(2):143–52.

parental nutrition should be administered until they recover and they should subsequently be on an extremely low-fat (total dietary fat <20 g/day) diet. In patients who have not reached lipid-lowering goals after diet and lifestyle intervention, lipid-lowering drugs may be used.

Patients with insulin resistance and diabetes mellitus should be treated with conventional therapies, including oral agents (metformin is the first-line drug) and insulin. Insulin therapy often provides the mainstay of treatment, and many patients require concentrated forms (eg, 500 U regular insulin) because of severe insulin resistance. Whether thiazolidinediones are particularly efficacious in patients with FPLD with *PPARG* mutations remains unclear. Simple sugars should be avoided in favor of high-fiber complex carbohydrates consumed throughout the day in combination with protein and/or fat, to avoid blood glucose spikes. The treatment goals are similar to patients with diabetes without lipodystrophy.

Hypertension, if uncontrolled, may be treated with angiotensin-converting enzyme inhibitors or angiotensin receptor blockers, because these medications also have favorable effects on proteinuria. No specific treatments have been shown to be particularly effective for hepatic steatosis or steatohepatitis associated with lipodystrophy.

Generalized lipodystrophies are characterized by extremely low serum leptin levels,[5] which led to research into recombinant human leptin (metreleptin) as a treatment option,[36] and since then several long-term studies have shown beneficial effects.[37–40]

Metreleptin therapy has been shown to improve metabolic abnormalities in patients with generalized lipodystrophy, including decreased serum triglyceride levels, increased insulin sensitivity, and reduced hepatic steatosis.[3] It is currently the only drug specifically approved for treatment of generalized lipodystrophy.[3] It is administered as a daily subcutaneous injection,[41] and dose adjustments are made every 3 to 6 months based on metabolic parameters and weight change. The most common side effects include hypoglycemia and injection site reactions, such as erythema and/or urticaria. The other side effects include development of neutralizing antibodies to metreleptin, and development of cutaneous T-cell lymphomas especially in patients with AGL.[42] The precise significance of neutralizing antibodies to leptin remains unclear at this time and some patients with AGL who have never received metreleptin therapy have also been reported to develop lymphomas. Because of paucity of data, approval of metreleptin for different types of lipodystrophy varies by country, depending on their regulatory boards (**Table 9**).

Change in body shape caused by lipodystrophy can often lead to psychological distress, and sometimes even physical discomfort, such as from absent fat pads on

Table 9
Approval and indications of metreleptin therapy

Type of Lipodystrophy	Approvals	Indications	Clinical Considerations
Generalized lipodystrophy (both CGL and AGL)	United States: approved as adjunct to diet for treatment of metabolic complications. Japan: approved Europe: available through compassionate care programs.	First-line drug treatment (after diet/exercise intervention) for metabolic and endocrine abnormalities. May prevent comorbidities and metabolic complications in young children.	Decreases hyperphagia, leading to weight loss. May need to be discontinued if excessive weight loss occurs.
Partial lipodystrophy (both FPLD and APL)	United States: not approved. Japan: approved as an adjunct to diet Europe: through compassionate care programs.	May be considered for patients with hypoleptinemia (leptin <4 ng/mL) who have severe metabolic abnormalities, such as HbA_{1c} >8% and/or triglycerides >500 mg/dL.	Clinical response not as good as in generalized lipodystrophy. Patients with lower leptin levels show the most benefit.

Abbreviations: APL, acquired partial lipodystrophy; HbA_{1c}, glycated hemoglobin.

the feet and buttocks. Patients should be referred to appropriate mental health providers for emotional distress. Plastic surgery may improve appearance in some people, although data are limited. Possible interventions include autologous fat transfer, dermal fillers, or muscle grafts to treat facial lipoatrophy; surgical reduction or liposuction of areas with excessive fat; and breast implants for improved cosmetics in women.

ACKNOWLEDGMENTS

The authors thank Pei-Yun Tseng, BS, for help with illustrations.

REFERENCES

1. Garg A. Acquired and inherited lipodystrophies. N Engl J Med 2004;350(12): 1220–34.
2. Garg A. Clinical review#: Lipodystrophies: genetic and acquired body fat disorders. J Clin Endocrinol Metab 2011;96(11):3313–25.
3. Brown RJ, Gorden P. Leptin therapy in patients with lipodystrophy and syndromic insulin resistance. In: Dagogo-Jack S, editor. Leptin: regulation and clinical applications. New York: Springer International Publishing; 2015. p. 225–36.
4. Handelsman Y, Oral EA, Bloomgarden ZT, et al. The clinical approach to the detection of lipodystrophy: an AACE consensus statement. Endocr Pract 2013; 19(1):107–16.
5. Haque WA, Shimomura I, Matsuzawa Y, et al. Serum adiponectin and leptin levels in patients with lipodystrophies. J Clin Endocrinol Metab 2002;87(5):2395.
6. Antuna-Puente B, Boutet E, Vigouroux C, et al. Higher adiponectin levels in patients with Berardinelli-Seip congenital lipodystrophy due to seipin as compared with 1-acylglycerol-3-phosphate-o-acyltransferase-2 deficiency. J Clin Endocrinol Metab 2010;95(3):1463–8.
7. Van Maldergem L, Magre J, Khallouf TE, et al. Genotype-phenotype relationships in Berardinelli-Seip congenital lipodystrophy. J Med Genet 2002;39(10):722–33.
8. Agarwal AK, Simha V, Oral EA, et al. Phenotypic and genetic heterogeneity in congenital generalized lipodystrophy. J Clin Endocrinol Metab 2003;88(10): 4840–7.
9. Magre J, Delepine M, Khallouf E, et al. Identification of the gene altered in Berardinelli-Seip congenital lipodystrophy on chromosome 11q13. Nat Genet 2001;28(4):365–70.
10. Agarwal AK, Arioglu E, De Almeida S, et al. AGPAT2 is mutated in congenital generalized lipodystrophy linked to chromosome 9q34. Nat Genet 2002;31(1): 21–3.
11. Kim CA, Delepine M, Boutet E, et al. Association of a homozygous nonsense caveolin-1 mutation with Berardinelli-Seip congenital lipodystrophy. J Clin Endocrinol Metab 2008;93(4):1129–34.
12. Hayashi YK, Matsuda C, Ogawa M, et al. Human PTRF mutations cause secondary deficiency of caveolins resulting in muscular dystrophy with generalized lipodystrophy. J Clin Invest 2009;119(9):2623–33.
13. Garg A. Gender differences in the prevalence of metabolic complications in familial partial lipodystrophy (Dunnigan variety). J Clin Endocrinol Metab 2000;85(5): 1776–82.
14. Garg A, Peshock RM, Fleckenstein JL. Adipose tissue distribution pattern in patients with familial partial lipodystrophy (Dunnigan variety). J Clin Endocrinol Metab 1999;84(1):170–4.

15. Subramanyam L, Simha V, Garg A. Overlapping syndrome with familial partial lipodystrophy, Dunnigan variety and cardiomyopathy due to amino-terminal heterozygous missense lamin A/C mutations. Clin Genet 2010;78(1):66–73.
16. Kobberling J, Dunnigan MG. Familial partial lipodystrophy: two types of an X linked dominant syndrome, lethal in the hemizygous state. J Med Genet 1986; 23(2):120–7.
17. Cao H, Hegele RA. Nuclear lamin A/C R482Q mutation in Canadian kindreds with Dunnigan-type familial partial lipodystrophy. Hum Mol Genet 2000;9(1):109–12.
18. Shackleton S, Lloyd DJ, Jackson SN, et al. LMNA, encoding lamin A/C, is mutated in partial lipodystrophy. Nat Genet 2000;24(2):153–6.
19. Speckman RA, Garg A, Du F, et al. Mutational and haplotype analyses of families with familial partial lipodystrophy (Dunnigan variety) reveal recurrent missense mutations in the globular C-terminal domain of lamin A/C. Am J Hum Genet 2000;66(4):1192–8.
20. Agarwal AK, Garg A. A novel heterozygous mutation in peroxisome proliferator-activated receptor-gamma gene in a patient with familial partial lipodystrophy. J Clin Endocrinol Metab 2002;87(1):408–11.
21. Semple RK, Chatterjee VK, O'Rahilly S. PPAR gamma and human metabolic disease. J Clin Invest 2006;116(3):581–9.
22. Gandotra S, Le Dour C, Bottomley W, et al. Perilipin deficiency and autosomal dominant partial lipodystrophy. N Engl J Med 2011;364(8):740–8.
23. Rubio-Cabezas O, Puri V, Murano I, et al. Partial lipodystrophy and insulin resistant diabetes in a patient with a homozygous nonsense mutation in CIDEC. EMBO Mol Med 2009;1(5):280–7.
24. Albert JS, Yerges-Armstrong LM, Horenstein RB, et al. Null mutation in hormone-sensitive lipase gene and risk of type 2 diabetes. N Engl J Med 2014;370(24): 2307–15.
25. Farhan SM, Robinson JF, McIntyre AD, et al. A novel LIPE nonsense mutation found using exome sequencing in siblings with late-onset familial partial lipodystrophy. Can J Cardiol 2014;30(12):1649–54.
26. George S, Rochford JJ, Wolfrum C, et al. A family with severe insulin resistance and diabetes due to a mutation in AKT2. Science 2004;304(5675):1325–8.
27. Garg A, Sankella S, Xing C, et al. Whole-exome sequencing identifies *ADRA2A* mutation in atypical familial partial lipodystrophy. JCI Insight 2016;1(9):e86870.
28. Misra A, Garg A. Clinical features and metabolic derangements in acquired generalized lipodystrophy: case reports and review of the literature. Medicine (Baltimore) 2003;82(2):129–46.
29. Misra A, Peethambaram A, Garg A. Clinical features and metabolic and autoimmune derangements in acquired partial lipodystrophy: report of 35 cases and review of the literature. Medicine (Baltimore) 2004;83(1):18–34.
30. Chen D, Misra A, Garg A. Clinical review 153: Lipodystrophy in human immunodeficiency virus-infected patients. J Clin Endocrinol Metab 2002;87(11):4845–56.
31. Grinspoon S, Carr A. Cardiovascular risk and body-fat abnormalities in HIV-infected adults. N Engl J Med 2005;352(1):48–62.
32. Hudon SE, Coffinier C, Michaelis S, et al. HIV-protease inhibitors block the enzymatic activity of purified Ste24p. Biochem Biophys Res Commun 2008;374(2): 365–8.
33. Lee H, Hanes J, Johnson KA. Toxicity of nucleoside analogues used to treat AIDS and the selectivity of the mitochondrial DNA polymerase. Biochemistry 2003; 42(50):14711–9.
34. Garg A. Lipodystrophies. Am J Med 2000;108(2):143–52.

35. Wilson DE, Chan IF, Stevenson KB, et al. Eucaloric substitution of medium chain triglycerides for dietary long chain fatty acids in acquired total lipodystrophy: effects on hyperlipoproteinemia and endogenous insulin resistance. J Clin Endocrinol Metab 1983;57(3):517–23.

36. Oral EA, Simha V, Ruiz E, et al. Leptin-replacement therapy for lipodystrophy. N Engl J Med 2002;346(8):570–8.

37. Chong AY, Lupsa BC, Cochran EK, et al. Efficacy of leptin therapy in the different forms of human lipodystrophy. Diabetologia 2010;53(1):27–35.

38. Javor ED, Cochran EK, Musso C, et al. Long-term efficacy of leptin replacement in patients with generalized lipodystrophy. Diabetes 2005;54(7):1994–2002.

39. Park JY, Javor ED, Cochran EK, et al. Long-term efficacy of leptin replacement in patients with Dunnigan-type familial partial lipodystrophy. Metabolism 2007; 56(4):508–16.

40. Simha V, Subramanyam L, Szczepaniak L, et al. Comparison of efficacy and safety of leptin replacement therapy in moderately and severely hypoleptinemic patients with familial partial lipodystrophy of the Dunnigan variety. J Clin Endocrinol Metab 2012;97(3):785–92.

41. Rodriguez AJ, Mastronardi CA, Paz-Filho GJ. New advances in the treatment of generalized lipodystrophy: role of metreleptin. Ther Clin Risk Manag 2015;11: 1391–400.

42. Brown RJ, Chan JL, Jaffe ES, et al. Lymphoma in acquired generalized lipodystrophy. Leuk Lymphoma 2016;57(1):45–50.

43. Shastry S, Delgado MR, Dirik E, et al. Congenital generalized lipodystrophy, type 4 (CGL4) associated with myopathy due to novel PTRF mutations. Am J Med Genet A 2010;152A(9):2245–53.

44. Rajab A, Straub V, McCann LJ, et al. Fatal cardiac arrhythmia and long-QT syndrome in a new form of congenital generalized lipodystrophy with muscle rippling (CGL4) due to PTRF-CAVIN mutations. PLoS Genet 2010;6(3):e1000874.

45. Simha V, Agarwal AK, Oral EA, et al. Genetic and phenotypic heterogeneity in patients with mandibuloacral dysplasia-associated lipodystrophy. J Clin Endocrinol Metab 2003;88(6):2821–4.

46. Novelli G, Muchir A, Sangiuolo F, et al. Mandibuloacral dysplasia is caused by a mutation in LMNA-encoding lamin A/C. Am J Hum Genet 2002;71(2):426–31.

47. Agarwal AK, Fryns JP, Auchus RJ, et al. Zinc metalloproteinase, ZMPSTE24, is mutated in mandibuloacral dysplasia. Hum Mol Genet 2003;12(16):1995–2001.

48. Garg A, Hernandez MD, Sousa AB, et al. An autosomal recessive syndrome of joint contractures, muscular atrophy, microcytic anemia, and panniculitis-associated lipodystrophy. J Clin Endocrinol Metab 2010;95(9):E58–63.

49. Agarwal AK, Xing C, DeMartino GN, et al. PSMB8 encoding the beta5i proteasome subunit is mutated in joint contractures, muscle atrophy, microcytic anemia, and panniculitis-induced lipodystrophy syndrome. Am J Hum Genet 2010;87(6): 866–72.

50. Thauvin-Robinet C, Auclair M, Duplomb L, et al. PIK3R1 mutations cause syndromic insulin resistance with lipoatrophy. Am J Hum Genet 2013;93(1):141–9.

51. Shastry S, Simha V, Godbole K, et al. A novel syndrome of mandibular hypoplasia, deafness, and progeroid features associated with lipodystrophy, undescended testes, and male hypogonadism. J Clin Endocrinol Metab 2010; 95(10):E192–7.

52. Weedon MN, Ellard S, Prindle MJ, et al. An in-frame deletion at the polymerase active site of POLD1 causes a multisystem disorder with lipodystrophy. Nat Genet 2013;45(8):947–50.

53. Graul-Neumann LM, Kienitz T, Robinson PN, et al. Marfan syndrome with neonatal progeroid syndrome-like lipodystrophy associated with a novel frameshift mutation at the 3' terminus of the FBN1-gene. Am J Med Genet A 2010;152A(11): 2749–55.

54. Garg A, Xing C. De novo heterozygous FBN1 mutations in the extreme C-terminal region cause progeroid fibrillinopathy. Am J Med Genet A 2014;164A(5):1341–5.

55. Garg A, Kircher M, Del Campo M, et al, University of Washington Center for Mendelian Genomics. Whole exome sequencing identifies de novo heterozygous CAV1 mutations associated with a novel neonatal onset lipodystrophy syndrome. Am J Med Genet A 2015;167A(8):1796–806.

56. Garg A, Subramanyam L, Agarwal AK, et al. Atypical progeroid syndrome due to heterozygous missense LMNA mutations. J Clin Endocrinol Metab 2009;94(12): 4971–83.

57. Merideth MA, Gordon LB, Clauss S, et al. Phenotype and course of Hutchinson-Gilford progeria syndrome. N Engl J Med 2008;358(6):592–604.

58. Savage DB, Semple RK, Clatworthy MR, et al. Complement abnormalities in acquired lipodystrophy revisited. J Clin Endocrinol Metab 2009;94(1):10–6.

Nutrition in Diabetes

Osama Hamdy, MD, PhD[a],*, Mohd-Yusof Barakatun-Nisak, PhD[b,c]

KEYWORDS

- Medical nutrition therapy • Nutrition • Diet • Glycemic index • Diabetes

KEY POINTS

- Medical nutrition therapy is effective in improving glycemic control, promoting weight loss, and modifying cardiovascular risk factors in patients with diabetes.
- Reduction of carbohydrate load, selection of low glycemic index food, and balancing macronutrients improve postprandial blood glucose levels.
- Selection of healthful dietary patterns, such as the Mediterranean diet or DASH diet, are beneficial in managing diabetes.

INTRODUCTION

Nutrition therapy is keystone of diabetes prevention and management and its importance has long been recognized before the era of modern scientific medicine.[1] Before insulin discovery, a starvation diet of very low caloric content (400–500 calories/day), known as the Allen diet, was commonly used to treat diabetes.[2] Another diet with extreme carbohydrate restriction to approximately 2% and very high fat to approximately 70% was used by Elliot P. Joslin for managing diabetes in the 1920s.[3] Although there was no clear distinction between what is known now as type 1 and type 2 diabetes (T2D), those eccentric diets were remarkably successful in managing diabetes and for even keeping patients with type 1 diabetes alive for a few years.[2,4] At that time, diabetes was commonly defined as carbohydrate-intolerance disease.[5] After insulin discovery, the amount of carbohydrates in the diabetes diet was increased to a maximum of 35% to 40% of the total daily caloric intake. By the late 1970s, a strong claim to reduce total fat and dietary saturated fat (SFAs) intake was made due to increased incidence of cardiovascular death, particularly in patients with diabetes.[6] Reduction of fat intake by approximately 10% required a compensatory increase in

Disclosure Statement: O. Hamdy is on the advisory board of Novo-Nordisk, Metagenics Inc, Astra Zeneca Inc, and Boeringher Inglehiem Inc, and is a consultant to Merck Inc. B.-N. Yusof has nothing to disclose.

[a] Department of Endocrinology, Joslin Diabetes Center, Harvard Medical School, One Joslin Place, Boston, MA 02481, USA; [b] Joslin Diabetes Center, Harvard Medical School, Boston, MA 02215, USA; [c] Department of Nutrition and Dietetics, Faculty of Medicine and Health Sciences, Universiti Putra Malaysia, Serdang, Selangor 43400, Malaysia
* Corresponding author.
E-mail address: Osama.hamdy@joslin.harvard.edu

other nutrients, and in this case it was dietary carbohydrates, which went up to approximately 55% to 60% (**Fig. 1**).[7]

Although a high carbohydrate diet has been frequently questioned as a major contributing factor to poor diabetes control and weight gain, little has changed for the past 3 decades.[8] Recently, the importance of specific foods and overall dietary patterns rather than a single isolated nutrient for managing diabetes and cardiovascular diseases (CVD) has emerged.[9,10] This review article discusses the current evidence around the role of nutrition in diabetes management.

MEDICAL NUTRITION THERAPY FOR DIABETES MANAGEMENT

In 1994, the American Dietetic Association used the term "medical nutrition therapy" (MNT) to better articulate appropriate nutrition care and process in diabetes management.[11] MNT can be described as intensive, focused, and structured nutrition therapy that helps in changing the eating behavior of patients with diabetes. Despite recent progress in pharmacologic management of diabetes, MNT remains a crucial tool for achieving optimal glycemic control.[12]

Although MNT is widely recognized by major diabetes organizations across the world, their dietary recommendations are slightly different (**Table 1**). In principle, the prime goal of MNT is to attain and maintain optimal glycemic control and metabolic improvement through healthy food choices while considering patients' personal needs, preferences, and lifestyle patterns.[13] Proper MNT was shown to reduce A1C by 0.5% to 2% in patients with T2D and by 0.3% to 1% in patients with type 1 diabetes.[14] MNT was also shown to be particularly beneficial after initial diabetes diagnosis and in patients with poor glycemic control. Nevertheless, its effectiveness is evident at any A1C level across the entire course of the disease.[13]

Practically, MNT remains the most challenging component of diabetes self-management by most patients. To enhance dietary adherence, an individualized MNT should be provided by registered dietitians or by health care providers who are well versed in nutrition. Comprehensive evaluation of the individual eating pattern, needs, nutrition status, weight history, and history of previous nutrition education are required before recommending an MNT plan.[12]

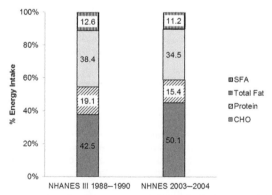

Fig. 1. Trend in macronutrient intake among adults with diabetes in the United States between 1988 and 2004. (*Data from* Oza-Frank R, Cheng YJ, Narayan KMV, et al. Trends in nutrient intake among adults with diabetes in the United States: 1988-2004. J Am Diet Assoc 2009;109(7):1173–8.)

Table 1
A comparison of key recommendation of medical nutrition therapy for people with type 2 diabetes

	ADA 2014/2016[1,12]	CDA 2013[17]	Joslin Guideline[16]
Calorie intake	Recommend reduced energy intake to promote weight loss in overweight/obese adults.	Recommend a nutritionally balanced calorie-reduced diet.	Recommend reduce daily caloric intake between 250 and 500 calories for overweight/obese individuals. Meal replacement that matches the nutrition guideline can be used to initiate and maintain weight loss.
Macronutrient distribution	No recommendation on specific macronutrient distribution. It should be individualized to meet calorie intake and metabolic goals.	Recommend 44%–60% carbohydrate, 15%–20% protein, 20%–35% total fat with consideration for individualization	Recommend 40%–45% carbohydrate, 20%–30% protein, and <35% total fat with adjustment should be made to meet the cultural and food preference of individual.
Eating pattern	Recommend a variety of eating patterns with consideration of personal preference.	Recommend a variety of dietary patterns with consideration on personal preference, values, and abilities.	Not available.
Dietary carbohydrate	Recommend carbohydrate intake from whole grains, vegetables, fruits, legumes, and dairy products with emphasis on foods lower in glycemic load.	Recommend food with a low GI value.	Recommend foods with a low GI value, such as whole grains, legumes, fruits, green salad with olive oil–based dressing and most vegetables. Limit consumption of refined carbohydrates, processed grains, and starchy foods, especially most pastas, white bread, white rice, low-fiber cereal, and white potatoes.
Dietary fiber	Emphasis on foods with higher fiber.	Recommend higher fiber/whole grains than general population (25–50 g per day or 15–25 per 1000 kcal).	Recommend ~14 g fiber/1000 calories (20–35 g) per day. If tolerated, ~50 g/d is effective in improving postprandial hyperglycemia and should be encouraged.
Sucrose and fructose	Recommend to limit intake of sucrose-containing foods and to avoid sugar-sweetened beverages.	Added sugar can be substituted for other carbohydrates in mixed meals up to maximum of 10% total caloric intake.	Recommend to limit consumption of sugar and sugary beverages.

(continued on next page)

Table 1
(continued)

	ADA 2014/2016[1,12]	CDA 2013[17]	Joslin Guideline[16]
Protein	Do not recommend reducing protein intake below daily allowance of 0.8 g/kg body weight including those with diabetes or kidney disease.	Recommend as for general population (1.0–1.5 g/kg body weight). Consider restricting to 0.8 g kg/body weight for those with chronic kidney disease.	Recommend protein intake of not <1.2 g/kg of adjusted body weight[a] for overweight/obese patients. Patients with signs of kidney disease should get a consult from nephrologist before increasing protein intake. Protein can be modified but not lowered to a level that may increase the risk of malnutrition or hypoalbuminemia.
Dietary fat	Recommend intake of total fat, SFA, cholesterol, and transfat as for the general population (total fat between 20% and 35%, SFA <10%). Support eating plan with key element of a Mediterranean-style diet over low in total fat and high in carbohydrates. Encourage eating food rich in long-chain omega 3 fatty acids but no support for omega-3 supplements.	Recommend SFA restriction to <7% and limit transfat to a minimum level. Encourage food rich in MUFA and PUFA up to 20% and 10%, respectively.	Emphasis on quality of fat rather than quantity. Recommend SFA to <7% and limit foods high in transfats. PUFA and MUFA should comprise the rest of fat intake.
Micronutrient supplements	No support for vitamin and mineral supplements.	No support for routine vitamin and mineral supplements.	No support for routine vitamin and mineral supplements.
Alcohol	Advised to drink in moderation. As alcohol may increase the risk for delayed hypoglycemia, education and awareness should be emphasized.	Advised as per general population with consideration on the same precautions.	Advise for moderate consumption. If consumed, no more than 1 drink[b] for women and no more than 2 drinks per day for men.

(continued on next page)

Table 1 (continued)			
	ADA 2014/2016[1,12]	CDA 2013[17]	Joslin Guideline[16]
Sodium	Recommend as for the general population (<2300 mg/d) with further reduction is to be individualized.	No specific cutoffs recommended but emphasized on DASH eating plan.	Recommend <2300 mg (~1 tsp of salt) per day.

Abbreviations: ADA, American Diabetes Association; CDA, Canadian Diabetes Association; DASH, Dietary Approach to Stop Hypertension; GI, glycemic index; MUFA, monounsaturated fatty acids; PUFA, polyunsaturated fatty acids; SFA, saturated fatty acids.
[a] Adjusted body weight = IBW (Ideal Body Weight) + 0.25 (Current Weight − IBW).[16]
[b] 1 drink is equal to 12 ounces of regular beer, 5 ounces of wine, or 1.5 ounces of 80-proof distilled alcohol.[16]

Macronutrient Recommendations

Dietary carbohydrates

There is no final or conclusive evidence for an ideal macronutrient proportion for all patients with T2D, but rather there is an emphasis on individualization of eating plan (see **Table 1**).[1,12,15] The Canadian Diabetes Association and the Joslin Nutrition Guidelines for overweight and obese patients with T2D provide some specific macronutrient distribution. Both point to the prime importance of macronutrient composition in a diabetes nutrition plan because carbohydrates, proteins, and fat have differential impact on blood glucose levels.

They recommended reduction in the total glycemic load (GL) of carbohydrates and their glycemic index (GI) (see **Table 1**).[16,17] Others also made a strong case for reducing carbohydrates in a diabetes diet.[8] Meanwhile, a recent randomized controlled study showed that A1C and weight reduction were comparable between calorie-restricted low-carbohydrate and high-carbohydrate diets at 24 and 52 weeks, but a low-carbohydrate diet, which was also high in unsaturated fat and low in saturated fat, achieved greater improvements in the lipid profile, blood glucose stability, and reductions in diabetes medications, suggesting it as an effective strategy for the optimizing T2D management.[18] Lowering GL by modest restriction of total carbohydrates to approximately 40% to 45% of the total daily caloric intake with favoring carbohydrates of lower GI also showed better effect on blood glucose levels in patients with T2D in comparison with conventional high-carbohydrate meal plans.[19,20] In the real world, foods with low GI property are often high in dietary fiber and whole grains, which also improve overall diet quality.[21]

Increased dietary fiber intake has been strongly recommended as part of diabetes management due to its benefit in inducing satiety,[22] increasing gastrointestinal transit time, and improving overall blood glucose level.[23] Approximately 14 g of fiber per 1000 calories or approximately 20 to 35 g per day is recommended (see **Table 1**). Approximately 50 g fiber per day, if tolerated, is effective in improving postprandial hyperglycemia.[16,17] Dietary fiber from unprocessed food, such as vegetables, fruits, seeds, nuts, and legumes, is preferred, but if needed, fiber supplement, such as psyllium, resistant starch, and β-glucan can be added to reach the total dietary fiber requirement.[16]

Limiting added sugars has been consistently recommended by most organizations (see **Table 1**).[12,16,17] Excessive intake of high-fructose sweetened beverages adversely influenced visceral fat deposition, lipid metabolism, blood pressure, insulin sensitivity, and de novo lipogenesis, in particular among overweight and obese patients.[24] The use of non-nutritive sweeteners may provide short-term benefits, but their long-term effects warrant future investigation.[25]

Dietary fats

In general, the type of fat is more important than the amount of fat intake. Now, it is clear that putting a limit on total fat (eg, <30%) and dietary cholesterol (<300 mg/d) have no substantial benefit on cardiovascular risk. This is in line with the recent recommendations of the Dietary Guideline for Americans,[26] American Diabetes Association,[12] and American Heart Association.[27] Although these organizations strongly support reduction in transfat from industrial hydrogenation of oils, the extent to which dietary saturated fatty acids (SFAs) increase CVD risk has become a controversial issue. Recent meta-analyses performed by De Sauza and colleagues,[28] and included 72 studies involving more than 600,000 participants from 18 countries, found no associations between dietary SFAs and all-cause mortality, CVD mortality, ischemic stroke, or T2D. Interestingly, O'Sullivan and colleagues[29] observed that food high in SFAs, including whole milk, cheese, butter, and other dairy products, were not associated with increased risk of mortality.

Increased consumption of fatty fish and long-chain omega 3 polyunsaturated fatty acids (PUFA) from vegetable oils (eg, canola, corn) and walnut were found to be protective against CVD mortality in patients with T2D. They improve lipid profile and modify platelet aggregation despite their lack of effect on glycemic control.[30] It was also found that supplementation of omega 3 PUFA does not offer any additional cardiovascular protection.[31]

Dietary protein

Dietary protein is important in nutrition management of diabetes. The current recommendations do not support protein restriction for adults with T2D.[12,16,17] Patients with diabetes, especially when they are poorly controlled, lose significant amount of their lean muscle mass as they age, and they lose it at a faster pace than individuals without diabetes.[32,33] Restricting protein intake, especially with lack of strength exercise, speeds lean muscle loss and may lead to profound sarcopenia.[34,35] Currently, several organizations do not recommend significant protein restriction below the recommended dietary allowance of 0.8 g/kg per day for patients with diabetic kidney disease who are not on dialysis.[12,16,17,36,37]

In the Modification of Diet in Renal Disease (MDRD) study, assignment to a low-protein diet of approximately 0.6 g/kg per day compared with the average protein diet of approximately 1.3 g/kg per day in patients with advanced kidney disease did not prevent the progressive decline in glomerular filtration rate (GFR) over 3 years.[38] Early findings from a meta-analysis of randomized clinical studies also did not show any beneficial renal effects from protein restriction in patients with diabetic nephropathy.[39] However, this is contradicted by another recent meta-analysis by Nezu and colleagues.[40] In the latter study, which has several limitations that may affect its quality, the effectiveness of a low-protein diet was mostly dependent on dietary adherence.[40]

For patients on a hypocaloric weight reduction diet, increasing absolute protein intake is important. Using fixed percentage (eg, 15%–20%) to estimate protein requirement in a hypocaloric diet may cause inadequate protein intake and put patients at risk of protein malnutrition and significant lean muscle mass loss during weight reduction. Joslin guidelines advocate a daily protein intake of not less than 1.2 g/kg of adjusted body weight, which is approximately equivalent to 20% to 30%

of total daily calories.[16] A higher protein intake reduces hunger, improves satiety, and minimizes lean muscle mass loss during weight reduction.[41]

Micronutrient recommendations There is no specific vitamin and mineral supplementation to recommend for patients with diabetes except for those with suspected deficiencies.[1] However, nutrient adequacy is important and should be achieved through a balance of high-quality dietary intake because poor glycemic control is usually associated with micronutrient deficiencies.[42] There are specific patients with diabetes who require additional supplementation, including those on calorie-restricted diets, elderly individuals, vegetarians, and pregnant and lactating women.[1]

Low serum vitamin D, measured as serum 25-hydroxy vitamin D, is common among the US population,[43] including patients with diabetes.[44,45] Vitamin D may modify diabetes risk through its effect on glucose homeostasis.[46] Longitudinal studies have universally shown an inverse association of vitamin D status with diabetes risk[44] and A1C level.[47] Low serum vitamin D concentration was shown to be associated with increased risk of macrovascular and microvascular complications in patients with T2D.[45] However, recent systematic review and meta-analyses that included 35 clinical trials reported that vitamin D_3 supplementation did not show any beneficial effect on glycemic outcomes or insulin sensitivity in the short term.[48] Longer clinical trials are lacking.

Patients who selected to have gastric bypass surgery for weight reduction are particularly at higher risk for vitamin and mineral deficiencies postsurgery.[49] Even before surgery, some patients were found to be depleted in iron, ferritin, and folic acid, to have anemia, and to have a high level of parathyroid hormone, indicating a low level of vitamin D.[50,51] Therefore, it is important to routinely screen patients before and after bariatric surgery for potential micronutrient deficiencies and supplement them with iron, vitamin B12, folic acid, and vitamin D in addition to adequate protein intake.

Diabetes-specific nutrition formula Diabetes-specific nutrition formula (DSNF) is usually used as part of MNT to facilitate initial weight reduction while improving glycemic control.[52,53] DSNFs provide approximately 190 to 350 calories per serving. They have balanced macronutrient composition, including fiber, and they are frequently fortified with vitamins and minerals. As these products are specifically designed for patients with diabetes, they contain low GI/GL carbohydrates, higher whey protein than casein, and contain unique blends of amino acids.[54–56] This combination has been consistently shown to improve postprandial plasma glucose and insulin response than standard formulas. In a meta-analysis by Elia and colleagues,[52] DSNF lowered postprandial plasma glucose by 18.5 mg/dL, reduced peak glucose excursion by 28.6 mg/dL, and reduced insulin requirement by 26% to 71% compared with standard formulas. Attenuating postprandial plasma glucose excursion is always a major clinical challenge and was found to contribute to cardiovascular complication in patients with diabetes.[57]

DSNF also improves glucagonlike peptide-1 (GLP-1) secretion. In response to food, patients with T2D frequently have lower GLP-1 response than healthy individuals.[58] GLP-1 hormone plays an important role in glucose homeostasis through stimulating insulin secretion, suppressing glucagon production, delaying gastric emptying, and enhancing satiety.[59]

Using DSNFs for tube feeding in hospitalized patients with diabetes was found to improve metabolic parameters, to reduce hospital length of stay, and to decrease the overall hospital cost in comparison with standard formulas.[60,61] As DSNFs are also fortified with vitamins and several micronutrients, their use for malnourished patients with T2D, especially for elderly patients, was found to improve overall nutritional status and optimize diabetes control.[61,62]

Dietary pattern Dietary pattern is an overall combination of beneficial foods that are habitually consumed, which together produce synergistic health effects.[26] Healthy dietary patterns are commonly rich in fruits, vegetables, nuts, legumes, fish, dairy products, and vegetable oils and low in red meat, processed red meat, refined grains, salt, and added sugar (**Table 2**).[9,10] This pattern is usually high in fiber, vitamins, antioxidants, minerals, polyphenols, and unsaturated fatty acids and is lower in GI/GL, sodium, and transfat.[15,63]

Ajala and colleagues[64] examined 20 RCTs that investigated the effect of different dietary patterns on glycemic control, lipid profile, and body weight in patients with T2D for 6 months or more. Six dietary patterns were included in this analysis: low carbohydrates, low GI, high fiber, high protein, vegetarian/vegan, and Mediterranean dietary patterns in comparison with the commonly used diabetes nutrition guidelines.[65] Low carbohydrates, low-GI, high-protein, and Mediterranean dietary patterns were found to be the most effective in diabetes management. The ultimate benefit on glycemic control was achieved with the Mediterranean dietary pattern (**Fig. 2**). These observations were also seen in 2 recent meta-analyses in which the Mediterranean dietary pattern reduced A1C by 0.30% to 0.47%.[66,67] The Mediterranean dietary pattern also has beneficial effects on cardiovascular risk factors.[64,67,68] In the PREDIMED trial, the subgroup of participants with T2D who followed a Mediterranean diet, even without caloric restriction, had a lower incidence of CVD after a median duration of 4.8 years when compared with those who followed a low-fat diet.[69] The combination of nutrient-rich foods in the Mediterranean diet might collectively induce favorable changes in cardio-metabolic risk factors, improve insulin sensitivity, and reduce oxidation and inflammation.[70] Such CVD benefits were not seen in the Women's Health Initiative study among participants who followed a low-fat diet,[71] which further supports the emerging role of dietary patterns in the primary prevention of CVD in patients with T2D.

The Dietary Approaches to Stop Hypertension (DASH) may be an ideal cardio-protective dietary pattern for patients with T2D.[72] Although the benefits of the DASH diet have been documented for hypertension management and for CVD risk reduction, little research was done in patients with T2D. In an 8-week small RCT of 44 participants withT2D, the DASH diet significantly improved glycemic control and cardio-metabolic parameters, and reduced inflammation markers.[73] Dietary quality also improved in those who followed the DASH diet in comparison with the control group. Their consumption of some minerals (calcium and potassium), fiber, fruits, vegetables, dairy, and whole grains were significantly increased.[73]

Vegetarian or vegan diets have also been tested in patients with diabetes. A recent meta-analysis of controlled clinical studied in patients with T2D for 4 weeks or more (n = 225) found a significant reduction in A1C by an average of 0.39%, but with no effect on fasting plasma glucose.[74] However, this beneficial effect is difficult to separate from the effect of weight loss, as many of these trials used calorie restriction, reduced dietary fat, or changed diabetes medications.[74–76]

SPECIFIC NUTRITION PLANS FOR PATIENTS WITH DIABETES
Nutrition Strategies for Weight Reduction in Type 2 Diabetes

Elliot P Joslin said "One of the first rules for the diabetic patient to learn is never to overeat."[5] Most patients with T2D are either overweight, obese, or severely obese. Weight

Table 2
Summary of studies on dietary pattern for diabetes management

| Diet-Style | Key Characteristic Inducing Benefits | Diabetes Management[Ref] | | |
		Glucose	Insulin	CVD Risk
Mediterranean diet	• Rich in whole grains, olive oil, fruits, vegetables, nuts, and legumes. • Low-to-moderate intake of dairy products, fish, poultry, and wine. • Low intake of red meat. • Very low sweets (only if desired).	↓[64,66,67]	↓[69]	↓[69]
DASH	• Rich in vegetables, fruits, whole grains, poultry, fish, nuts, and low-fat dairy products. • Low in red meat, sweets, and sugar-containing beverages. • Emphasize keep saturated fats and sodium to a very minimum level.	↓[73]	[a]↓[99]	↓[73]
Vegetarian an vegan	• Vegan: eliminate all animal-derived products. • Vegetarian: eliminate some animal products, including lacto-avo (eat dairy or egg only), pesco (eat fish, egg, or dairy), semi (eat all but no red meat and poultry).	[b]↓[74]	NA	NA
Dietary Guideline for America (AHEI)	AHEI is an index based on food and nutrients to predict chronic disease risk. • High-quality diet is those rich in whole grains, fruits, vegetables, nuts, legumes, long-chain omega 3 fatty acids, and PUFAs. • Low in sugar-sweetened beverages, fruits juices, red meats, processed meats, and foods high in sodium and transfat. • Moderate alcohol consumption.	NA		
Prudent/Paleo	• Rich in whole grains, fruits, vegetables, legumes, and vegetable fats. • Low in red meats, refined grains, and sugared soft drinks.	NA		
Lower carbohydrates diet	• Low-to-moderate carbohydrate (<40% carbohydrate from energy) • High in plant-based protein and fat.	↓[8,18,64]	[c]↓[18]	[c]↓[18]

Abbreviations: ↓, reduced; AHEI, Alternate Healthy Eating Index; CVD, cardiovascular disease; DASH, Dietary Approach to Stop Hypertension; NA, not available; PUFAs, polyunsaturated fatty acids.
[a] May reduce insulin levels.[99]
[b] Results were not consistent and cofounded by calorie-restricted diet that induced weight loss in the study.[74]
[c] Individual study finding.

management is crucial for diabetes management in those patients. Any degree of weight loss improves diabetes prognosis.[77,78] A modest weight reduction of 5% to 10% of the initial body weight is frequently recommended. This amount of weight reduction is realistic and is clinically meaningful.[79,80] It has been shown to improve

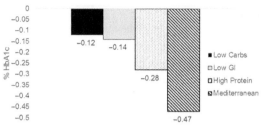

Fig. 2. Difference in A1C response to various dietary patterns when compared with standard diabetes nutrition guideline. (*Data from* Ajala O, English P, Pinkney J. Systematic review and meta-analysis of different dietary approaches to the management of type 2 diabetes. Am J Clin Nutr 2013;97(3):505–16.)

glycemic control and other diabetes-related outcomes, including reduced need for antihyperglycemic medications. In the Action for Health in Diabetes (Look AHEAD) study that included overweight and obese patients with T2D, participants in the intensive lifestyle intervention arm had greater weight loss than those in the diabetes support and education arm (8.6% vs 0.7% at 1 year, 6.0% and 3.5% at 9.6 years of follow-up).[77,81] This magnitude of weight reduction was associated with improvement in glycemic control, CVD risk factors,[77,79] sleep apnea,[82] and urinary continence.[83] It was also associated with reduction in medications used for diabetes and CVD risk management.[81] Additional benefits of weight reduction in the same study included improvement in fitness and health-related quality of life.[84]

Despite the impressive improvement in glycemic control and other diabetes-related outcomes,[77] intensive lifestyle intervention did not show any pertinent benefit in reducing cardiac events in comparison with the control group.[79] The unexpected reduction in the incidence of cardiovascular events among US adults during the same period might deteriorate the study power to detect its primary endpoint.[85] Increased use of cardio-protective drugs by the control group might also contribute to the lack of difference between the 2 arms. Patients in the control group also lost some weight probably after observing the announced short-term benefits of intensive lifestyle intervention.

Translating these findings into real-world practice settings is challenging. Patients with T2D may not receive a comparable degree of support to promote weight loss as participants in the Look AHEAD study due to limited time and resources.[86] However, successful implementation of the Weight Achievement and Intensive Treatment (Why WAIT) program at Joslin Diabetes Centre had shown the feasibility of successful adoption of intensive lifestyle intervention in routine clinical practices.[87] The 12-week multidisciplinary program has demonstrated 11.1% weight reduction sustained for 1 year in obese participants with T2D. This weight loss was associated with improved glycemic control and reduction in cardiovascular risk factors. A small proportion of participants were able to achieve partial or complete diabetes remission at 1 year.[78]

To achieve a weight loss goal, structured modified dietary intervention with hypocaloric diet is recommended to create negative energy balance.[87] In the Why WAIT program, the daily calorie goal was identified by reducing daily caloric intake by approximately 250 to 500 calories and rounding it to the nearest level of 1200, 1500, or 1800 calories.[87] In general, most men consumed 1800 kcal/d and most women consumed 1500 kcal/d with few exceptions (**Table 3**). As outlined previously, DSNFs can be used as a meal replacement (MR) to enhance weight reduction.[53] MRs

Table 3
Daily calorie needs for weight loss management

Gender	Weight Reduction (kilocalorie/d)	Weight Maintenance (kilocalorie/d)
Men	1800	1800–2200
Women	1500	1500–2000
Women height <150 cm (59 inches)	1200	1500

Data from Joslin Diabetes Centre, Joslin Clinic. Clinical nutrition guideline for overweight and obese adults with type 2 diabetes, prediabetes or those at high risk of developing type 2 diabetes 08 07 2011. Boston: 2011. Available at: https://www.joslin.org/bin_from_cms/Nutrition_Guidelines-8.22.11(1).pdf.

can be consumed in the form of ready-to-drink shakes, ready-to-mix powders, or bars. The common nutrition information of the ready-to-drink shakes has been summarized elsewhere.[53] MRs help patients to adhere to their energy-restricted meal plan and control portion size. Frequency of MRs was also shown to be associated with the magnitude of weight loss. In the Look AHEAD study, participants in the highest quartile or MR usage (~2 per day) had a higher percentage of weight reduction (11.2%) than the lowest quartile of usage (5.9%) at 1 year (**Fig. 3**).[88] In the Why WAIT program, participants were instructed to consume 2 MRs (each of 190 calories) and 2 snacks of 100 to 200 calories for their breakfast and lunch and a healthy choice from dinner menus for 12 weeks. However, patients on MRs should carefully monitor their blood glucose to reduce risk of hypoglycemia.[89]

Weight reduction through a low-calorie diet is always associated with reduction in several micronutrients, including B vitamins, iron, calcium, and magnesium, which are essential for metabolism, energy, and bone health.[90] DSFs may maintain nutrient adequacy during weight loss by calorie-restricted diets.[53] In an RCT, participants who followed a low-calorie diet of only traditional food had a significantly lower level of 9 essential vitamins and minerals than those who used traditional food and DSF after 1 year despite equal macronutrient composition.[91]

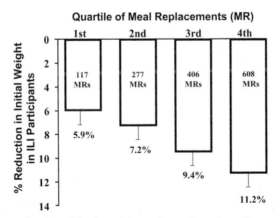

Fig. 3. Percentage reduction of body weight at 1 year based on the quartiles of meal replacements. (*Data from* Wadden TA, West DS, Neiberg RH, et al. One-year weight losses in the Look AHEAD study: factors associated with success. Obesity (Silver Spring) 2009;17(4):713–22.)

Eating Plan for Type 1 Diabetes

Carbohydrate counting has been the mainstay for determining mealtime insulin requirements in patients with type 1 diabetes.[12] It was initially thought that only carbohydrates affect postprandial hyperglycemia; however, introduction of continuous glucose monitoring showed that dietary fat, protein, and GI have a significant effect on postprandial glycemic excursion.[92]

Consumption of a high-fat meal results in sustained late postprandial hyperglycemia. This effect is caused by delayed gastric emptying, which in turn delays peak postprandial glycemic excursion.[93] Adding 35 g of fat (approximately 7 teaspoons) increased postprandial plasma glucose by 2.3 mmol/L at 5 hours. Wolpert and colleagues[94] observed that 50 g fat (10 teaspoons) caused significant hyperglycemia over 5 hours even when additional insulin was injected. Protein intake also induces a late excursion in postprandial plasma glucose. However, its effect varies according

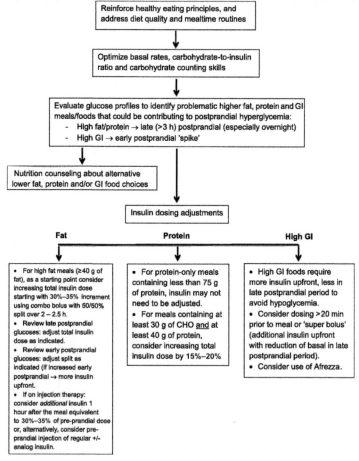

Fig. 4. Clinical application on the effect of fat, protein, and glycemic index on postprandial glycemic control. (*Data from* Bell KJ, Smart CE, Steil GM, et al. Impact of fat, protein, and glycemic index on postprandial glucose control in type 1 diabetes: implications for intensive diabetes management in the continuous glucose monitoring era. Diabetes Care 2015;38(6):1008–15.)

to the amount of concomitant carbohydrates.[92] Adding 35 g protein (~1 oz) to 30 g carbohydrates (2 carbs exchanges) increased blood glucose concentration by 2.6 mmol/L at 5 hours.[95] Eating 12.5 to 50.0 g (0.5–1.5 oz) of protein alone did not affect postprandial glycemia. However, increasing protein intake to 75 to 100 g (2.5–3.3 oz) significantly increased postprandial plasma glucose.[96] Thus, a meal high in fat and protein may require a higher insulin dose to control late postprandial hyperglycemia than a lower fat and protein meal even if combined with the same amount of carbohydrates.[94–96]

At a similar amount of carbohydrates, a low GI meal results in lower glycemic response than a high GI meal.[92] Studies suggested that risk of mild hypoglycemia may increase when low GI food is ingested in comparison with high GI food.[97,98] For this reason, more upfront insulin may be needed to cater the effect of higher GI food.[97,98]

These observations indicate that the premeal insulin dose should be adjusted based on the overall meal composition rather than on only calculating the carbohydrate content of the meal.[92] The empirical approach for clinical application on the effects of fat, protein, and GI on postprandial glycemic excursion, adapted from Bell and colleagues,[92] is shown in **Fig. 4**.

FUTURE CONSIDERATION

Although macronutrient composition of diet is important, it is difficult to separately examine the effects of individual dietary components on plasma glucose because diet is a complex entity with extensive interaction between foods. This is highly relevant, as people eat food rather than individual nutrients, such as carbohydrate, protein, or fat for diabetes management.

REFERENCES

1. Evert AB, Boucher JL, Cypress M, et al. Nutrition therapy recommendations for the management of adults with diabetes. Diabetes Care 2013;36(11):3821–42.
2. Allen F. Studies concerning diabetes. J Am Med Assoc 1914;LXIII(11):939.
3. Hockaday TDR. Should the diabetic diet be based on carbohydrate of fat restriction?. In: Turner M, Thomas B, editors. Nutrition and diabetes. London : Libbey; 1981. p. 23–32.
4. Joslin EP. The Treatment of Diabetes Mellitus. Can Med Assoc J 1924;14(9): 808–11.
5. Joslin EP. 5th edition. A diabetic manual for the mutual use of doctor and patient, vol. 26. Philadelphia: Lea & Febiger; 1934.
6. Kannel WB, McGee DL. Diabetes and glucose tolerance as risk factors for cardiovascular disease: the Framingham study. Diabetes Care 1979;2(2):120–6.
7. Oza-Frank R, Cheng YJ, Narayan KMV, et al. Trends in nutrient intake among adults with diabetes in the United States: 1988-2004. J Am Diet Assoc 2009; 109(7):1173–8.
8. Feinman RD, Pogozelski WK, Astrup A, et al. Dietary carbohydrate restriction as the first approach in diabetes management: critical review and evidence base. Nutrition 2014;31(1):1–13.
9. Mozaffarian D. Dietary and policy priorities for cardiovascular disease, diabetes, and obesity: a comprehensive review. Circulation 2016;133(2):187–225.
10. Ley SH, Hamdy O, Mohan V, et al. Prevention and management of type 2 diabetes: dietary components and nutritional strategies. Lancet 2014;383(9933): 1999–2007.

11. Identifying patients at risk: ADA's definitions for nutrition screening and nutrition assessment. J Am Diet Assoc 1994;94(8):838–9.
12. American Diabetes Association. 3. Foundations of care and comprehensive medical evaluation. Diabetes Care 2016;39(Suppl 1):S23–35.
13. Pastors JG, Warshaw H, Daly A, et al. The evidence for the effectiveness of medical nutrition therapy in diabetes management. Diabetes Care 2002;25(3):608–13.
14. Franz MMJ, Powers MA, Leontos C, et al. The evidence for medical nutrition therapy for type 1 and type 2 diabetes in adults. J Am Diet Assoc 2010;110(12): 1852–89.
15. Wheeler ML, Dunbar SA, Jaacks LM, et al. Macronutrients, food groups, and eating patterns in the management of diabetes: a systematic review of the literature, 2010. Diabetes Care 2012;35(2):434–45 [systematic review and meta-analyses].
16. Joslin Diabetes Centre, Joslin Clinic. Clinical nutrition guideline for overweight and obese adults with type 2 diabetes, prediabetes or those at high risk of developing type 2 diabetes 08 07 2011. Boston: 2011. Available at: https://www.joslin. org/bin_from_cms/Nutrition_Guidelines-8.22.11(1).pdf.
17. Canadian Diabetes Association Clinical Practice Guidelines Expert Committee. Canadian Diabetes Association clinical practice guidelines for the prevention and management of diabetes in Canada. Can J Diabetes 2013;37(Suppl 1):S1–212.
18. Tay J, Luscombe-Marsh ND, Thompson CH, et al. Comparison of low- and high-carbohydrate diets for type 2 diabetes management: a randomized trial. Am J Clin Nutr 2015;102(4):780–90.
19. Jenkins DJA, Kendall CWC, McKeown-Eyssen G, et al. Effect of a low-glycemic index or a high-cereal fiber diet on type 2 diabetes: a randomized trial. JAMA 2008;300(23):2742–53.
20. Ma Y, Olendzki BC, Merriam PA, et al. A randomized clinical trial comparing low-glycemic index versus ADA dietary education among individuals with type 2 diabetes. Nutrition 2008;24(1):45–56.
21. Barakatun Nisak MY, Ruzita AT, Norimah AK, et al. Improvement of dietary quality with the aid of a low glycemic index diet in Asian patients with type 2 diabetes mellitus. J Am Coll Nutr 2010;29(3):161–70.
22. Slavin J, Green H. Dietary fibre and satiety. Nutr Bull 2007;32(s1):32–42.
23. Post RE, Mainous AG, King DE, et al. Dietary fiber for the treatment of type 2 diabetes mellitus: a meta-analysis. J Am Board Fam Med 2012;25(1):16–23.
24. Stanhope KL, Schwarz JM, Keim NL, et al. Consuming fructose-sweetened, not glucose-sweetened, beverages increases visceral adiposity and lipids and decreases insulin sensitivity in overweight/obese humans. J Clin Invest 2009; 119(5):1322–34.
25. Gardner C, Wylie-Rosett J, Gidding SS, et al. Nonnutritive sweeteners: current use and health perspectives: a scientific statement from the American Heart Association and the American Diabetes Association. Diabetes Care 2012;35(8): 1798–808.
26. USDA. Scientific report of the 2015 dietary guidelines advisory committee. Diet Guidel Advis Comm; 2015. Available at: https://health.gov/dietaryguidelines/ 2015-scientific-report/.
27. Fox CS, Golden SH, Anderson C, et al. Update on prevention of cardiovascular disease in adults with type 2 diabetes mellitus in light of recent evidence: a scientific statement from the American Heart Association and the American Diabetes Association. Diabetes Care 2015;38(9):1777–803.
28. de Souza RJ, Mente A, Maroleanu A, et al. Intake of saturated and trans unsaturated fatty acids and risk of all cause mortality, cardiovascular disease, and type

2 diabetes: systematic review and meta-analysis of observational studies. BMJ 2015;351:h3978.

29. O'Sullivan TA, Hafekost K, Mitrou F, et al. Food sources of saturated fat and the association with mortality: a meta-analysis. Am J Public Health 2013;103(9): e31–42 [systematic review and meta-analyses].

30. McEwen B, Morel-Kopp M-C, Tofler G, et al. Effect of omega-3 fish oil on cardiovascular risk in diabetes. Diabetes Educ 2010;36(4):565–84.

31. Rizos EC, Ntzani EE, Bika E, et al. Association between omega-3 fatty acid supplementation and risk of major cardiovascular disease events: a systematic review and meta-analysis. JAMA 2012;308(10):1024–33 [systematic review and meta-analyses].

32. Lee JSW, Auyeung TW, Leung J, et al. The effect of diabetes mellitus on age-associated lean mass loss in 3153 older adults. Diabet Med 2010;27(12):1366–71.

33. Leenders M, Verdijk LB, van der Hoeven L, et al. Patients with type 2 diabetes show a greater decline in muscle mass, muscle strength, and functional capacity with aging. J Am Med Dir Assoc 2013;14(8):585–92.

34. Kalyani RR, Corriere M, Ferrucci L. Age-related and disease-related muscle loss: the effect of diabetes, obesity, and other diseases. Lancet Diabetes Endocrinol 2014;2(10):819–29.

35. Paddon-Jones D, Rasmussen BB. Dietary protein recommendations and the prevention of sarcopenia. Curr Opin Clin Nutr Metab Care 2009;12(1):86–90.

36. KDOQI. KDOQI Clinical practice guidelines and clinical practice recommendations for diabetes and chronic kidney disease. Am J Kidney Dis 2007;49(2 Suppl 2):S12–154.

37. Tuttle KR, Bakris GL, Bilous RW, et al. Diabetic kidney disease: a report from an ADA Consensus Conference. Diabetes Care 2014;37(10):2864–83.

38. Modification of Diet in Renal Disease (MDRD) Study Group, Levey AS, Adler S, et al. Effects of dietary protein restriction on the progression of moderate renal disease in the Modification of Diet in Renal Disease Study. J Am Soc Nephrol 1996;7(12):2616–26 [Erratum appears in J Am Soc Nephrol 1997;8(3):493].

39. Pan Y, Guo LL, Jin HM. Low-protein diet for diabetic nephropathy: a meta-analysis of randomized controlled trials. Am J Clin Nutr 2008;88(3):660–6 [systematic review and meta-analyses].

40. Nezu U, Kamiyama H, Kondo Y, et al. Effect of low-protein diet on kidney function in diabetic nephropathy: meta-analysis of randomised controlled trials. BMJ Open 2013;3(5) [pii:e002934]. [systematic review and meta-analyses].

41. Hamdy O, Horton ES. Protein content in diabetes nutrition plan. Curr Diab Rep 2011;11(2):111–9.

42. Mooradian A, Morley J. Micronutrient status in diabetes mellitus. Am J Clin Nutr 1987;45(5):877–95.

43. Forrest KYZ, Stuhldreher WL. Prevalence and correlates of vitamin D deficiency in US adults. Nutr Res 2011;31(1):48–54.

44. Mitri J, Muraru MD, Pittas AG. Vitamin D and type 2 diabetes: a systematic review. Eur J Clin Nutr 2011;65(9):1005–15 [systematic review and meta-analyses].

45. Herrmann M, Sullivan DR, Veillard A-S, et al. Serum 25-hydroxyvitamin D: a predictor of macrovascular and microvascular complications in patients with type 2 diabetes. Diabetes Care 2015;38(3):521–8.

46. Mitri J, Pittas AG. Vitamin D and diabetes. Endocrinol Metab Clin North Am 2014; 43(1):205–32 [systematic review and meta-analyses].

47. Kositsawat J, Freeman VL, Gerber BS, et al. Association of A1C levels with vitamin D status in U.S. adults: data from the National Health and Nutrition Examination Survey. Diabetes Care 2010;33(6):1236–8.

48. Seida JC, Mitri J, Colmers IN, et al. Clinical review: Effect of vitamin D3 supplementation on improving glucose homeostasis and preventing diabetes: a systematic review and meta-analysis. J Clin Endocrinol Metab 2014;99(10):3551–60 [systematic review and meta-analyses].

49. Mechanick JI, Youdim A, Jones DB, et al. Clinical practice guidelines for the perioperative nutritional, metabolic, and nonsurgical support of the bariatric surgery patient–2013 update: cosponsored by American Association of Clinical Endocrinologists, the Obesity Society, and American Society for Metabolic & Bariatric Surgery. Endocr Pract 2013;19(2):337–72.

50. Schweiger C, Weiss R, Berry E, et al. Nutritional deficiencies in bariatric surgery candidates. Obes Surg 2010;20(2):193–7.

51. Flancbaum L, Belsley S, Drake V. Preoperative nutritional status of patients undergoing Roux-en-Y gastric bypass for morbid obesity. J Gastrointest Surg 2006; 10(7):1033–7.

52. Elia M, Ceriello A, Laube H, et al. Enteral nutritional support and use of diabetes-specific formulas for patients with diabetes: a systematic review and meta-analysis. Diabetes Care 2005;28(9):2267–79 [systematic review and meta-analyses].

53. Hamdy O, Zwiefelhofer D. Weight management using a meal replacement strategy in type 2 diabetes. Curr Diab Rep 2010;10(2):159–64.

54. Vanschoonbeek K, Lansink M, van Laere KMJ, et al. Slowly digestible carbohydrate sources can be used to attenuate the postprandial glycemic response to the ingestion of diabetes-specific enteral formulas. Diabetes Educ 2009;35(4): 631–40.

55. van Loon LJC, Kruijshoop M, Menheere PPCA, et al. Amino acid ingestion strongly enhances insulin secretion in patients with long-term type 2 diabetes. Am J Clin Nutr 2003;26(3):625–30.

56. Mortensen LS, Hartvigsen ML, Brader LJ, et al. Differential effects of protein quality on postprandial lipemia in response to a fat-rich meal in type 2 diabetes: comparison of whey, casein, gluten, and cod protein. Am J Clin Nutr 2009;90(1):41–8.

57. Ceriello A. Postprandial hyperglycemia and diabetes complications: is it time to treat? Diabetes 2004;54(1):1–7.

58. Vilsbøll T, Krarup T, Deacon CF, et al. Reduced postprandial concentrations of intact biologically active glucagon-like peptide 1 in type 2 diabetic patients. Diabetes 2014;50(March 2001):609–13.

59. Flint A, Raben A, Astrup A, et al. Glucagon-like peptide 1 promotes satiety and suppresses energy intake in humans. J Clin Invest 1998;101(3):515–20.

60. Hamdy O, Ernst FR, Baumer D, et al. Differences in resource utilization between patients with diabetes receiving glycemia-targeted specialized nutrition vs standard nutrition formulas in U.S. hospitals. JPEN J Parenter Enteral Nutr 2014;38(2 Suppl):86S–91S.

61. Gosmanov AR, Umpierrez GE. Medical nutrition therapy in hospitalized patients with diabetes. Curr Diab Rep 2012;12(1):93–100.

62. de Luis D a, Izaola O, Aller R, et al. A randomized clinical trial with two enteral diabetes-specific supplements in patients with diabetes mellitus type 2: metabolic effects. Eur Rev Med Pharmacol Sci 2008;12:261–6.

63. Mozaffarian D, Appel LJ, Van Horn L. Components of a cardioprotective diet: new insights. Circulation 2011;123(24):2870–91.

64. Ajala O, English P, Pinkney J. Systematic review and meta-analysis of different dietary approaches to the management of type 2 diabetes. Am J Clin Nutr 2013; 97(3):505–16 [systematic review and meta-analyses].

65. American Diabetes Association. Evidence-based nutrition principles and recommendations for the treatment and prevention of diabetes and related complications. Diabetes Care 2002;25(Suppl 1):S50–60.

66. Huo R, Du T, Xu Y, et al. Effects of Mediterranean-style diet on glycemic control, weight loss and cardiovascular risk factors among type 2 diabetes individuals: a meta-analysis. Eur J Clin Nutr 2015;69(11):1200–8 [systematic review and meta-analyses].

67. Esposito K, Maiorino MI, Bellastella G, et al. A journey into a Mediterranean diet and type 2 diabetes: a systematic review with meta-analyses. BMJ Open 2015; 5(8):e008222 [systematic review and meta-analyses].

68. Yao B, Fang H, Xu W, et al. Dietary fiber intake and risk of type 2 diabetes: a dose-response analysis of prospective studies. Eur J Epidemiol 2014;29(2):79–88.

69. Estruch R, Ros E, Salas-Salvadó J, et al. Primary prevention of cardiovascular disease with a Mediterranean diet. N Engl J Med 2013;368(14):1279–90.

70. Jacobs DR, Gross MD, Tapsell LC. Food synergy: an operational concept for understanding nutrition. Am J Clin Nutr 2009;89(5):1543S–8S.

71. Howard BV, Van Horn L, Hsia J, et al. Low-fat dietary pattern and risk of cardiovascular disease: the Women's Health Initiative Randomized Controlled Dietary Modification Trial. JAMA 2006;295(6):655–66.

72. Clark AL. Use of the Dietary Approaches to Stop Hypertension (DASH) eating plan for diabetes management. Diabetes Spectr 2012;25(4):244–52.

73. Azadbakht L, Fard NRP, Karimi M, et al. Effects of the Dietary Approaches to Stop Hypertension (DASH) eating plan on cardiovascular risks among type 2 diabetic patients: a randomized crossover clinical trial. Diabetes Care 2011;34(1):55–7.

74. Yokoyama Y, Barnard ND, Levin SM, et al. Vegetarian diets and glycemic control in diabetes: a systematic review and meta-analysis. Cardiovasc Diagn Ther 2014; 4(5):373–82.

75. Barnard ND, Cohen J, Jenkins DJA, et al. A low-fat vegan diet and a conventional diabetes diet in the treatment of type 2 diabetes: a randomized, controlled, 74-wk clinical trial. Am J Clin Nutr 2009;89(5):1588S–96S.

76. Barnard ND, Scialli AR, Turner-McGrievy G, et al. The effects of a low-fat, plant-based dietary intervention on body weight, metabolism, and insulin sensitivity. Am J Med 2005;118(9):991–7.

77. Wing RR. Long-term effects of a lifestyle intervention on weight and cardiovascular risk factors in individuals with type 2 diabetes mellitus: four-year results of the Look AHEAD trial. Arch Intern Med 2010;170(17):1566–75.

78. Mottalib A, Sakr M, Shehabeldin M, et al. Diabetes remission after nonsurgical intensive lifestyle intervention in obese patients with type 2 diabetes. J Diabetes Res 2015;2015:468704.

79. Wing RR, Bolin P, Brancati FL, et al. Cardiovascular effects of intensive lifestyle intervention in type 2 diabetes. N Engl J Med 2013;369(2):145–54.

80. Hamdy O. Nonsurgical diabetes weight management: be prepared for sustainable and practical interventions. Curr Diab Rep 2011;11(2):75–6.

81. The Look AHEAD Research Group. Reduction in weight and cardiovascular disease risk factors in individuals with type 2 diabetes: one-year results of the Look AHEAD trial. Diabetes Care 2007;30(6):1374–83.

82. Foster GD, Borradaile KE, Sanders MH, et al. A randomized study on the effect of weight loss on obstructive sleep apnea among obese patients with type 2 diabetes: the Sleep AHEAD study. Arch Intern Med 2009;169(17):1619–26.

83. Phelan S, Kanaya AM, Subak LL, et al. Weight loss prevents urinary incontinence in women with type 2 diabetes: results from the Look AHEAD trial. J Urol 2012; 187(3):939–44.

84. Rubin RR, Wadden TA, Bahnson JL, et al. Impact of intensive lifestyle intervention on depression and health-related quality of life in type 2 diabetes: the Look AHEAD Trial. Diabetes Care 2014;37(6):1544–53.

85. Gerstein HC. Do lifestyle changes reduce serious outcomes in diabetes? N Engl J Med 2013;369(2):189–90.

86. Forman-Hoffman V, Little A, Wahls T. Barriers to obesity management: a pilot study of primary care clinicians. BMC Fam Pract 2006;7:35.

87. Hamdy O. Diabetes weight management in clinical practice—the why WAIT model. US Endocrinol 2008;4(2):49–54.

88. Wadden TA, West DS, Neiberg RH, et al. One-year weight losses in the Look AHEAD study: factors associated with success. Obesity (Silver Spring) 2009; 17(4):713–22.

89. Hamdy O, Goebel-Fabbri A, Carver C, et al. Why WAIT program: a novel model for diabetes weight management in routine clinical practice. Obes Manag 2008; 4(4):176–83.

90. Gardner CD, Kim S, Bersamin A, et al. Micronutrient quality of weight-loss diets that focus on macronutrients: results from the A TO Z study. Am J Clin Nutr 2010;92(2):304–12.

91. Ashley JM, Herzog H, Clodfelter S, et al. Nutrient adequacy during weight loss interventions: a randomized study in women comparing the dietary intake in a meal replacement group with a traditional food group. Nutr J 2007;6(1):12.

92. Bell KJ, Smart CE, Steil GM, et al. Impact of fat, protein, and glycemic index on postprandial glucose control in type 1 diabetes: implications for intensive diabetes management in the continuous glucose monitoring era. Diabetes Care 2015;38(6):1008–15 [systematic review and meta-analyses].

93. Lodefalk M, Aman J, Bang P. Effects of fat supplementation on glycaemic response and gastric emptying in adolescents with type 1 diabetes. Diabet Med 2008;25(9):1030–5.

94. Wolpert HA, Atakov-Castillo A, Smith SA, et al. Dietary fat acutely increases glucose concentrations and insulin requirements in patients with type 1 diabetes: implications for carbohydrate-based bolus dose calculation and intensive diabetes management. Diabetes Care 2013;36(4):810–6.

95. Smart CEM, Evans M, O'Connell SM, et al. Both dietary protein and fat increase postprandial glucose excursions in children with type 1 diabetes, and the effect is additive. Diabetes Care 2013;36(12):3897–902.

96. Paterson MA, Smart C, McElduff P, et al. Influence of pure protein on postprandial blood blucose levels in individuals with type 1 diabetes mellitus. In: 2014 Conference ADA. Diabetes 2014;63:A15. Available at: http://www.mdlinx.com/endocrinology/conference-abstract.cfm/16262/?conf_id=34530&searchstring=&coverage_day=0&nonus=0&page=2.

97. Mohammed NH, Wolever TMS. Effect of carbohydrate source on post-prandial blood glucose in subjects with type 1 diabetes treated with insulin lispro. Diabetes Res Clin Pract 2004;65(1):29–35.

98. Nansel TR, Gellar L, McGill A. Effect of varying glycemic index meals on blood glucose control assessed with continuous glucose monitoring in youth with type 1 diabetes on basal-bolus insulin regimens. Diabetes Care 2008;31(4):695–7.

99. Shirani F, Salehi-Abargouei A, Azadbakht L. Effects of Dietary Approaches to Stop Hypertension (DASH) diet on some risk for developing type 2 diabetes: a systematic review and meta-analysis on controlled clinical trials. Nutrition 2013; 29(7–8):939–47 [systematic review and meta-analyses].

Metformin
From Research to Clinical Practice

Meng H. Tan, MD[a],*, Hussain Alquraini, MD[a], Kara Mizokami-Stout, MD[a], Mark MacEachern, MLIS[b]

KEYWORDS

- Metformin • Glucose-lowering drug • Type 2 diabetes mellitus
- Polycystic ovary syndrome • Delaying onset of type 2 diabetes mellitus
- Gestational diabetes

KEY POINTS

- Metformin is the first-line glucose-lowering drug to control hyperglycemia in type 2 diabetes mellitus (T2DM); an insulin sensitizer, it decreases hepatic gluconeogenesis and increases glucose disposal in skeletal muscles.
- Metformin is safe (small risk for hypoglycemia, weight neutral, and some gastrointestinal [GI] adverse events), is inexpensive, reduces microvascular complication risk, and lowers cardiovascular mortality compared with sulfonylurea therapy.
- Metformin-induced lactic acidosis is rare; metformin-associated lactic acidosis (MALA) is often caused by other conditions.
- Guidelines for metformin's use in T2DM patients with mild to moderate renal impairment and congestive heart failure have changed.
- Metformin is also used to delay the onset of T2DM, in treating gestational diabetes mellitus (GDM) (especially outside the United States), and in women with polycystic ovary syndrome (PCOS).

INTRODUCTION

Many professional diabetes organizations recommend metformin (provided there are no contraindications for its use) as the first glucose-lowering drug (GLD) to be initiated when lifestyle therapies for T2DM do not achieve glycemic target.[1–4] Metformin has emerged as the preferred first GLD as new knowledge on T2DM and metformin is

The authors have nothing to disclose.
[a] Division of Metabolism, Endocrinology and Diabetes, Department of Internal Medicine, University of Michigan, Ann Arbor, MI, USA; [b] Taubman Health Sciences Library, University of Michigan, Ann Arbor, MI, USA
* Corresponding author. Division of Metabolism, Endocrinology and Diabetes, Department of Internal Medicine, University of Michigan, 24 Frank Lloyd Wright Drive, Lobby G, Suite 1500, Ann Arbor, MI 48106.
E-mail address: mengt@med.umich.edu

Endocrinol Metab Clin N Am 45 (2016) 819–843
http://dx.doi.org/10.1016/j.ecl.2016.06.008

uncovered by research and translated into clinical practice. This article's aim is to review selected aspects of this new knowledge (identified in a literature search of PubMed, Embase, and Cochrane Central Register of Controlled Trials in November 2015) reported since 2000. Specifically, the focus is on

1. Use in T2DM
2. Use in other diseases and conditions
3. Current research that may lead to more pleiotropic effects

This review discusses some old concepts of this 59-year-old (as of 2016) GLD that have changed, yielding to new ones.

USE IN TYPE 2 DIABETES MELLITUS
Drug Development

Metformin (dimethylguanidine) has its roots in a plant, *Galega officinalis* (French lilac, Goat's rue, or Spanish sainfoin), rich in guanidine. An outline of the events from 1918, when guanidine was shown to lower blood glucose in animals, to its launch as an oral GLD in 1957 and beyond is shown in **Table 1**.[5]

The First-Line Oral Glucose-Lowering Drug for Type 2 Diabetes Mellitus

The only approved indication for metformin use is as "an adjunct to diet and exercise to improve glycemic control in adults and children with type 2 diabetes mellitus."[6] The package insert reports the clinical trials results that led to this indication. Meta-analysis and systematic reviews of metformin monotherapy (**Table 2**) support its glucose-lowering effect in T2DM patients.[7–10]

Table 1	
Development of metformin from plant to glucose-lowering drug	
Year	**Drug Development Events**
Late 1800s	*Galega officinalis* — rich in guanidine
1918	Guanidine lowers blood glucose in animals
1920s	Guanidine is toxic; isoamylene guanidine less toxic
1920s–early 1930s	Synthalin A (decamethylene diguanide) and synthalin B (dodecamethylene diguanide) synthesized
1929	Flumamine (dimethylbiguanide) synthesized and used for treating influenza in the Philippines. This intrigued clinical pharmacologist Jean Sterne in France to investigate the glucose-lowering effect of this drug.
1957	Sterne published article on the glucose-lowering properties of dimethylbiguanide and proposed the name Glucophage (glucose eater) for metformin.
1958	Metformin launched in United Kingdom
1957 and 1958	Clinical trials with more potent biguanides phenformin and buformin reported.
1970s	Both phenformin and buformin withdrawn because of their association with lactic acidosis.
1972	Metformin launched in Canada
1995	Metformin launched in the US
2004	Metformin ER available
2016	DR metformin acts in ileum and lowers blood glucose.

Table 2
Meta-analyses and systematic reviews for metformin monotherapy

Type of Study	Hemoglobin A_{1c} (%)
Meta-analysis 11 RCTs 1957–1994 Minimum duration of study 6 wk[7]	−1.2% (Absolute) from baseline (−12.5% relative from baseline)
Meta-analysis 16 RCTs[8]	−0.88% (Absolute) compared with placebo
Systematic review and meta-analysis 12 RCTs 1980–2008[9]	∼1% (Absolute) compared with placebo
Meta-analysis 19 RCTs 1950–2010 Minimum duration of study 12 wk[10]	−1.12% (Absolute) from baseline

Abbreviation: RCT, randomized controlled trial.

Physicians can choose from 9 different classes of oral GLDs[9,11–13] to manage T2DM when pharmacotherapy is needed (**Table 3**). In monotherapy versus placebo, the glucose-lowering effect ranges from −0.5% to −1.25% hemoglobin A_1 (HbA_{1c}), with 4 classes (metformin, sulfonylureas, α-glucosidase inhibitors, and thiazolidinediones) from −1% to −1.25%.

In choosing an oral GLD for T2DM, in addition to glucose lowering, other aspects of the drug (safety profile, impact on microvascular and macrovascular complications, cardiovascular and total mortality, cost, and disruption of lifestyle) should be considered by the physician and patient in their joint decision.[14–16] Prescribed since 1957, metformin is safe (small risk for hypoglycemia and weight neutral and can be associated with weight loss and some GI adverse events), is inexpensive, can reduce microvascular complication risk by improving glycemic and blood pressure control,[17] and has a lower cardiovascular mortality compared with sulfonylurea therapy.[18]

Every drug has a primary and secondary failure rate. The primary failure rate for metformin during the first year of therapy was 55% (7%–81%) in UK primary care settings.[19] The secondary failure rate for metformin was 42% during 2 to 5 years of follow-up in a Kaiser Permanente cohort.[20] Failure was higher in those who are younger at diabetes onset, and those who had longer duration of disease and higher HbA_{1c} at initiation of therapy.

To achieve glycemic target at secondary failure, a second oral or injectable GLD is added to initiate dual therapy.[1–4] **Table 4** shows the additional glycemic improvement.[21–23] Some combination therapy (metformin plus thiazolidinediones, sulfonylureas, glinides, and basal and biphasic insulins) are associated with weight gain. Others (metformin plus glucagon-like peptide [GLP]-1 receptor agonists, α-glucosidase, and dipeptidyl peptidase [DPP]-4 inhibitors) are associated with weight loss or no weight change.[22,23] The risk for hypoglycemia in combination therapy is increased with biphasic insulin, basal insulin, sulfonylurea, and glinides. The best option for a second GLD (risks/benefits, cost, and so forth) is currently being studied in Glycemia Reduction Approaches in Diabetes: A Comparative Effectiveness Study.[24] When indicated, triple therapy is then initiated followed by combination injectable therapies.[1–4] In all combination therapies, metformin is used unless there are contraindications to using it or a patient cannot tolerate it. Each combination has its own benefits and risks and physicians have to consider what is best for their patients.

With metformin used in monotherapy and combination therapy for T2DM, the number of its prescriptions in the United States has increased from 2008 to 2014, from 51.6 million to 76.9 million prescriptions.[25,26] Metformin, the top prescribed GLD, was the seventh most prescribed drug in the United States in 2014.

Table 3
Decrease in hemoglobin A_{1c} by 9 classes of glucose-lowering medications

Drug	Sheifali et al,[9] 2010 (Hemoglobin A_{1c} Absolute Decrease vs Placebo)	Kaur et al,[11] 2015 (Hemoglobin A_{1c} Absolute Decrease vs Placebo)	DeFronzo,[12] 2011 (Hemoglobin A_{1c} Absolute Decrease vs Placebo)	Zieve et al,[13] 2007 (Hemoglobin A_{1c} Absolute Decrease vs Placebo)
α-Glucosidase inhibitors	~1%; 15 acarbose and 6 miglitol RCTs, >150 mg daily	—	—	—
Biguanides	~1%; 7 IM and 5 ER RCTs up to 1500 mg daily;	—	—	—
DPP-4 inhibitors	~0.75%; 19 sita and 7 vilda RCT; 100 mg daily	—	—	—
Meglitinides	~0.75%; 8 nate and 1 repa; 360 mg daily	—	—	—
Sulfonylureas	~1.25%; 2 glim RCT; ≥8 mg daily	—	—	—
Thiazolidinediones	~1.25%; 17 Rosi RCT; 8 mg daily ~1%; 10 Pio RCT; 30 mg daily	—	—	—
SGLT2 inhibitors	—	~0.77%; 4 Cana RCTs; 300 mg daily	—	—
Bromocryptine	—	—	~0.56%; 1 RCT; 4.8 mg daily	—
Bile acid resin binders	—	—	—	−0.5%; 1 RCT; 3.75 g daily

Abbreviations: cana, canagliflozin; glim, glimepiride; IM, immediate release; nate, nateglinide; pio, pioglitazone; RCT, randomized controlled trial; repa, repaglinide; Rosi, rosiglitazone; SGLT2, sodium/glucose cotransporter-2; sita, sitagliptin; vilda, vildagliptin.

Table 4
Meta-analysis of metformin plus another glucose-lowering drug on glycemic control in type 2 diabetes mellitus patients

Variable	Monami et al,[21] 2008	Phung et al,[22] 2010	Liu et al,[23] 2012
Type of analysis	Meta-analysis	Meta-analysis	Network meta-analysis
Studies	27 CTs	27 RCTs	39 RCTs
	HbA1c reduction	*HbA1c reduction*	*HbA1c reduction*
SU	−0.85% (−0.78 to −0.94)	−0.79% (−1.15 to −0.43)	−0.82% (−0.95 to −0.70)
AGI	−0.61% (−0.55 to −0.67)	−0.65% (−1.11 to −0.19)	−0.66% (−0.90 to −0.42)
TZDs	−0.42% (−0.40 to −0.44)	−1.00% (−1.62 to −0.38)	−0.82% (−0.98 to −0.66)
Glinides	—	−0.71% (−1.24 to −0.18)	−0.71% (−1.01 to −0.43)
DPP-4 inhibitors	—	−0.79% (−0.94 to −0.63)	−0.69% (−0.79 to −0.61)
GLP-1 RA	—	−0.99% (−1.19 to −0.78)	−1.02% (−1.17 to −0.86%)
Basal insulin	—	—	−1.07% (−1.46 to −0.69%)
Biphasic insulin	—	—	−0.88% (−1.21 to −0.56)

Abbreviations: AGI, α-glucosidase inhibitor; DPP-4, dipeptidyl peptidase-4; GLP-1 RA, glucagon like peptide-1 receptor agonist; SU, sulfonylurea; TZDs, thiazolidinediones.

Formulations and Costs

Metformin is available as tablet and liquid formulations. Metformin tablet formulations are either immediate release (IR) or extended release (ER).[6] The ER formulation (metformin hydrochloride combined with a drug-controlling polymer) differs from the IR formulation in that it is released and absorbed more slowly.[27–30] Patients adhere to the ER formulation better because it is taken once daily and has fewer GI adverse events. The ER formulation, however, is more expensive. A new formulation, delayed-release (DR) metformin, recently reported its phase II study.[31]

The costs of metformin tablets vary (depending on brand name vs generic, IR vs ER formulation, manufacturer, and pharmacy). In the United States, the retail price for 60 tablets of 500-mg metformin (presumably IR and generic) varies from no charge in one pharmacy to $15.09 in another, with a wide range—5 pharmacies approximately $4, 4 pharmacies approximately $5, and 1 pharmacy approximately $10.[32] For metformin ER, for 60 tablets of 500-mg dose, the cost ranges from $4.00 to $21.18 with the pharmacy's free coupon.[33] Liquid metformin, Riomet, is much more expensive — for 300 mL of 500 mg/5 mL of Riomet, the cost (with a free coupon) varies from $398.20 to $419.53 per month.[34]

Absorption and Excretion

The area under the curve for the time and plasma concentration for metformin ER, 2000 mg once daily, versus metformin IR, 1000 mg twice daily, are similar. Whereas food decreases the absorption of metformin IR (Glucophage product insert), it increases the bioavailability of metformin ER. After repeated administration, metformin IR accumulates in plasma (<5 ug/mL).

Although absorbed mainly in the proximal small intestine, a significant percent of the metformin dose is delivered to the distal small intestine where it accumulates in the mucosa.[35] The bioavailability of metformin IR and metformin ER is approximately

50%. Organic cation transporters (OCTs) play a major role in the absorption and disposal of metformin. In the intestines, plasma membrane monoamine transporter may be the major transporter responsible for the uptake of metformin. The OCTs 1 and 3 transport metformin in the liver, skeletal muscle, and kidney (where OCT2 also plays a role).

Metformin, not bound to plasma protein, is excreted unchanged by the kidneys; the hepatic and biliary systems are not involved. This has clinical implications for patients with impaired renal function — in the product label, metformin was contraindicated in men and women with a serum creatinine level greater than 1.5 mg/dL and greater than 1.3 mg/dL, respectively[6] (discussed later).

Mechanism of Action

Metformin improves glycemic control in T2DM by increasing insulin sensitivity in the liver and peripheral organs. This leads to decreased hepatic glucose production (the main effect) and increased glucose disposal in skeletal muscles. A systematic review of in vivo studies in humans[36] showed metformin enhances insulin suppression of endogenous hepatic glucose production and clearance of glucose in the fasting state, but it did not enhance insulin-mediated glucose uptake in peripheral tissues.

Metformin improves glycemic control through its action in the liver,[37–41] small intestines,[31,42,43] and skeletal muscles[44,45] (**Fig. 1**).

Adverse Effects

Gastrointestinal

The most common adverse effects of metformin are GI (nausea, abdominal cramps, and diarrhea). Approximately 30% of patients on metformin IR, especially at initiation of therapy and on doses above 2000 mg, experience them, in particular diarrhea. Metformin ER causes fewer GI adverse effects than metformin IR. A possible cause is the release of 5-hydroxytryptamine in the duodenum.[46] Recently, a cobiotic was reported to improve GI tolerability of metformin.[47]

Lactic acidosis

The most severe adverse effect is MALA, highlighted as a black box warning in the metformin product insert.[6] It is rare, however, with many studies[48–60] showing the incidence to be less than 10/100,000 patient years, 10-fold less than phenformin-associated lactic acidosis (**Table 5**). MALA mortality rate was approximately 50% between 1960 and 2000, but, it has since decreased to approximately 25%. A systematic review reported no difference in incidence of lactic acidosis associated with metformin compared with other oral GLDs (4.3 cases/100,000 patient years versus 5.4 cases/100,000 patient years).[56]

T2DM patients have measurable plasma lactate irrespective of whether they are on metformin or other GLDs. Plasma lactate increases when there is an overproduction (sepsis, hypoxia, dehydration, congestive heart failure, metformin, and so forth) and/or clearance (hepatic dysfunction leads to decreased lactate clearance). Lactic acidosis in a patient on metformin does not imply metformin causality. There is a difference between the 2 groups of patients with lactic acidosis — MALA and metformin-induced lactic acidosis. In acute metformin overdose cases, the lactic acidosis is most likely induced by metformin[61] because other risk factors are absent and metformin is elevated. In many reported cases of MALA, the diagnosis was questioned. Misbin and colleagues[51] reported only 47 of the 66 cases of MALA were confirmed. Of these, 43 had other risk factors, leaving only 4 cases of truly related with metformin. A review of 839 MALA cases indicated only approximately 14% met the criteria of MALA, which

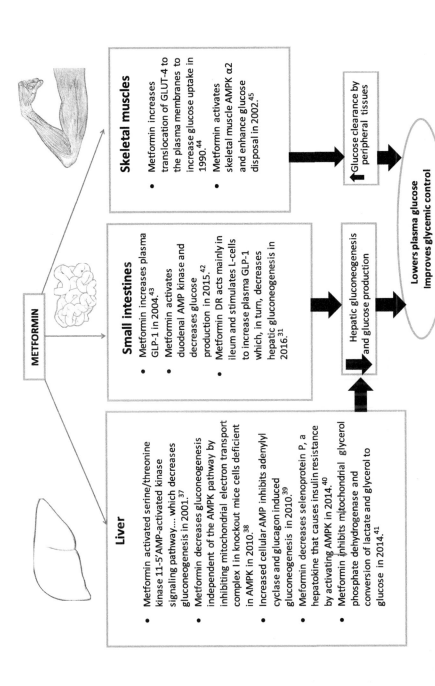

Liver

- Metformin activated serine/threonine kinase 11-5'AMP-activated kinase signaling pathway.... which decreases gluconeogenesis in 2001.[37]
- Metformin decreases gluconeogenesis independent of the AMPK pathway by inhibiting mitochondrial electron transport complex I in knockout mice cells deficient in AMPK in 2010.[38]
- Increased cellular AMP inhibits adenylyl cyclase and glucagon induced gluconeogenesis in 2010.[39]
- Metformin decreases selenoprotein P, a hepatokine that causes insulin resistance by activating AMPK in 2014.[40]
- Metformin inhibits mitochondrial glycerol phosphate dehydrogenase and conversion of lactate and glycerol to glucose in 2014.[41]

Small intestines

- Metformin increases plasma GLP-1 in 2004.[43]
- Metformin activates duodenal AMP kinase and decreases glucose production in 2015.[42]
- Metformin DR acts mainly in ileum and stimulates L-cells to increase plasma GLP-1 which, in turn, decreases hepatic gluconeogenesis in 2016.[31]

Skeletal muscles

- Metformin increases translocation of GLUT-4 to the plasma membranes to increase glucose uptake in 1990.[44]
- Metformin activates skeletal muscle AMPK α2 and enhance glucose disposal in 2002.[45]

Glucose clearance by peripheral tissues

Hepatic gluconeogenesis and glucose production

**Lowers plasma glucose
Improves glycemic control**

METFORMIN

Fig. 1. Metformin — mechanisms and sites of action.

Table 5
Incidence of metformin-associated lactic acidosis

Study, Reference, Year	Incidence of Metformin-associated Lactic Acidosis (Cases/100,000 Patient Years)
Wiholm & Myrhed,[48] 1993	2.4 (1987–1991)
DeFronzo et al,[49] 1995	0
Brown et al,[50] 1998	9.7
Misbin et al,[51] 1998	5
UKPDS 34,[17] 1998	0
Salpeter et al,[52] 2003	8.1–9.9
Stang et al,[53] 1999	9
Cryer et al,[54] 2005	0
Bodmer et al,[55] 2008	3.3
Salpeter et al,[56] 2010	4.3
Eppenga et al,[57] 2014	7.4
Richy et al,[58] 2014	10.4
Huang et al,[59] 2015	2.3

included a pH less than 7.35, blood lactate greater than 5 mmol/L (45 mg/dL), and a detectable (not elevated) plasma metformin level.[62]

Several groups have questioned the risk of lactic acidosis in metformin users T2DM.[63,64]

Other metformin-associated adverse effects are found in its product monograph.[6]

Contraindications

Impaired renal function

Until April 2016, metformin was contraindicated in T2DM men and women whose serum creatinine level was greater than 1.5 mg/dL and greater than 1.3 mg/dL, respectively, to reduce the risk for lactic acidosis.[6] Clearance of metformin and lactate decreased with reduction of creatinine clearance.[65] Many cases of reported lactic acidosis are seen in patients with impaired renal function.[57]

Metformin use in T2DM patients with severe renal failure (stage 5) is associated with increased total mortality[66] and should be contraindicated. The restricted use of metformin in T2DM patients with mild to moderate renal impairment, however, has been challenged.[67] New research suggests no significant risk of lactic acidosis in these patients.[68] A less restrictive use of metformin in T2DM patients and using estimated glomerular filtration rate (eGFR) to guide clinicians in using metformin in them were recently approved by the Food and Drug Administration.[69] It was estimated that 465,000 T2DM patients with mild or moderate renal failure can be using metformin if its use in these patients is less restrictive.[70]

Although no randomized controlled clinical trials on the safety of metformin use in T2DM patients with mild/moderate stable renal insufficiency have been reported, there are clinical practice guidelines for such use.[2,71] Metformin has been used in these patients in the real world.[70,72] Physicians should know the serum creatinine/eGFR to decide what dose to initiate, monitor these variables regularly to adjust the dose, and stop metformin when indicated (**Table 6**). The eGFR may be a more relevant marker than serum creatinine, especially in the elderly.

Recently, the American College of Radiology updated their guidelines (based on eGFR ≥ 30 or <30 mL/min/1.73 m^2) on the use intravenous contrast in patients on

Table 6
Recommendations for metformin use based on estimated glomerular filtration rate

Estimated Glomerular Filtration Rate (mL/min per 1.73 m²)	Recommendation Lipska et al,[67] 2011 and ADA/ EASD position paper	Recommendation NICE
—		
≥60	No renal contraindication for metformin use Monitor renal function annually.	Step up metformin over weeks to minimize risk for GI side-effects. Try metformin ER if GI intolerance is a problem.
<60 and ≥45	Continue metformin use if tolerated. Monitor renal function every 3–6 mo.	
<45 and >30	Prescribe metformin with caution. Use lower dose (50% maximal dose). Monitor renal function every 3 mo.	Review metformin dose if eGFR <45 mL/min/1.73 m².
<30	Stop metformin.	Stop metformin if eGFR <30 mL/min/1.73 m².
Caution	"Required in those at risk of for acute kidney injury or with anticipated fluctuations in renal status."	"Prescribe metformin with caution for those at risk of a sudden deterioration in kidney function."

Abbreviations: ADA, american diabetes association; EASD, european association for the study of diabetes; NICE, national institute for health and care excellence.
   Data from Refs.[2,67,71]

metformin.[73] They stated that patients on metformin do not have a higher risk for post-contrast acute renal injury than other patients.

Congestive heart failure

Metformin was contraindicated in T2DM patients with congestive heart failure. Despite this, metformin was used by many (approximately 11%) patients with T2DM with heart failure.[74] This contraindication has been challenged because several observational studies report metformin use in T2DM patients with heart failure is associated with lower mortality risk.[75–78] Compared with sulfonylurea use in T2DM patients with heart failure, metformin use was associated with lower morbidity and mortality.[77,78] Prospective randomized controlled clinical trials are needed to verify these findings from observational studies. T2DM patients on metformin have lower concentrations of N-terminal prohormone of brain natriuretic peptide (NT-proBNP).[79] Congestive heart failure was not a contraindication in the 2009 Glucophage product insert.[6]

Precautions and Warnings

Excessive alcohol use

Ethanol inhibits lactate clearance; but the hyperlactenemia is mild.[80] Metformin can cause mild fasting hyperlactenemia.[81] Diabetes patients on metformin should be informed of these if they abuse alcohol.

Impaired hepatic function

Lactic acidosis has been reported in T2DM patients on metformin with hepatic impairment.[82] Because lactate is mainly cleared by the liver, there is a theoretic increased risk of lactic acidosis in patients with impaired hepatic function using metformin.[82] Hence, in these patients, metformin should be avoided. A recent retrospective cohort study reports, however, that metformin may be safely used in T2DM with cirrhosis.[83] Furthermore, there was improved survival with 57% reduction in all-cause mortality in metformin users compared with nonmetformin users. These findings need to be further evaluated in larger cohorts or randomized controlled clinical trials.

Many T2DM patients have nonalcoholic fatty liver disease with elevated liver enzymes. Metformin use in these patients are discussed later.

Metformin-induced liver injury (hepatocellular damage with cholestasis) is rare, but it has been described.[84,85]

Vitamin B_{12} deficiency

Metformin treated T2DM patients may be at risk of developing vitamin B_{12} deficiency.[86] Prevalence of vitamin B_{12} deficiency varies depending on the study and cutoff of vitamin B_{12} level used. The drop in vitamin B_{12} was estimated to be approximately 7% is a randomized placebo controlled clinical trials.[87] Patients on sulfonylurea plus metformin have higher incidence of vitamin B_{12} deficiency than those on insulin plus metformin therapy.[88] The higher the dose of sulfonylurea, the greater is the effect. Dose of metformin and duration of treatment influence the vitamin B_{12} deficiency.[88,89] Metformin when combined with histamine H_2-receptor antagonists or proton pump inhibitors can cause vitamin B_{12} deficiency and neuropathy.[90] When indicated, vitamin B_{12} level should be measured in T2DM patients on metformin.

Drug-drug interactions

The Glucophage package insert lists several drug-drug interactions between metformin and other drugs, including glyburide, furosemide, nifedipine, and cimetidine.[6]

Metformin use in older patients

For older T2DM patients, metformin is also the first-line oral GLD when lifestyle therapies fail and there are no contraindications to using it. Because hypoglycemia can do more harm in these older patients who also have greater risk for impaired renal function and cardiovascular disease, physicians should be more vigilant when prescribing metformin.[1]

USE IN OTHER DISEASES AND CONDITIONS
Delaying or Preventing the Onset of Type 2 Diabetes Mellitus

The personal and societal burden of T2DM is increasing, with an estimated 415 million people affected globally in 2015.[91] Another estimated 318 million people globally have impaired glucose tolerance (IGT).[91] One way to reduce the health and economic burden of T2DM is to delay the progression of prediabetes to T2DM. Lifestyle, pharmacotherapy, and bariatric surgery intervention strategies have been reported to be effective.[92] Metformin delays the development of or prevents new-onset T2DM (**Table 7**).[93–97] Compared with placebo, metformin reduced the development of T2DM by 31%.[93] In 2005, implementation of the Diabetes Prevention Program was reported to be cost effective with a cost per quality-adjusted life year of $31,000 for the metformin intervention.[98] Since then, the cost-effectiveness of the metformin intervention has been updated.[99] Although not officially approved to slow the progression of prediabetes to T2DM, metformin is currently used off-label for this purpose.

Table 7
Randomized clinical trials using metformin to prevent or delay the new onset of type 2 diabetes mellitus

Study, Reference, Year	Type	Metformin Dose	Duration	Outcome (New-Onset Diabetes)
Knowler et al,[93] 2002	RCT (North Americans; metformin = 1073 and placebo = 1082)	850 mg bid	2.8 y	Metformin = 21.7% Placebo = 28.9% (31% lower risk in metformin group)
Ramachandran et al,[94] 2006	RCT (Indians; placebo n = 136 and metformin n = 133)	250 mg bid	2.5 y	Control = 55.0% Metformin = 40.5% RRR = 26.4 (19.4–35.1)
Li et al,[95] 1999	RCT (Chinese; metformin n = 33 and placebo = 37)	250 mg tid	12 mo	Metformin = 1 (3%) Placebo = 6 (16.2%)
Yang et al,[96] 2001	RCT (Chinese; metformin n = 88; control n = 85)	250 mg tid	3 y	Control = 11.4% Metformin = 4.0%

Abbreviations: RCT, randomized controlled trials; RRR, relative risk reduction.

Polycystic Ovary Syndrome

PCOS affects 6% to 21% of reproductive age women.[100] The key features of this disorder include insulin resistance, hyperandrogenism, and ovarian dysfunction, resulting in a variety of metabolic abnormalities, hirsutism, infertility, and an increased risk of endometrial hyperplasia.[101] Therapy for PCOS focuses on treatment primarily for hirsutism, oligomenorrhea and infertility, and correction of cardiometabolic abnormalities and includes both lifestyle interventions as well as pharmacotherapy.[102] Metformin is often prescribed to treat these women (**Table 8**).

Gestational Diabetes Mellitus

GDM is associated with a variety of adverse maternal and fetal outcomes, including increased risk of abortions, congenital abnormalities, macrosomia, shoulder dystocia, neonatal hypoglycemia, and respiratory distress.[117] The risk of adverse outcomes increases with maternal hyperglycemia; thus, the goals of treatment are to achieve and maintain euglycemia.[118] Insulin has been the mainstay of therapy for GDM. Oral GLDs (metformin and glyburide), however, are increasingly used, especially outside the United States.[117–124] Metformin, a category B drug in pregnancy,[6] crosses the placenta. It seems safe and effective, however, for use in pregnancy.[119] Currently, the American College of Obstetricians and Gynecologists and the UK National Institute for Health and Care Excellence recommend that insulin, metformin, and glyburide can be considered first-line GLDs when pharmacotherapy is needed.[117,120] The American Diabetes Association recommends that pregnant patients treated with metformin should be informed that it crosses the placenta and long-term studies are needed although no adverse effects on the fetus have been demonstrated.[1] Caution in the interpretation of studies thus far and longer-term follow-up of infants of these women are suggested (**Table 9**).[125]

CURRENT RESEARCH ON POSSIBLE NEW USES FOR METFORMIN
Metformin Use in Type 2 Diabetes Mellitus Patients with Cancer

Several studies and meta-analyses established an association between diabetes and cancer.[126] This association can be explained by hyperinsulinemia, hyperglycemia, and

Table 8
Metformin use in patients with polycystic ovary syndrome

Clinical Problem	Comment (References)	Studies (References)
Insulin resistance	Affects ~65%–70% of women with PCOS[103] Hyperinsulinemia results in hyperandrogenism. Prevalence of IGT is 30%–40% and of T2DM is 5%–10%.[104]	Metformin decreases fasting insulin levels, fasting glucose levels, triglycerides, and insulin resistance as measured by the HOMA index.[105,106]
Obesity	Common but not required to diagnose PCOS	Metformin caused weight loss or potentiated weight loss in combination with a low-calorie diet in women with PCOS.[107] Meta-analysis of metformin vs lifestyle interventions demonstrated similar outcomes on body mass index at 6 mo.[108]
Hirsutism	Present in ~65%–75% of women with PCOS[109]	Meta-analysis reported total testosterone, free testosterone, and androstenedione levels decreased with metformin use compared with placebo.[110] Meta-analysis reported no significant benefit was observed on hirsutism as measured by the Ferriman-Gallwey score.[111] Metformin was ineffective for treatment of hirsutism vs placebo and lifestyle interventions in systematic review.[112] Endocrine Society guidelines: OCPs as first-line therapy for hirsutism with antiandrogen therapy used as an adjunct[102]
Infertility	Metformin used as a treatment of infertility based on early trials demonstrating induction of ovulation.[29–31]	Metformin in combination with gonadotropins for ovulation induction — meta-analysis reported an increased pregnancy and live birth rates.[113] ESHRE/ASRM group recommended against the routine use of metformin for anovulatory infertility except in women with glucose intolerance[114] and clomiphene citrate is considered the first-line agent.[102]
Pregnancy complications	Higher rates of pregnancy complications — GDM, pregnancy-induced hypertension, preeclampsia, preterm birth, and neonatal morbidity[38,39] The risk of GDM is doubled in women with PCOS.	Meta-analysis reported a decreased risk of miscarriage as well as lower rates of preterm labor.[115] Metformin does not significantly decrease the incidence of GDM.[115,116] Metformin use throughout pregnancy similarly does not seem to reduce the risk of preeclampsia.[115]

Abbreviations: ASRM, american society of reproductive medicine; ESHRE, european society of human reproduction and embryology; HOMA, homeostatic model assessment.

Table 9
Metformin use in gestational diabetes mellitus

Study/Meta-analysis/Guidelines	Comments
Prospective study	Nearly one-half of women treated with metformin during their pregnancy require supplemental insulin, although at slightly lower doses compared with those on insulin only.[121]
Systematic review meta-analysis	No evidence of significant difference in maternal and neonatal outcomes between metformin vs insulin in GDM[122] Meta-analysis — compared with insulin, women who used metformin in GDM experienced several benefits, including less maternal weight gain, less pregnancy-induced hypertension, less severe neonatal hypoglycemia, and higher patient satisfaction. Risk for preterm birth was higher.[123]
Guidelines	American College of Obstetricians and Gynecologists[120] and the UK National Institute for Health and Care Excellence recommend that metformin, glyburide, or insulin can be used in GDM.[117] The American Diabetes Association recommends that pregnant patients treated with metformin should be informed that it crosses the placenta and long-term studies are needed although no adverse effects on the fetus have been demonstrated.[1]
Metformin vs glyburide	GDM women on metformin had less maternal weight gain and babies have less macrosomia although higher treatment failure and higher fasting blood glucose.[123] Babies of metformin-treated GDM mothers had lower weight and Ponderal index but higher BG at 1 h and 3 h after birth compared with babies of glyburide-treated GDM mothers.[124]

chronic inflammation in T2DM patients, with insulin-stimulating growth of cancerous cells and enhancing mitogenesis. Recently, new observations suggest that metformin may possibly play a role in cancer treatment and prevention.[127] Proposed mechanisms for metformin's anticancer effects includes metformin activation of AMP-activated protein kinase (AMPK)and suppression of mammalian target of rapamycin resulting in inhibition of tumor cell growth and induction of tumor cell death.[128,129] **Table 10** summarizes systematic reviews and meta-analyses of mainly observational studies, showing a significant reduction in cancer risk and mortality with metformin use.[126,130–143] A large number of these observational studies, however, suffered from methodological shortcomings (heterogeneity in several studies) and time-related biases.[144] Randomized clinical trials failed to show consistent benefit with metformin related to cancer outcomes.[126,127]

Metformin has also been evaluated as an adjunct to chemotherapy and radiation therapy in the treatment of different tumors, including breast,[145] glioblastoma,[146] bladder,[147] and liver cancer,[148] and the results suggest that metformin has a potential role as an adjunct therapy in cancer treatment. When accessed on March 07, 2016, there were approximately 150 clinical trials on metformin and cancer listed in www.clinicaltrials.gov.

Metformin Use in Patients with Nonalcoholic Fatty Liver Disease

Nonalcoholic fatty liver disease (NAFLD), the most common liver disease,[149] is strongly associated with insulin resistance, obesity, and T2DM. Lifestyle modification with diet and exercise is the first line of treatment. Pharmacologic therapy and bariatric surgery have also been studied. Drugs studied include insulin sensitizers (metformin

Table 10
Systematic reviews and meta-analysis of effect of metformin on cancer in patients with type 2 diabetes mellitus

First Author, Reference, Year	Cancer Type	Number and Type of Studies	Summary of Results
Yang et al,[130] 2015	Breast	18 (10 CCs, 8 cohorts)	Metformin associated with significant reduction in all-cause mortality (RR, 0.652; 95% CI, 0.488–0.873; $P = .004$). No reduction in incidence.
Wu et al,[131] 2015	Prostate	10 (6 Cohorts, 4 CCs)	Metformin is not significantly associated with reduction in prostate CA risk.
Raval et al,[132] 2015	Prostate	9 (8 Retrospective cohorts, 1 CC)	Metformin use was marginally associated with reduction in the risk of biochemical recurrence (pooled HR 0.82; 95% CI, 0.67–1.01; $P = .06$). Metformin use was not significantly associated with reduction in metastases or all-cause and prostate cancer-specific mortality.
Deng et al,[133] 2015	Prostate	13 (8 Cohorts, 5 CCs)	Metformin therapy was associated with significantly decreased incidence of prostate cancer (RR 0.88; 95% CI [0.78, 0.99]; $P = .03$.) Metformin therapy was not associated with decreased all-cause mortality or decreased recurrence of prostate cancer.
Yu et al,[134] 2014	Prostate	21 (16 Cohorts, 5 CCs)	Metformin use was significantly associated with a decreased cancer risk (OR 0.91; 95% CI, 0.85–0.97) and biochemical recurrence (HR 0.81; 95% CI, 0.68–0.98) of prostate cancer. The association of metformin use with all-cause mortality of patients with prostate cancer, however, was not significant.
Nie et al,[135] 2014	Lung	15 (11 Cohorts; 4 CCs)	No significant association between metformin use and cancer
Wang et al,[136] 2013	Lung	6 CCs	Risk of lung cancer was lower in metformin users than in those without metformin (OR 0.55; 95% CI, 0.35–0.85; $P<.001$)
Singh et al,[137] 2014 (abstract)	Colorectal	8	In patients with DM, use of metformin (vs nonuse) was associated with decreased all-cause mortality (6 studies; adjusted HR 0.63; 95% CI, 0.49–0.81) and colorectal cancer-specific mortality (3 studies; adjusted HR 0.66; 95% CI, 0.50–0.87)

(continued on next page)

Table 10
(continued)

First Author, Reference, Year	Cancer Type	Number and Type of Studies	Summary of Results
Mei et al,[138] 2014	Colorectal	6 Retrospective cohorts	Pooled HR favoring metformin users was 0.56 for overall survival (95% CI, 0.41–0.77) and 0.66 for colorectal cancer-specific survival (95% CI, 0.50–0.87)
Singh et al,[139] 2013	Colorectal	15 (5 CC, 8 cohorts, 2 RCTs)	Meta-analysis of observational studies shows 11% reduction in colorectal cancer risk associated with metformin use (n 9 studies; OR 0.89; 95% CI, 0.81–0.99).
Gandini et al,[140] 2014	Multiple	47 (11 Prospective cohorts, 16 CCs, 14 Retrospective cohorts, 6 clinical trials)	Overall cancer incidence was reduced by 31% (SRR 0.69; 95% CI, 0.52–0.90). Cancer mortality was reduced by 34% (SRR, 0.66; 95% CI, 0.54–0.81).
Stevens et al,[126] 2012	Multiple	13 Clinical trials	No statistically significant beneficial effect of metformin on cancer outcomes
DeCensi et al,[141] 2010	Multiple	11 (4 Cohorts, 7 CCs)	31% Reduction in overall summary (RR 0.69; 95% CI, 0.61–0.79) was found in subjects taking metformin compared with other antidiabetic drugs.
Noto et al,[142] 2012	Multiple	24 (11 Cohorts, 10 CCs, and 3 RCTs)	Risks of cancer among metformin users were significantly lower than those among nonmetformin users: the pooled RRs (95% CI) were 0.66 (0.49–0.88) for cancer mortality, 0.67 (0.53–0.85) for all-cancer incidence, 0.68 (0.53–0.88) for colorectal cancer, 0.20 (0.07–0.59) for hepatocellular cancer, and 0.67 (0.45–0.99) for lung cancer.
Zhang et al,[143] 2013	Multiple	37 (16 CCs, 21 cohorts)	Among metformin users compared with nonusers, the SRR for overall cancer incidence was 0.73 (95% CI, 0.64–0.83) and that for mortality was 0.82 (95% CI, 0.76–0.89).

Abbreviations: CC, case control; CI, confidence interval; DM, diabetes mellitus; HR, hazard ratio; OR, odds ratio; RCT, randomized control trials; RR, relative risk, SRR, summary relative risk.

and thiazolidinediones), among others.[150] Metformin reduces aspartate aminotransferase and alanine aminotransferase significantly in patients with NAFLD but does not improve histologic changes.[151] Metformin also decreases hepatic fat content in patients with NAFL. Two meta-analyses concluded that metformin is ineffective for treating NAFLD.[152,153] Based on available evidence, current guidelines do not recommend metformin as a treatment of NAFLD.[154,155] In T2DM patients with NAFLD, however, metformin can be used to control hyperglycemia.

Metformin Use in Patients with Dementia and Alzheimer Disease

There is epidemiologic evidence that T2DM and Alzheimer disease are associated.[156] Possible mechanisms linking the 2 diseases are also available.[157,158] Mechanisms on how metformin can decrease dementia have been proposed. Clinical studies on metformin and dementia, however, reported conflicting results.[159–162]

SUMMARY

In closing, new knowledge uncovered by research, especially during the past 2 decades, has changed the understanding and use of metformin in the management of T2DM. Although metformin's cellular and molecular mechanisms of action continue to evolve, how it improves glycemic control is better understood. As the recommended first-line oral GLD to control hyperglycemia in T2DM, and its continued use in combination therapy, metformin is now the most prescribed GLD in the United States. Metformin is safe (small risk for hypoglycemia, inexpensive [generic metformin IR], and weight neutral and can be associated with weight loss but has some GI adverse events), can reduce microvascular complication risk by improving glycemic and blood pressure control, and has a lower cardiovascular mortality compared with sulfonylurea therapy. Metformin-induced lactic acidosis is rare. Guidelines for its use in T2DM patients with mild to moderate renal impairment and congestive heart failure have changed. The Food and Drug Administration recently revised its warnings on the use of metformin in T2DM patients with mild to moderate renal impairment. Metformin is also used to prevent/delay the onset of T2DM globally and in treating GDM, especially outside the United States. Its use in women with PCOS is one of its pleiotropic effects. Current research may lead to more pleiotropic effects. As research uncovers new knowledge, even the new concepts can be challenged.[163]

REFERENCES

1. American Diabetes Association. Approaches to glycemic treatment. Diabetes Care 2016;39(Suppl 1):S52–9.
2. Inzucchi SE, Bergenstal RM, Buse JB, et al. Management of hyperglycemia in type 2 diabetes, 2015: a patient-centered approach. Update to a position statement of the American Diabetes Association and the European Association for the Study of Diabetes. Diabetes Care 2015;38:140–9.
3. Garber AJ, Abrahamson MJ, Barsilay JI, et al. Consensus Statement by the American Association of Clinical Endocrinologists and American College of Endocrinology on the comprehensive type 2 diabetes management algorithm – 2016 Executive Summary. Endocr Pract 2016;22:84–113.
4. Clement M, Goldenberg R, Hanna A, et al. Canadian Diabetes Association 2013 Clinical Practice Guidelines for the Prevention and Management of Diabetes in Canada: Pharmacologic Management of type 2 diabetes. Can J Diabetes 2013; 37(Suppl 1):S61–8.
5. Bailey CJ, Day C. Metformin: its botanical background. Pract Diab Int 2004;21: 115–7.
6. Bristol-Myers [product insert] Squibb Company Glucophage® and Glucophage® XR.
7. Campbell IW, Howlett HCS. World wide experience of metformin as an effective glucose-lowering agent: a meta-analysis. Diabetes Metab Rev 1995;11:S57–62.
8. Saenz A, Fernandez-Esteban I, Mataix A, et al. Metformin monotherapy for type 2 diabetes mellitus. Cochrane Database Syst Rev 2005;(3):CD002966.

9. Sherifali D, Nerenberg K, Pullennayegum E, et al. The effect of oral antidiabetic agents on A1c levels – a systematic review and met-analysis. Diabetes Care 2010;33:1859–64.

10. Hirst JA, Farmer AJ, Ali R, et al. Quantifying the effect of metformin treatment and dose on glycemic control. Diabetes Care 2012;35:446–54.

11. Kaur K, Likar N, Dang SA, et al. Efficacy and safety of canagliflozin among patients with type 2 diabetes mellitus: a systematic review and meta-analysis. Indian J Endocrinol Metab 2015;19:705–21.

12. DeFronzo RA. Bromocryptine: a Sympatholytic, D2-Dopamine agonist for the treatment of Type 2 diabetes. Diabetes Care 2011;34:789–94.

13. Zieve FJ, Kalin MF, Schwartz SL, et al. Results of the Glucose-Lowering Effect of WelChol Study (GLOWS): A Randomized, Double-Blind, Placebo-Controlled Pilot Study Evaluating the Effect of Colesevelam Hydrochloride on Glycemic Control in subjects with Type 2 Diabetes. Clin Ther 2007;29:74–83.

14. Bolen S, Feldman L, Vassy J, et al. Systematic review: comparative effectiveness and safety of oral medications for type 2 diabetes mellitus. Ann Intern Med 2007;147:386–99.

15. Bennett WL, Maruthur NM, Singh S, et al. Comparative effectiveness and safety of medications for type 2 diabetes: an update including new drugs and 2-drug combinations. Ann Intern Med 2011;154:602–13.

16. Pogach LM. Doctor, how certain are we that this diabetes medication is best for me? Ann Intern Med 2007;147:428–30.

17. Effect of intensive blood-glucose control with merformin on complications in overweight patients with type 2 diabetes (UKPDS 34). UK Prospective Diabetes Study (UKPDS) Group. Lancet 1998;352:854–65.

18. Roumie CL, Hung AM, Greevy RA, et al. Comparative Effectiveness of Sulfonylurea and Metformin Monotherapy on Cardiovascular Events in Type 2 Diabetes Mellitus - A Cohort Study. Ann Intern Med 2012;157(9):601–10.

19. Cook MN, Girman CJ, Stein PP, et al. Initial monotherapy with either metformin or sulphonylureas often fails to achieve or maintain current glycaemic goals in patients with type 2 diabetes in UK primary care. Diabet Med 2007;24:350–8.

20. Brown J, Conner C, Nichols GA. Secondary failure of metformin monotherapy in clinical practice. Diabetes Care 2010;33:501–6.

21. Monami M, Lamanna C, Marchionni N, et al. Comparison of different drugs as add-on treatments to metformin in type 2 diabetes: a meta-analysis. Diabetes Res Clin Pract 2008;79:196–203.

22. Phung OJ, Scholle JM, Talwar M, et al. Effect of noninsulin antidiabetic drugs added to metformin therapy on glycemiic control, weight gain, and hypoglycemia in type 2 diabetes. JAMA 2010;303:1410–8.

23. Liu SC, Tu YK, Chien MN, et al. Effect of antidiabetic agents added to metformin on glycaemic control, hypoglycemia and weight change in patients with type 2 diabetes: a network meta-analysis. Diabetes Obes Metab 2012;14:810–20.

24. Nathan DM, Buse JB, Kahn SE, et al. Rationale and Design of the Glycemia Reduction Approaches in Diabetes: A Comparative Effectiveness Study (GRADE). Diabetes Care 2013;36:2254–61.

25. Available at: www.statista.om/statistics/233986/top-us-pharma-products-by-prescriptions/. Accessed February 24, 2016.

26. Available at: www.imshealth.com../us_Top_Medicine_Disp. Accessed February 24, 2016.

27. Chacra AR. Evolving metformin treatment strategies in type-2 diabetes: from immediate-release metformin monotherapy to extended-release combination therapy. Am J Ther 2014;21:198–210.

28. Schwartz S, Fonseca V, Berner B, et al. Efficacy, tolerability, and safety of a novel once-daily extended-release metformin in patients with type 2 diabetes. Diabetes Care 2006;29:759–64.

29. Donnelly LA, Morris AD, Pearson ER. Adherence in patients transferred from immediate release metformin to a sustained released formulation: a population-base study. Diabetes Obes Metab 2009;11:338–42.

30. Fujii RK, Restrepo M, Fernandes RA, et al. Efficacy and safety of an extended-release metformin Formulation In type-2 diabetes mellitus treatment: a systematic review. Value Health 2015;1:A56.

31. Buse J, DeFronzo RA, Rosenstock J, et al. The primary glucose-lowering effect of metformin resides in the gut, not the circulation: results from short-term pharmacokinetic and 12-week dose-ranging studies. Diabetes Care 2016;39: 198–205.

32. Available at: http://www.goodrx.com/metformin. Accessed January 23, 2016.

33. Available at: http://www.goodrx.com/metformin-er-glucophage-xr. Accessed January 23, 2016.

34. Available at: http://www.goodrx.com/riomet?gclid=CLQnYn7wMoCFQuSa QodGh4Nig. Accessed January 23, 2016.

35. Graham GC, Punt J, Arora M, et al. Clinical Pharmacokinetics of metformin. Clin Pharmacokinet 2011;50:81–98.

36. Natali A, Ferrannini E. Effects of metformin and thiazolidinediones on suppression of hepatic glucose production and stimulation of glucose uptake in type 2 diabetes: a systematic review. Diabetologia 2006;49:434–41.

37. Zhou GC, Myers R, Li Y, et al. Role of AMP-activated protein kinase in mechanism of metformin action. J Clin Invest 2001;108:1167–74.

38. Foretz M, Hebrard S, Leclerc J, et al. Metformin inhibits hepatic gluconeogenesis in mice independently of the LKB1/AMPK pathway via a decrease in hepatic energy state. J Clin Invest 2010;120:2355–69.

39. Miller RA, Chu QW, Xie JX, et al. Biguanides suppress hepatic glucagon signaling by decreasing production of cyclic AMP. Nature 2013;494:256–61.

40. Takayam H, Misu H, Iwama H, et al. Metformin Suppresses Expression of the Selenoprotein P Gene vis an AMP-activated Kinase (AMPK)/Fox3a Pathway in H4IIEC3 Hepatocytes. J Biol Chem 2014;289:335–45.

41. Madiraju AK, Erion DM, Rahimi Y, et al. Metformin suppresses gluconeogenesis by inhibiting mitochondrial glycerophosphate dehydrogenase. Nature 2014; 510:542–6.

42. Duca FA, Cote CD, Rasmussen BA, et al. Metformin activates a duodenal AMPK-dependent pathway to lower hepatic glucose production. Nat Med 2015;21:506–14.

43. Manucci E, Tesi F, Bardini G, et al. Effects of metformin on glucagon-like peptide-1 levels in obese patients with and without type 2 diabetes. Diabetes Nutr Metab 2004;17:336–42.

44. Klip A, Leiter LA. Cellular mechanism of action of metformin. Diabetes Care 1990;13:696–704.

45. Musi N, Hirshman MF, Nygren J, et al. Metformin Increases AMP-activated protein kinase activity in skeletal muscle of subjects with type 2 diabetes. Diabetes 2002;51:2074–81.

46. Cubeddu LX, Bonisch H, Gothert M, et al. Effects of metformin on intestinal 5-hydroxytrytamine (5-HT) release and on 5-HT$_3$ receptors. Naunyn Schmiedebergs Arch Pharmacol 2000;361:85–91.

47. Greenway F, Wang S, Heiman M. A novel cobiotic containing a probiotiuc and an antioxidant augments the glucose control and gastrointestinal tolerability of metformin: a case report. Benef Microbes 2014;5:29–32.

48. Wiholm BE, Myrhed M. Metformin-associated lactic acidosis in Sweden 1977-1991. Eur J Clin Pharmacol 1993;44:589–91.

49. DeFronzo RA, Goodman AM, Multicenter Metformin Study Group. Efficacy of metformin in patients with non-insulin-dependent diabetes mellitus. N Engl J Med 1995;333:541–9.

50. Brown JB, Oedula K, Barzilay J, et al. Lactic acidosis rates in type 2 diabetes. Diabetes Care 1998;21:1659–63.

51. Misbin RI, Green L, Stadel BV, et al. Lactic acidosis in patients with diabetes treated with metformin. N Engl J Med 1998;338:265–6.

52. Salpeter SR, Greyber E, Paternade GA, et al. Risk of fatal and nonfatal lactic acidosis with metformin use in type 2 diabetes mellitus. Arch Intern Med 2003;163:2594–602.

53. Stang MR, Wysowski DK, Butler-Jones D. Incidence of lactic Acidosis in metformin users. Diabetes Care 1999;22:925–7.

54. Cryer DR, Nichlas SP, Henry DH, et al. Comparative outcomes study of metformin intervention versus conventional approach: the COSMIC approach study. Diabetes Care 2005;28:539–43.

55. Bodmer M, Meier C, Krahenbuhl S, et al. Metformin, sulfonylureas, or other antidiabetics drugs and the risk of lactic acidosis or hypoglycemia. Diabetes Care 2008;31:2086–91.

56. Salpeter SR, Greyber E, Pasternak GA, et al. Risk of fatal and nonfatal lactic acidosis with metformin use in type 2 diabetes mellitus [Review]. The Cochrane Library 2010;(4):CD002967.

57. Eppenga WL, Lalmohamed A, Geerts A, et al. Risk of lactic acidosis or elevated lactate concentrations in metformin users with renal impairment: a population-based cohort study. Diabetes Care 2014;37:2218–24.

58. Richy FF, Sabido-Espin M, Guedes S, et al. Incidence of lactic acidosis in patients with type 2 diabetes with and without renal impairment treated with metformin: a retrospective cohort study. Diabetes Care 2014;37:2291–5.

59. Huang WY, Castelino RL, Peterson GM. Adverse event notifications implicating metformin with lactic acidosis in Australia. J Diabetes Complications 2015;29:1261–5.

60. Kajbaf F, Lalau JD. Mortality rate in so-called "metformin-associated lactic acidosis": a review of the data since the 1960s. Pharmacoepidemiol Drug Saf 2014;23:1123–7.

61. Dell'Aglio DM, Perino LJ, Kazzi Z, et al. Acute metformin overdose: Examining serum pH, lactate level and metformin concentrations in survivors versus non-survivors: a systematic review of the literature. Ann Emerg Med 2009;54:818–23.

62. Kajbaf F, Lalau JD. The criteria for metformin-associated lactic acidosis: the quality of reporting in a large pharmacovigilance database. Diabet Med 2013;30:345–8.

63. Stacpole PW. Metformin and lactic acidosis: guilt by association? Diabetes Care 1998;21:1587–8.

64. Mathieu C. Metformin-associated lactic acidosis: time to let it go? J Diabetes Complications 2015;29:974–5.

65. Tucker GT, Casey C, Phillips PJ, et al. Metformin kinetics in healthy subjects and in patients with diabetes mellitus. Br J Clin Pharmacol 1981;12:235–46.

66. Hung SC, Chang YK, Liu JS, et al. Metformin use and mortality in patients with advanced chronic kidney disease: national, retrospective, observational, cohort study. Lancet Diabetes Endocrinol 2015;3:605–14.

67. Lipska KJ, Bailey CJ, Inzucchi SE. Use of metformin in the setting of mild-to-moderate renal insufficiency. Diabetes Care 2011;34:1431–7.

68. Inzucchi SE, Lipska KL, Mayo H, et al. Metformin in patients with type 2 diabetes and kidney disease: a systematic review. JAMA 2014;312:2668–75.

69. US Food and Drug Administration. Drug Safety Communication: FDA revises warnings regarding use of the diabetes medication metformin in certain patients with reduced kidney function. April 8, 2016. UCM 494140. Available at: http://www.fda.gov/Drugs/DrugSafety/ucm493244.htm. Accessed June 16, 2016.

70. Flory JH, Hennessy S. Metformin use reduction in mild to moderate renal impairment: possible inappropriate curbing of use based of food and drug administration contraindications. JAMA Intern Med 2015;175:458–9.

71. Type 2 diabetes in adults: management. NICE guidelines [NG 28]. 2015. Available at: http://www.nice.org.uk/guidance/ng28.

72. Schorr M, Hemmelgarn BR, Tonelli M, et al. Assessment of serum creatinine and kidney function among incident metformin users. Can J Diabetes 2013;37:226–30.

73. ACR Committee of Drugs and Contrast Media. Metformin. American College of Radiology; ACR Manual on contrast Media. Version 10.1. 2015. p. 45–46. Available at: http://www.acr.org/~/media/37D84428BF1D4E1B9A3A2918DA9E27A3.pdf.

74. Masoudi FA, Wang YF, Inzucchi SE, et al. Metformin and thiazolidinedione use in medicare patients with heart failure. JAMA 2003;290:81–5.

75. Fung CSC, Wan EYF, Wong CKH, et al. Effect of metformin monotherapy on cardiovascular diseases and mortality: a retrospective cohort study on Chinese type 2 diabetes patients. Cardiovasc Diabetol 2015;14:137.

76. Aguilar D, Chan W, Bozkurt B, et al. Metformin Use and mortality in ambulatory patients with diabetes and heart failure. Circ Heart Fail 2011;4:53–8.

77. Andersson C, Olesen JB, Hansen PR, et al. Metformin treatment is associated with a low risk of mortality in diabetic patients with heart failure: a retrospective nationwide cohort study. Diabetologia 2010;53:2546–53.

78. Eurich DT, Majumdar SR, McAlister FA, et al. Improved clinical outcomes associated with metformin in patients with diabetes and heart failure. Diabetes Care 2005;28:2345–51.

79. Rosiak M, Postula M, Kaplon-Cieslicka A, et al. Metformin treatment may be associated with decreased levels of NT-proBNP in patients with type 2 diabetes. Adv Med Sci 2013;58:362–8.

80. Kreisberg R. Lactate homeostasis and lactic acidosis. Ann Intern Med 1980;92:227–37.

81. Davis TME, Jackson D, Davis WA, et al. The relationship between metformin therapy and the fasting plasma lactate in type 2 diabetes: the freemantle diabetes study. Br J Clin Pharmacol 2001;52:137–44.

82. Bailey CJ. Biguanides and NIDDM. Diabetes Care 1992;15:755–72.

83. Zhang X, Harmsen WS, Mettler TA, et al. Continuation of metformin use after a diagnosis of cirrhosis significantly improves survival of patients with diabetes. Hepatology 2014;60:2008–16.

84. Zheng L. Metformin as a rare cause of drug-induced liver injury. a case report and literature review. Am J Ther 2016;23(1):e315–7.

85. Saadi T, Waterman M, Yassin H, et al. Metformin-induced mixed hepatocellular and cholestatic hepatic injury: case report and literature review. Int J Gen Med 2013;6:703–6.
86. Niafar M, Hai F, Porhomayon J, et al. The role of metformin on vitamin B12 deficiency: a meta-analysis review. Intern Emerg Med 2015;10:93–102.
87. de Jager J, Kooy A, Lehert P, et al. Long term treatment with metformin in patients with type 2 diabetes and risk of vitamin B-12 deficiency: randomized placebo controlled trial. BMJ 2010;340:c2181.
88. Kang DH, Yun JS, Ko SH, et al. Higher Prevalence of metformin-induced vitamin B12 deficiency in sulfonylurea combination compared with insulin combination in patients with type 2 diabetes: a cross-sectional study. PLoS One 2014;9: e109878.
89. Beulens JWJ, Hart HE, Kuijs R, et al. Influence of duration and dose of metformin on cobalamin deficiency in type 2 diabetes patients using metformin. Acta Diabetol 2015;52:47–53.
90. Zdilla MJ. Metformin with either histamine h2-receptor antagonists or proton pump inhibitors: a polypharmacy recipe for neuropathy via vitamin B12 depletion. Clin Diabetes 2015;33:90–5.
91. Available at: www.idfdiabetsatlas. Accessed March 4, 2015.
92. Merlotti C, Morbito A, Pontiroli AE. Prevention of type 2 diabetes: a systematic review and met-analysis of different intervention strategies. Diabetes Obes Metab 2014;16:719–27.
93. Knowler WC, Barrett-Connor E, Fowler SE, et al, Diabetes Prevention Program Research Group. Reduction in the incidence of type 2 diabetes with lifestyle intervention or Metformin. N Engl J Med 2002;346:393–403.
94. Ramachandran A, Snehalatha C, Mary S, et al, Indian Diabetes Prevention Programme (IDPP). The Indian Diabetes Programme shows that lifestyle modification and metformin prevent type 2 diabetes in Asian Indian subjects with impaired glucose tolerance (IDDP-1). Diabetologia 2006;49:289–97.
95. Li CL, Pan CY, Lu JM, et al. Effect of metformin on patients with impaired glucose tolerance. Diabet Med 1999;16:477–81.
96. Yang WY, Lin LX, Qi JW, et al. The preventive effect of Acarbose and Metformin on the IGT population from becoming diabetes mellitus: A 3-year multi-centre prospective study. Chin J Endocrinol Metab 2001;17:131–4.
97. Knowler WC, Fowler SE, Hamman RF, et al, for the Diabetes Prevention Program Research Group. 10-year follow-up of diabetes incidence and weight loss in the Diabetes Prevention Program Outcomes Study. Lancet 2009;374:1677–86.
98. Herman WH, Hoerger TJ, Brandle M, et al. The Cost-effectiveness of lifestyle modification or metformin in preventing type 2 diabetes in adults with impaired glucose tolerance. Ann Intern Med 2005;142:323–32.
99. Herman WH. The cost-effectiveness of diabetes prevention: results from the Diabetes Prevention Program and the Diabetes Prevention Program Outcomes Study. Clin Diabetes Endocrinol 2015;1:9, 1–10.
100. Joham AE, Teede HJ, Ranasinha S, et al. Prevalence of infertility and use of fertility treatment in women with polycystic ovary syndrome: data from a large community-based cohort study. J Womens Health (Larchmt) 2015;24:299–307.
101. Johnson NP. Metformin use in women with polycystic ovary syndrome. Ann Transl Med 2014;2:56.
102. Legro RS, Arslanian SA, Ehrmann DA, et al. Diagnosis and treatment of polycystic ovary syndrome: endocrine society clinical practice guideline. J Clin Endocrinol Metab 2013;98:4565–92.

103. DeUgarte CM, Bartolucci AA, Azziz R. Prevalence of insulin resistance in the polycystic ovary syndrome using the homeostasis model assessment. Fertil Steril 2005;83:1454–60.

104. Legro RS, Kunselman AR, Dodson WC, et al. Prevalence and predictors of risk for type 2 diabetes mellitus and impaired glucose tolerance in polycystic ovary syndrome: a prospective, controlled study in 254 affected women. J Clin Endocrinol Metab 1999;84:165–9.

105. Costello MF, Shrestha B, Eden J, et al. Metformin versus oral contraceptive pill in polycystic ovary syndrome: a cochrane review. Hum Reprod 2007;22:1200–9.

106. Salpeter SR, Buckley NS, Kahn JA, et al. Meta-analysis: metformin treatment in persons at risk for diabetes mellitus. Am J Med 2008;121:149–57.

107. Pasquali R, Gambineri A, Biscotti D, et al. Effect of long-term treatment with metformin added to hypocaloric diet on body composition, fat distribution, and androgen and insulin levels in abdominally obese women with or without the polycystic ovary syndrome. J Clin Endocrinol Metab 2000;85:2767–77.

108. Naderpoor N, Shorake S, de Courten B, et al. Metformin and lifestyle modification in polycystic ovary syndrome: systematic review and meta-analysis. Hum Reprod Update 2015;21:560–74.

109. Azziz R, Sanchez LA, Knochenhauer ES, et al. Androgen excess in women: experience with over 1000 consecutive patients. J Clin Endocrinol Metab 2004;89:453–62.

110. Tang T, Norman RJ, Balen AH, et al. Insulin-sensitizing drugs (metformin, troglitazone, rosiglitazone, pioglitazone, D-chiro-inositol) for polycystic ovary syndrome [Review]. Cochrane Database Syst Rev 2003;(2):CD003053.

111. Cosma M, Swiglo BA, Flynn DN, et al. Insulin Sensitizers for the treatment of hirsutism: a systematic review and meta-analysis of randomized controlled trials. J Clin Endocrinol Metab 2008;93:1135–42.

112. Cahill DJ, O'Brien K. Polycystic ovary syndrome (PCOS): metformin. BMJ Clin Evid 2015;1408.

113. Palomba S, Falbo A, La Sala GB. Metformin and gonadotropins for ovulation induction in patients with polycystic ovary syndrome: a systematic review with meta-analysis of randomized controlled trials. Reprod Biol Endocrinol 2014;12:3.

114. The Thessaloniki ESHRE/ASRM-Sponsored PCOS Consensus Workshop Group. Consensus on infertility treatment related to polycystic ovary syndrome. Fertil Steril 2008;89:505–22.

115. Feng L, Lin XF, Wan ZH, et al. Efficacy of metformin on pregnancy complications in women with polycystic ovary syndrome: a meta-analysis. Gynecol Endocrinol 2015;31:893–9.

116. Roos N, Kieler H, Sahlin L, et al. Risk of adverse pregnancy outcomes in women with polycystic ovary syndrome: population based cohort study. BMJ 2011;343: d6309.

117. Holt RIG, Lambert KD. The use of oral hypoglycemic agents in pregnancy. Diabet Med 2014;31:282–91.

118. The HAPO Study Cooperative Research Group. Hyperglycemia and adverse pregnancy outcomes. N Engl J Med 2008;358:1991–2002.

119. Lautatzis ME, Goulis DG, Vrontakis M. Efficacy and safety of metformin during pregnancy in women with gestational diabetes mellitus or polycystic ovary syndrome: a systematic review. Metabolism 2013;62:1522–34.

120. Committee on Practice Bulletins-Obstetrics. Practice Bulletin No. 137: Gestational diabetes mellitus. Obstet Gynecol 2013;122:406–16.

121. Rowan JA, Hague WM, Gao WZ, et al. Metformin versus insulin for the treatment of gestational diabetes. N Engl J Med 2008;358:2003–15.

122. Nicholson W, Bolen S, Witkop CT, et al. Benefits and risks of oral diabetes agents compared with insulin in women with gestational diabetes. Obstet Gynecol 2009;113:193–205.

123. Balsells M, Garcia-Patterson A, Sola I, et al. Glibenclamide, metformin, and insulin for the treatment of gestational diabetes: a systematic review and meta-analysis. BMJ 2015;350:h102.

124. Silva JC, Fachin DRRN, Coral ML, et al. Perinatal impact of the use of metformin and glyburide for the treatment of gestational diabetes. J Perinat Med 2012;40: 225–8.

125. Feig D. Review: Oral drugs for gestational diabetes do not increase adverse maternal and neonatal outcomes more than insulin. Ann Intern Med 2009;150: JC4–9.

126. Stevens R, Ali R, Bankhead C, et al. Cancer outcomes and all-cause mortality in adults allocated to metformin: Systematic review and collaborative meta-analysis of randomized clinical trials. Diabetologia 2012;55:2593–603.

127. Kordes S, Pollak M, Zwinderman A, et al. Metformin in patients with advanced pancreatic cancer: a double-blind, randomized, placebo-controlled phase 2 trial. Lancet Oncol 2015;16:839–47.

128. Riedmaier AE, Fisel P, Nies AT, et al. Metformin and cancer: from the old medicine cabinet to pharmacological pitfalls and prospects. Trends Pharmacol Sci 2013;34:126–35.

129. Morales DR, Morris AD. Metformin in cancer treatment and prevention. Annu Rev Med 2015;66:17–29.

130. Yang T, Yang Y, Liu SC. Association between metformin therapy and breast cancer incidence and mortality: evidence from a meta-analysis. J Breast Cancer 2015;18:264–70.

131. Wu GF, Zhang XL, Luo ZG, et al. Metformin therapy and prostate cancer risk: a meta-analysis of observational studies. Int J Clin Exp Med 2015;8:13089–98.

132. Raval AD, Thakker D, Vyas A, et al. Impact of metformin on clinical outcomes among men with prostate cancer: a systematic review and meta-analysis. Prostate Cancer Prostatic Dis 2015;18:110–21.

133. Deng D, Yang Y, Tang XJ, et al. Association between metformin therapy and incidence, recurrence and mortality of prostate cancer: evidence from a meta-analysis. Diabetes Metab Res Rev 2015;31:595–602.

134. Yu HL, Jiang XS, Sun XJ, et al. Effect of Metformin on Cancer Risk and Treatment Outcome of Prostate Cancer: A Meta-Analysis of Epidemiological Observational Studies. PLoS One 2014;9:e116327, 1–14.

135. Nie SP, Chen H, Zhuang MQ, et al. Anti-diabetic medications do not influence risk of lung cancer in patients with diabetes mellitus: a systematic review and meta-analysis. Asian Pac J Cancer Prev 2014;15:6863–9.

136. Wang L, Song Y, Wu GN, et al. Association of the metformin with the risk of lung cancer: a meta-analysis. Transl Lung Cancer Res 2013;2:259–63.

137. Singh P, Singh S, Gonsalves W, et al. Association of metformin with reduced mortality in patients with colorectal cancer. J Clin Oncol 2014;32:3(suppl 3).

138. Mei ZB, Zhang ZJ, Liu CY, et al. Survival benefits of metformin for colorectal cancer patients with diabetes: a systematic review and meta-analysis. PLoS One 2014;9:e91818.

139. Singh S, Singh H, Singh PP, et al. Antidiabetic medications and the risk of colorectal cancer in patients with diabetes mellitus: a systematic review and meta-analysis. Cancer Epidemiol Biomarkers Prev 2013;22:2258–68.

140. Gandini S, Puntoni M, Heckman-Stoddard BM, et al. Metformin and Cancer Risk and Mortality: A Systematic Review and meta-analysistaking into account Biases and Confounders. Cancer Prev Res (Phila) 2014;7:867–85.

141. DeCensi A, Puntoni M, Goodwin P, et al. Metformin and cancer risk in diabetic patients: a systematic review and meta-analysis. Cancer Prev Res (Phila) 2010; 3:1451–61.

142. Noto H, Goto A, Tsujimoto T, et al. Cancer risk in diabetic patients treated with metformin: a systematic review and meta-analysis. PLoS One 2012;7:e33411.

143. Zhang PP, Li H, Tan XH, et al. Association of metformin use with cancer incidence and mortality: a meta-analysis. Cancer Epidemiol 2013;37:207–18.

144. Suissa S, Azoulay L. Metformin and the risk of cancer: time-related biases in observational studies. Diabetes Care 2012;35:2665–73.

145. Kim J, Lim W, Kim E, et al. Phase II randomized trial of neoadjuvant metformin plus letrozole versus placebo plus letrozole for estrogen receptor positive postmenopausal breast cancer (METEOR). BMC Cancer 2014;14:170.

146. Sesen J, Dahan P, Scotland S, et al. Metformin inhibits growth of human glioblastoma cells and enhances therapeutic response. Alonso MM, ed. PLoS One 2015;10:e0123721.

147. Wang D, Wu X. In vitro and in vivo targeting of bladder carcinoma with metformin in combination with cisplatin. Oncol Lett 2015;10:975–81.

148. Kim E, Kim M, Cho C, et al. Low and high linear energy transfer radiation sensitization of HCC cells by metformin. J Radiat Res 2014;55:432–42.

149. Tolman KG, Dalpiaz AS. Treatment of non-alcoholic fatty liver disease. Ther Clin Risk Manag 2007;3:1153–63.

150. Hardy T, Anslee QM, Day CP. Nonalcoholic fatty liver disease: new treatments. Curr Opin Gastroenterol 2015;31:175–83.

151. Than NN, Newsome PN. A concise review of non-alcoholic fatty liver disease. Atherosclerosis 2015;239:192–202.

152. Musso G, Gambino R, Cassader M, et al. A meta-analysis of randomized trials for the treatment of nonalcoholic fatty liver disease. Hepatology 2010;52:79–104.

153. Tang WJ, Xu QY, Hong T, et al. Comparative efficacy of anti-diabetic agents on non-alcoholic liver disease in patients with type 2 diabetes: a systematic review and meta-analysis of randomized and non-randomized studies. Diabetes Metab Res Rev 2016;32:200–16.

154. Chalasani N, Younossi Z, Lavine JE, et al. The diagnosis and management of non-alcoholic fatty liver disease: practice guideline by the american association for the study of liver diseases, American College of Gastroenterology, and the American Gastroenterological Association. Hepatology 2012;55:2005–23.

155. LaBrecque D, Abbas Z, Anania F, et al. World Gastroenterology Organization Global Guidelines: Nonalcoholic fatty liver disease and nonalcoholic steatohepatitis. J Clin Gastroenterol 2014;4:467–73.

156. Li X, Song D, Leng SX. Link between type 2 diabetes and Alzheimer's disease: from epidemiology to mechanism and treatment. Clin Interv Aging 2015;10: 549–60.

157. Patrone C, Eriksson O, Lindholm D. Diabetes drugs and neurological disorders: new views and therapeutic possibilities. Lancet Diabetes Endocrinol 2014;2: 256–62.

158. Hettich MM, Matthes F, Ryan DP, et al. The anti-diabetic drug metformin reduces bace1 protein level by interfering with the MD1 complex. PLoS One 2014;9: e102420.

159. Dominguez RO, Marschoff ER, Gonzalez SE, et al. Type 2 diabetes and/or its treatment leads to less cognitive impairment in Alzheimer's disease patients. Diabetes Res Clin Pract 2012;98:68–74.

160. Hsu CC, Wahlqvist ML, Lee MS, et al. Incidence of dementia is increased in type 2 diabetes and reduced by the use of sulfonylureas and metformin. J Alzheimers Dis 2011;24:485–93.

161. Imfeld P, Bodmer M, Jick SS, et al. Metformin, other antidiabetic drugs, and risk of Alzheimer's disease: a population-based case-control study. J Am Geriatr Soc 2012;60:916–21.

162. Ng TP, Feng L, Yap KB, et al. Long-term metformin usage and cognitive function among older adults with diabetes. J Alzheimers Dis 2014;41:61–8.

163. Boussageon R, Gueyffier F, Cornu C. Metformin as first line treatment for type 2 diabetes: are we sure? BMJ 2016;352:h6748.

Insulin

Making Sense of Current Options

Alissa R. Segal, PharmD, CDE, CDTC, FCCP[a,b,*], Tejaswi Vootla, MD[b],
Richard S. Beaser, MD[b]

KEYWORDS

- Insulin • Glargine U-300 • Insulin degludec • Basaglar • Lispro U-200 • Afrezza
- Regular U-500 • Insulin therapy

KEY POINTS

- The evolution of insulin replacement products has sought to advance insulin replacement designs to mimic natural insulin secretory patterns with increasing accuracy.
- Newer insulins include longer acting basal insulins with reduced day-to-day variability, and concentrated and inhaled prandial insulins to more effectively cover postprandial insulin needs.
- Combination products are also evolving, including combinations of the longer-acting basal insulins with rapid-acting or glucagonlike protein-1 receptor agonists, to allow further individualization of therapies.
- These newer insulin products can be integrated and used with existing insulin replacement program designs that consider patient physiologic needs, self-care abilities, comorbidities, and cost.

THE HISTORY AND EVOLUTION OF INSULIN

Insulin was discovered in 1921 by the team of Drs. Frederick G. Banting, Charles Best, and James Collip at the University of Toronto. Although insulin was first extracted from a dog's pancreas, public demand necessitated the use of porcine and bovine sources.[1] These early insulins had a relatively short duration of action and needed to be injected multiple times each day. The high antigenicity of these products also resulted in great interpatient and intrapatient variability in action, both peaking and duration.

Subsequent development of newer insulins sought to prolong the time action profile to extend the duration of action and with the goal of reducing the number of daily injections. It was not until the mid 20th century that further understanding of the natural physiologic insulin secretory pattern lead to the realization that mimicking those patterns was a more appropriate goal of therapy than reducing the number of daily

The authors have nothing to disclose.
[a] Department of Pharmacy Practice, MCPHS University, 179 Longwood Avenue, Boston, MA 02115, USA; [b] Joslin Diabetes Center, 1 Joslin Place, Boston, MA 02215, USA
* Corresponding author.
E-mail address: alissa.segal@mcphs.edu

Endocrinol Metab Clin N Am 45 (2016) 845–874
http://dx.doi.org/10.1016/j.ecl.2016.06.009
0889-8529/16/© 2016 Elsevier Inc. All rights reserved.

injections. Natural physiologic insulin secretion is characterized by basal insulin release throughout the day, with additional rapid release of insulin in response to carbohydrate ingestion (prandial insulin release).

In the early 1980s, to overcome the disadvantages of insulin from porcine, bovine, and combinations of both, and to help with the animal source supply problem associated with increasing incidence of diabetes, biosynthetic insulin was developed using recombinant DNA technology. These insulins were identical in amino acid sequence to human insulin and were first approved by the US Food and Drug Administration (FDA) in 1982.[2]

The problems with the action profiles and extreme variability of the early insulin preparations have largely been addressed by progressive improvements in formulations. When combined with the knowledge of physiologic insulin secretion, we evolved into the use of regimens that incorporate both the basal and bolus insulin. The first recombinant DNA human insulin analog, insulin lispro (Humalog, Eli Lilly, Indianapolis, IN) a rapid-acting bolus insulin, was approved by the FDA in 1996,[3] followed by the approval of the basal analog glargine (Lantus; Sanofi-Aventis, Bridgewater, NJ) in 2000.[4] The more predictable action profiles of the long-acting analog insulins (insulin glargine and detemir) are associated with lower rates of hypoglycemia, particularly nocturnal hypoglycemia, than NPH.[5] Less hypoglycemia can also reduce weight gain.[6] These advances, coupled with improvement in both needle devices and insulin delivery systems such as pens, continued to facilitate the use of insulin therapy.[7]

In 2016, we now fully embrace the need for insulin products that match the secretion of the endogenous insulin as closely as possible. The Diabetes Control and Complications Trial (DCCT), and the follow-up study, Epidemiology of Diabetes Interventions and Complications, which clearly showed that physiologic insulin replacement for type 1 diabetes reduces microvascular and neuropathic complications of diabetes, and the impact of early intervention with physiologic insulin replacement was seen for many years.[8] In truth, the DCCT was conducted before the insulin analogs were developed, and physiologic control was achieved using combinations of regular, NPH, Lente, and Ultralente insulins. The basal analogs that we have had since 2000, although an improvement, still do not create a smooth ideal basal insulin action, because they do seem to have a peak effect and uneven action over 24 hours, leading to problems such as hypoglycemia and hyperglycemia as late effects.[9] The aim of the newer basal insulins that are being introduced into the market is to have a truly basal effect with a flat activity profile and increased duration of action to mimic endogenous basal insulin secretion as closely as possible. As the duration of insulin activity increases, being able to provide basal insulin action reliably for a full 24 hours with 1 daily injection may lead to better patient adherence and reduce some of the hesitation to initiate insulin therapy. The relative time action profiles for the various types of insulins currently available are illustrated in **Fig. 1**.[10]

BASAL INSULINS

Long-acting (basal) insulin analogs have contributed significantly to the advancement of diabetes management. The initial long-acting basal insulin analogs that have been available in the market, insulins glargine and detemir, were developed to mimic the peakless and continuous kinetic profile of physiologic basal insulin secretion. The advantages of early long-acting analogs (insulin detemir and insulin glargine 100 U/mL or U-100) over NPH are a reduced incidence of nocturnal and overall hypoglycemia as well as a better ability to mimic endogenous basal insulin production.[5] However, clamp studies and clinical data show that the glucose-lowering effect of these early

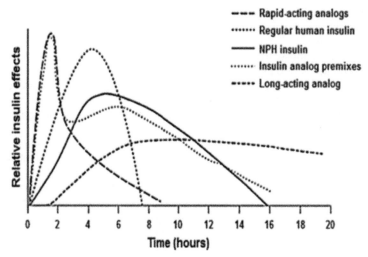

Fig. 1. Comparisons of the time action profiles for the various types of insulins that have been available for the last few years. These have been the staples of current insulin replacement treatment design. NPH, neutral protamine hagadorn. (*From* Eliaschewitz FG, Barreto T. Concepts and clinical use of ultra-long basal insulin. Diabetol Metab Syndr 2016;8.)

basal insulin analogs tend to wax and wane considerably over 24 hours with once-daily dosing.[9] The mean duration of action of both glargine and detemir fall slightly short of 24 hours at clinically relevant doses. This is of importance in treating people with type 1 diabetes and also people with type 2 diabetes who have lost a considerable degree of their endogenous insulin secretion and need full 24-hour basal coverage,[11] resulting in the need for some people to take twice daily injections to cover their basal insulin requirements. The impact of erratic glycemic patterns is also seen, including sporadic hypoglycemia resulting from variability in the peak effects and hyperglycemia late in the expected action profile owing to variability in the duration of action. This prompted the continued efforts to develop a basal insulin with an even flatter and longer profile of action, which might further improve safety and action reliability. The latest generation of long-acting insulins, which some refer to as "ultra"–long-acting insulins, are an attempt to meet this need.

INSULIN GLARGINE 300 U/mL (TOUJEO)

It has long been known from the experience with U-500 regular insulin that altering the concentration of insulin can impact the time–action profile for a given amount of units, or the measure of biologic activity.[12] Based on this principle, insulin glargine 300 U/mL, or glargine U-300, was developed to address the duration concerns seen with the early basal analogs. Increasing the concentration from 100 to 300 U/mL lead to a lower injection volume and formation of a smaller subcutaneous depot, which results in slower and more prolonged insulin activity.[13] In addition, glargine U-300 demonstrated less within-day and within-subject variability, thus providing more consistent basal activity compared with the glargine U-100 formulation.[14]

  The EDITION (6-Month, Multicenter, Randomized, Open-label, Parallel-group Study Comparing the Efficacy and Safety of a New Formulation of Insulin Glargine and Lantus Both Plus Mealtime Insulin in Patients With Type 2 Diabetes Mellitus With a

6-month Safety Extension Period) series of open-label, noninferiority trials compared the clinical efficacy of glargine U-300 with glargine U-100 in types 1 and 2 diabetes mellitus populations.[15-19] Glargine U-300 was shown to be consistently noninferior to glargine-100 in these trials when comparing the mean change in hemoglobin A1C, although the U-300 arm frequently required higher doses of insulin to achieve the same glycemic change. Lower incidence of hypoglycemic events, primarily nocturnal, was noted with glargine U-300 compared with glargine U-100.[20] Another interesting observation from these trials was the trend of less weight gain seen in the participants on glargine U-300.[21]

As with all new concentrated insulin, glargine U-300 is only available in a prefilled pen calibrated for the higher concentration, so no dose conversions calculations are required. This reduces the potential for dosing errors. Doses are dialed in 1-U increments up to a maximum of 80 U in a single injection.[22] Patients requiring higher doses of insulin will still require multiple injections to receive their entire dose of this formulation. Glargine U-300 improved on prior basal analogs with its more stable, consistent, prolonged profile allowing for achievement of comparable glycemic targets with less hypoglycemia.

FOLLOW-ON BIOLOGIC INSULIN GLARGINE (BASAGLAR)

Insulin is considered to be a biological product because it is manufactured through biotechnology using bacteria or yeast.[23] Several of the early insulin analogs (insulin lispro, aspart, and glargine) have lost their patent exclusivity. Thus, the opportunity to develop similar products at a lower cost for our patients seems to be at hand. However, when these insulins were approved by the FDA, there was not a separate approval process for biological products. Unlike other biologics, insulin is regulated under the Food, Drug and Cosmetic Act rather than the Public Health Service Act.[24] Because the term biosimilar is limited to highly similar agents to those approved through the Public Health Service Act, similar insulin products are referred to as follow-on biologics rather than biosimilars. Even though they are approved though the Food, Drug and Cosmetic Act, follow-on biologics, unlike generic drugs, are not considered bioequivalent to their reference product given the complexity in the production of these products, but have been shown to have no clinically meaningful differences from the reference product in terms of mechanism of action, safety profile, and administration.[24]

The first follow-on biologic insulin was approved by the FDA in 2015 for insulin glargine. Basaglar was approved through an abbreviated new drug application.[25] The preclinical pharmacokinetic/pharmacodynamic studies were clamp studies were done in small populations of healthy subjects and those with type 1 diabetes demonstrated comparable effects with its reference product, glargine U-100 (Lantus).[26,27] Two phase III randomized trials compared Basaglar with glargine U-100 (Lantus). One study population had type 1 diabetes and the other population had type 2 diabetes. Both insulin glargine products provided effective and comparable glucose control with similar safety profiles.[28,29] Owing to patent litigation agreements, Basaglar will not be available in the United States until December of 2016. Basaglar can be dosed and adjusted similarly to its reference product. It will only be available via a prefilled KwikPen.[30]

With the advent of follow-on biologic insulins, there is a much needed potential to reduce diabetes treatment costs and increase the accessibility and variety of insulins available to even those with insurance coverage. Although the cost of Basaglar in the United States is unknown as of this writing, based the costs of biosimilar insulin in

Europe and an analysis of potential cost savings in the United States, a 15% lower cost could translate into a cost savings of $2 or $3 billion per year.[31]

As a clinician prescribing a follow-on biologic insulin, several factors need to be taken into consideration. These are not generic medications and may not perform exactly the same as the parent or the reference product. In some areas, such as manufacturing process and quality, including batch-to-batch, variability there is no opportunity to monitor their performance because nothing in this area appears in the public domain. Clinicians need to rely on their regulators and the reputation of the manufacturers as to the reliability of the manufacturing and quality monitoring.[32] Postmarketing pharmacovigilance is recommended, but this has its own flaws; adverse events maybe seriously underreported. Follow-on biologics have the same nonproprietary name as their reference products, so reports need to include the product's national drug code and/or proprietary name. Accordingly, there will likely be a need for longer term clinical studies and interchangeability or switching studies of insulin in practice, as well as comprehensive pharmacovigilance and postmarketing surveillance, to provide further parameters to help clinicians use these products.

INSULIN DEGLUDEC (TRESIBA, INSULIN DEGLUDEC U-100, INSULIN DEGLUDEC U-200, RYZODEG-INSULIN DEGLUDEC/INSULIN ASPART 100 U/mL)

Insulin degludec is a long-acting insulin analog that has been available outside of the United States for several years and was approved by the US FDA in September 2015.[33] It is currently available in 2 forms, a 100 U/mL concentration and a 200 U/mL concentration.[33] A fixed-dose combination with the rapid acting insulin aspart (Ryzodeg, Novo Nordisk, Plainsboro, NJ), containing 70% degludec and 30% aspart at a concentration of 100 U/mL, is approved by the FDA,[34] but the date for its introduction onto the US market has not been determined at the time of this writing. In addition, a fixed-dose combination of insulin degludec and liraglutide is under review by the FDA.

Insulin degludec exists in insulin dimers self-associating into a multihexamers after the subcutaneous injection from which monomers slowly dissociate.[34] Owing to this process, the resulting pharmacodynamics demonstrate a protracted activity profile with almost equal effects across an individual (24-hour) dosing interval.[35,36] The consistency of the pharmacodynamic profile at steady state is apparent even as doses increase in patients with type 2 diabetes, but not in type 1 diabetes at higher doses (**Fig. 2**).[37] The duration of action is greater than 42 hours,[38] offering a basal insulin option for more flexible dosing than every 24 hours without adverse effecting glycemic control.[39] This flat pharmacodynamic profile is more consistent both within and between individuals when compared with equivalent doses of insulin glargine 100 U/mL in patients with type 1 diabetes.[38]

Insulin degludec has been extensively studied in comparison to glargine U-100 and insulin detemir in patients with types 1 and 2 diabetes in the BEGIN trials (A Trial Assessing the Implications of Switching From Insulin Glargine to Insulin Degludec in Subjects With Type 2 Diabetes Mellitus). These noninferiority studies evaluated usage as a once daily injection, thrice weekly, or flexible dosing (8–40 hours between doses) over 26 to 52 weeks.[40,41] The primary objectives of the trials were to confirm the efficacy based on change in hemoglobin A1C and rates of hypoglycemia in addition to various regimens from prandial insulin to oral agents. All trials were randomized, controlled, parallel-group, multicenter, multinational, and treat-to-target designs in which degludec was compared with an active comparator. A metaanalysis of 7 of these trials found that degludec was noninferior to glargine U-100 in patients with

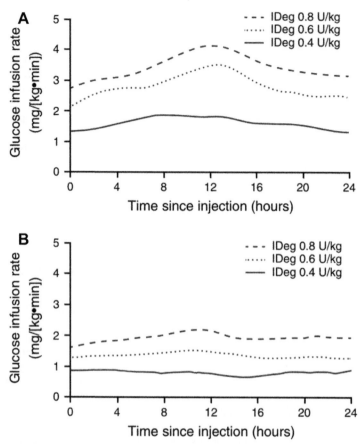

Fig. 2. Glucose infusion rates (GIR) over time for various dosing levels of insulin degludec (IDeg) in subjects with (*A*) type 1 diabetes and (*B*) type 2 diabetes. The GIR reflects the glucose lowering effect of an insulin. These curves demonstrate that there is minimal peaking in people with type 1 diabetes and even less so with type 2 diabetes. (*From* Haahr H, Heise T. A review of the pharmacological properties of insulin degludec and their clinical relevance. Clin Pharmacokinet 2014;53:791; with permission.)

types 1 and 2 diabetes on basal/bolus insulin regimens, as well as with patients with type 2 diabetes who were naïve to insulin therapy.[41] Of note, the participants in these studies experienced fewer hypoglycemic episodes (particularly those episodes that occurred overnight) and a lower total daily dose of insulin was required for participants with type 1 diabetes or those with type 2 diabetes naïve to insulin.[40–42] In addition, participants in the various BEGIN trials tended to gain either similar amounts of weight or less weight than those on the active comparators.[41–44]

One initial concern was a possible increased cardiovascular risk found in a metaanalysis during the initial FDA review. Although degludec did not impact any classic cardiovascular risk parameters (low-density lipoprotein cholesterol, high-density lipoprotein cholesterol, or blood pressure), with the mandate for trials of diabetes mediations to look at actual cardiovascular outcomes rather than just risk parameters, there was a request for additional evaluation.[44] A double blind randomized crossover study (the DEVOTE [A Trial Comparing Cardiovascular Safety of Insulin Degludec

Versus Insulin Glargine in Subjects With Type 2 Diabetes at High Risk of Cardiovascular Events] trial) is expected to be completed in the middle of 2016.[45] Presentation of a preplanned interim analysis from this trial led to the FDA approval of degludec U-100 and 2 other formulations, degludec U-200 and Ryzodeg.[46]

Insulin Degludec 200 U/mL (Degludec U-200)

To accommodate patients with higher insulin requirements to minimize the number of injections needed degludec was simultaneously developed in double (200 U/mL) the typical concentration. A double-blind, crossover, randomized glucose clamp study in patients with type 1 diabetes demonstrated bioequivalence in the pharmacokinetic and pharmacodynamic properties of the 100 and 200 U/mL formulations.[47] Three clinical trials were conducted evaluating degludec U-200. The first 2 trials were the BEGIN COMPARE (vs degludec U-100 over 22 weeks) and BEGIN LOW VOLUME (vs Glargine U-100 over 26 weeks) trials. These trials found degludec U-200 had similarly efficacy as both active comparators, but lower rates of hypoglycemia compared with glargine U-100.[48,49] The third trial evaluated the use of degludec U-200 compared with glargine U-100 in participants requiring higher doses (>81 U/d) of basal insulin using a crossover design with participants receiving each treatment for a period of 16 weeks. This study confirmed similar efficacy with participants requiring similar daily doses of both treatments; however, rates of nocturnal hypoglycemia and weight gain were lower with degludec U-200.[50]

There are important considerations when choosing degludec U-200 for a patient. First, degludec U-100 and degludec U-200 have the same proprietary name, thus mistakes may be made during prescribing or dispensing of these insulins.[14] In addition, similar to degludec U-100, degludec U-200 is only available in a prefilled pen with dosing based on actual units of insulin up to a maximum single dose of 160 units.[33] Although this delivery system avoids any possible issues with dose conversion errors and allows for single injections for those requiring larger doses, the dosing increments for the 2 devices are different (1-U dosing increment for degludec U-100 vs 2-U dosing increments for degludec U-200), so education must be provided if individuals are switching from 1 concentration to the other.[21]

Insulin degludec (70%)/insulin aspart (30%) 100 U/ml (IDegAsp, Ryzodeg)

The premixed formulation of the long-acting insulin degludec (70%) and rapid-acting insulin aspart (30%; Ryzodeg) is a new insulin analog formulation coformulated into a single injection.[34] Premixtures of the other basal insulins were not possible because either unstable hybrid hexamers were formed or the acidity of the basal insulin formulation was not conducive to mixture with the neutral solution of the rapid-acting insulin formulation. In these instances, neither the rapid or long-acting action profile would have been preserved.[51]

In this premixed formulation, insulin degludec continues to exist in a stable dihexameric state when mixed with insulin aspart without any interaction and the distinct pharmacokinetic/pharmacodynamic profiles of the 2 analogs remains intact upon subcutaneous injection.[43] The resulting pharmacodynamic profile of IDegAsp reflects the action profiles of the rapid-acting insulin aspart and the long-acting insulin degludec (**Fig. 3**).[34] The median onset of appearance for the insulin aspart component was 14 minutes after injection with a peak concentration after 72 minutes. The degludec component reached a steady state after 3 to 4 days with a half-life of about 25 hours.[34]

The primary studies evaluating IDegAsp were noninferiority trials in participants with type 2 diabetes, compared with glargine U-100 + oral treatment(s) or insulin protaminated aspart/aspart 70/30, and in participants with type 1 diabetes with prandial

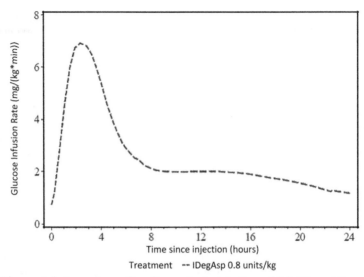

Fig. 3. Glucose infusion rate profile after a single injection of 0.8 U/kg of the premixed formulation of the long-acting insulin degludec (70%) and rapid-acting insulin aspart (30%; Ryzodeg) in 640 subjects with type 1 diabetes. IDegAsp, degludec (70%)/insulin aspart (30%) 100 U/mL. (*From* Ryzodeg [package insert]. Plainsboro, NJ: Novo Nordisk, Inc; 2015; with permission.)

insulin aspart at other meals compared with insulin detemir and prandial insulin aspart, for 16 to 26 weeks.[51] All trials demonstrated the noninferiority of the ability of IDegAsp to improve glycemic control effectively compared with the active comparator. They also found lower rates of hypoglycemia and in most of the trials participants required lower basal insulin doses with the exception of the trial conducted in Japanese patients with type 2 diabetes.[52–55]

IDegAsp offers a new option for patients to either decrease the number of daily injections when incorporated into a basal/bolus insulin regimen or a single injection option when a patient with type 2 diabetes is not achieving glucose goals with basal insulin.

Insulin degludec/liraglutide (IDegLira, Xultophy)
Insulin degludec is also formulated into a mixture with the glucagonlike protein-1 receptor agonist (GLP-1 RA) liraglutide, which is available in many countries outside of the United States, and has been submitted for review to the FDA. The formulation contains 100 U/mL of insulin degludec and 3.6 mg/mL of liraglutide. Each dosing increment contains 1 U of insulin degludec with 0.036 mg of liraglutide up to a maximum dose of 50 U of insulin degludec with 1.8 mg of liraglutide.[56] The goal of this formulation seeks to use the benefits of a GLP-1 receptor agonist to reduce the fasting and the postprandial blood glucose excursions, while providing the stable basal insulin activity of insulin degludec in a single injection. This formulation increases adherence with a single injection, while also controlling glucose levels and minimizing weight gain with insulin therapy.

The DUAL (A Trial Comparing Sequential Addition of Insulin Aspart Versus Further Dose Increase With Insulin Degludec/Liraglutide in Subjects With Type 2 Diabetes Mellitus, Previously Treated With Insulin Degludec/Liraglutide and Metformin and in

Need of Further Intensification) series of trials were completed to evaluate this formulation in patients with type 2 diabetes. Participants included patients naïve to insulin (DUAL I,[57] DUAL III,[58] and DUAL IV[59]), as well as those experienced with insulin therapy (DUAL II[60] and DUAL V[61]) for 26 weeks. The IDegLira combination lowered hemoglobin A1C levels greater than all comparators, including insulin degludec, insulin glargine, liraglutide, and placebo. IDegLira enabled more participants to achieve target hemoglobin A1C levels than all comparators and resulted in less weight gain when compared with insulin degludec or insulin glargine.[57-61]

This unique formulation offers another treatment option for those patients requiring basal insulin therapy while minimizing weight gain. It is likely that patients may be more adherent to a single injection of IDegLira and may offer some cost savings (single insurance copayment) over separate injections of insulin degludec and liraglutide. However, owing to the coformulation that caps the daily liraglutide dose at 1.8 mg, which is the maximum daily dose used for diabetes treatment currently in the individual delivery formulation, use of this treatment is limited to those patients who require less than or equal to 50 U of basal insulin. As with any combination product, dosing flexibility is limited, and in this instance they may not achieve maximum efficacy of liraglutide unless they require the maximum dose (50 U) of degludec.

PRANDIAL INSULINS

It has been known for many years that in a person who does not have diabetes, normal insulin secretion in response to increasing glucose levels is biphasic.[62] In these individuals, the first phase of pancreatic insulin secretion rapidly increases at the start of food consumption. That rapid increase reaches half-maximum levels in about 16 to 18 minutes after a carbohydrate meal, and then peaks at about 30 to 45 minutes.[63,64] The person with early type 2 diabetes has reduced first phase insulin release in that first 30-minute time period, whereas the second phase, occurring over the next 2 hours, can be normal or augmented.[65] This reduction in first phase insulin release has been identified as a key early defect with type 2 diabetes, and the second phase, although augmented, is often still insufficient to reduce elevated glucose levels in the face of insulin resistance, thus leading to the glycemic manifestations of type 2 diabetes.

The significance of this postprandial hyperglycemia in the pathophysiology of type 2 diabetes and its complications has been discussed for some time, and although that is beyond the scope of this review, it was demonstrated years ago that as you get closer to targeted hemoglobin A1C levels, much of the contribution to that hemoglobin A1C elevation is postprandial glycemia.[66] Thus, from a clinical perspective and in consideration of the pathophysiologic changes occurring with type 2 diabetes, one cannot only replace basal insulin and expect to optimally control glycemia when postprandial hyperglycemia is also a significant contributor. At some point, targeting postprandial glycemia becomes necessary, both in the selection of antidiabetes medications, and in the context of this current discussion, moving from a program using only basal insulin replacement to those that include prandial insulin coverage.

Keeping in mind the timing of the first and second phase insulin releases, one can appreciate the impact of evolving insulins available for prandial coverage. Regular insulin, peaking at about 3 hours and with persistent action lasting, in reality, a number of hours afterward, missed that first phase insulin defect and much of the early food absorption, but often caused hypoglycemia hours later, before the next meal or at bedtime. Rapid-acting analogs came next and were more aligned with the timing of food absorption in their replacement of mealtime insulin requirements.[67] We recently added to the armamentarium inhaled technosphere insulin, which works even faster,[68] and the more concentrated lispro U-200,[3] providing additional treatment options. There are more options that are likely to be available in the future. Thus, with this evolution of insulins, we now have additional flexibility in how we match insulin to our patients' needs and requirements.[67] The clinical indications for advancing to the use of these prandial insulins are discussed elsewhere in this article.

INSULIN LISPRO 200 U/mL (LISPRO U-200, HUMALOG)

Lispro U-100 was the first rapid acting analog to be approved by the FDA in 1996.[3] It can be taken 15 minutes before a meal with an onset of action within 15 minutes, peak effects in 30 to 90 minutes, and rapid clearance within 5 hours of the initial injection.[69] Because of its fairly rapid action, it is aimed to control the postprandial increase in glucose and the rapid clearance from the blood stream will lead to a decrease in hypoglycemia as a late effect. Lispro U-100 underwent an extensive clinical trial to establish its safety, efficacy, and action profile.[3]

As the prevalence of obesity has been increasing in the last 2 decades,[70] so is the percentage of population with diabetes who are obese. There is a well-established symbiotic association between obesity and insulin resistance.[71] This has led to a significant percentage of the diabetic population who are highly insulin resistant necessitating the need for a higher insulin requirement.[72]

Lispro U-200 was introduced as new formulation of the insulin lispro in 2015. The pharmacodynamics were shown to be bioequivalent to lispro U-100 in healthy subjects (**Fig. 4**).[3,73] Since bioequivalence was demonstrated, the safety and efficacy data established for the lispro U-100 can be extrapolated to lispro U-200; thus, no clinical trials were required to compare lispro U-200 with the other rapid-acting analogs.

Similar to other new concentrated insulin formulations, lispro U-200 is only available in a calibrated prefilled pen (Kwikpen), which holds double the units (600 vs 300 U) as the lispro U-100 pen. With the similarity of lispro U-200 to lispro U-100 and as it is dosed in actual units by 1-U increments up to a maximum of 60 U in a single injection,[3] it could be used in either type 1 or type 2 diabetes. Its primary benefit is less waste with

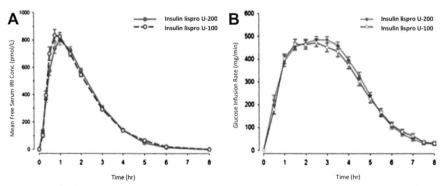

Fig. 4. (*A, B*) Comparison of the mean free serum insulin concentration and glucose infusion rate for insulin lispro U-100 versus U-200, demonstrating comparable pharmacokinetic and pharmacodynamics profiles of these 2 different concentrations. (*From* de la Peña A, Seger M, Soon D, et al. Bioequivalence and comparative pharmacodynamics of insulin lispro 200 u/ml relative to insulin lispro (humalog) 100 u/ml. Clin Pharmacol Drug Dev 2016;5:72; with permission.)

fewer pens required each month. If an individual requires more than 60 U for their prandial dose, multiple injections will be required.

As the market continues to expand with numerous insulins of varying action profile and concentrations, confusion regarding insulin increases. The potential for medication prescribing and dispensing errors further increases with multiple concentrations of an insulin with the same proprietary name.[21] The likelihood for dosing errors is decreased with the correct use of the prefilled pens. In the unlikely situation that a patient draws insulin out of the pen, the patient must account for the differences in concentration by dose reduction to prevent resulting hypoglycemia. To ensure appropriate use, patients should be provided with prescriptions for the pen needles required to appropriately use the pen along with any prescription for insulin and counseled on the risks of incorrect use.

INSULIN HUMAN INHALATION POWER (TECHNOSPHERE INSULIN, AFREZZA)

The ability to administer insulin via an alternative route other than subcutaneous injection is much sought after to decrease barriers to insulin therapy. Inhalable products are the first to achieve marketed products. The first inhaled insulin, Exubera, was available on the US market from 2006 to 2007.[74] Despite similar efficacy to those patients with type 2 diabetes taking subcutaneous insulin and initial excitement regarding the ability to dose prandial insulin without injections, this product faced several obstacles to successful use. The inhaler was cumbersome to use and doses were available in a limited selection of fixed dose powder packets that required dose conversions (units to milligrams) made use of this treatment impractical for many patients.[74] Residual concerns remained regarding adverse pulmonary effects after the product was removed from the market owing to lack of commercial success.[74–76]

In June of 2014, the FDA approved a new inhaled insulin (Afrezza).[77] The active compound is an inhalation powder formulation of monomers of regular human insulin and fumaryl diketopiperazine, a pharmaceutical excipient to which proteins adsorb that allow for the pulmonary delivery of these proteins and then excreted unchanged.[78] Because the active ingredients are monomers of regular insulin, this insulin is classified as a rapid-acting prandial insulin with an onset of about 12 to 15 minutes, peaking at 60 minutes with a total duration of action of 2.5 to 3 hours.[77,79] Inhalation should occur at the beginning of a meal using a single inhalation per cartridge, although a second inhalation immediately after the meal may improve control for large or higher fat meals. Single-use cartridges are available in fixed doses of 4, 8, and 12 U. If the dose required is in between or greater than the fixed dose in the cartridge, additional inhalations of other or similar strength cartridges may be necessary. It is important to note that a new inhaler must be used after every 15 days of use.[77]

The role of this inhaled insulin in managing patients with type 1 diabetes was evaluated in a 24-week, noninferiority trial (Affinity 1 trial [Comparison of Technosphere® Insulin Versus Technosphere Powder (Placebo) in Insulin-Naive Subjects With Type 2 Diabetes Mellitus]) involving 344 patients comparing the addition of inhaled insulin and insulin aspart with basal insulin. Although the difference in the A1C reduction met the criteria to be considered noninferior to insulin aspart, fewer participants achieved a hemoglobin A1C of less than 7% with inhaled insulin. Of note, fewer participants using inhaled insulin experienced hypoglycemia compared with insulin aspart; however, more patients experienced a cough, which led 5.7% to discontinue treatment.[80]

One study using the currently marketed inhaler was conducted in patients with type 2 diabetes. A 24-week placebo-controlled study (Affinity 2 trial) was conducted in 353 adults with type 2 diabetes whose were inadequately controlled with maximally tolerated doses of oral antidiabetes medications. At week 24, treatment with inhaled insulin plus oral antidiabetes medications provided a significantly greater mean reduction in hemoglobin A1C levels compared with the placebo inhalation.[81]

The most common adverse reactions (≥2%) associated with insulin human inhalation powder include hypoglycemia, cough, and throat pain or irritation. To assess for the presence of chronic lung conditions and owing to concerns of diminished pulmonary function, it is recommended to assess pulmonary function (eg, forced expiratory volume in 1 second) before treatment initiation, after 6 months of therapy, and annually thereafter. Inhaled insulin is contraindicated in patients with chronic lung disease, such as asthma or chronic obstructive pulmonary disease.[82] A boxed warning regarding the risk of acute bronchospasm was issued owing to events observed in patients with asthma and chronic obstructive pulmonary disease who use the insulin human inhalation powder. Afrezza is also not recommended for patients who smoke or have recently stopped smoking (within the last 6 months).[77] The FDA has a Risk Evaluation and Mitigation Strategy program, which is essentially designed to determine if the clinical benefits outweigh the risks.[83] A Risk Evaluation and Mitigation Strategy study for Afrezza is being undertaken owing to the risk of acute bronchospasm in patients with chronic lung disease to assess this risk and reinforce appropriate patient selection and evaluation before therapy initiation.[84]

What Are the Current Barriers Associated with Insulin and What Do We Do to Overcome Them?

Before addressing the practical application of these newer insulins to the clinical design of insulin replacement programs, one must consider the many challenges and barriers to doing so. A goal of having these newer insulins is that they will help to address these challenges and barriers. It will remain to be seen if, in fact, they succeed.

Insulin replacement therapy is an imperfect treatment. It must be administered by patients and thus requires skill training for those patients by the health care provider. That, in and of itself, makes it more challenging to having someone take a pill. It is also trying to replicate a natural physiologic function using imperfect replacement strategies. However, as we look at the evolution of insulins over the years, each step does move incrementally closer to a more idealized insulin replacement system, overcoming—or at least lowering—some of those barriers to treatment.

Barriers can be thought of in 3 categories, those emanating from the patient, those emanating from the health care provider, and those that are a result of imperfect health care delivery systems.[85] Strategies exist to address these barriers.[86] Patient barriers include issues such as social stigma attached to using insulin, and their perception that using insulin reflects a personal failure that they are not in control of their diabetes. Such issues are often addressed through education about the natural progression of diabetes and that at some point the use of insulin is inevitable. The need to use insulin should never be presented as a threat. Many people believe that insulin is not effective and could cause complications, having seen friends and relatives start insulin in the context of bad events happening. Patients perceive that the administration of insulin is as painful as other inoculations and feel that using insulin will dramatically impact their lifestyle. Supportive education can help, including explanations about the newer insulin pens and the size of the insulin needles. A self-demonstration of the dry air injection by the provider could ease some of the fear about starting insulin therapy. Education regarding alternative methods of insulin administration, fixed basal patch pumps, or inhaled insulin, may also ease concerns regarding the lifestyle impact of this therapy. While discussing insulin therapy, patients should be educated about the possible side effects such as weight gain and hypoglycemia, and strategies to minimize them. Having open, nonjudgmental discussions of the patients' concerns and using a multidisciplinary approach could alleviate some of the patient fears, such as meal plans and carbohydrate counting demonstrated by a dietitian or the correct method of insulin delivery shown by a clinical pharmacist. Some of the advantages of the newer insulins, as discussed elsewhere in this article, may help to address these issues as well. Finally, today we always have to consider cost. Sometimes, explaining to the patients that in the long run insulin could be less expensive than using multiple oral medications, but when faced with high copays or coverage refusals, this is small consolation. Industry copay cards and other savings programs can help. The use of less physiologic insulin regimens, premixed insulins, or older insulin products may be short-term solutions, but may come with compromises.

Barriers emanating from providers also must be considered. Gaps in familiarity with how to design, implement, and monitor complex insulin treatment programs, particularly when some of the newer insulins may be involved, can limit treatment efficacy and slow treatment advancement. The use of outsourced expert resources to help in this regard relies on coordination of the health care delivery system. Being able to refer to diabetes specialists, or have access to Certified Diabetes Educators, including nurses, dietitians, exercise physiologists, and clinical pharmacists, can be effective, because dealing with some of the patient barriers can be time consuming for care providers and having educators available with time to devote to these issues can improve efficiency and care efficacy. Medicare and Medicaid have begun to reimburse such services. Endocrine/diabetes specialty practices can build communication bridges to area primary care providers to expedite this care sharing.[85,86]

As recommended by American Diabetes Association and American Association of Clinical Endocrinologists setting individualized goals[87,88] and designing an appropriate insulin regimen needs to be done for better patient adherence while maintaining glycemic targets and minimizing the side effect profile. This is where the knowledge of these new insulins that are becoming available is helpful and allows clinicians to add to their armamentarium of available insulin therapies.

Insulin Design in Clinical Practice: Evolving Strategies and Role of These Newer Insulins

How do the new insulins that have become available in the last few years impact our approach to the design of insulin replacement programs? And how is their availability impacting the traditional barriers to insulin therapy that we have just discussed? There is something of a "chicken and egg" issue here—were the new insulins designed to meet perceived gaps in the tools we have available to us for the design of optimized insulin replacement treatments, or did the development of new insulins stimulate creative new treatment designs now that new tools were available? The truth is likely some of both, but recognizing that helps us to understand how the evolution of insulin treatment has occurred. We can look at these new tools and apply them to the current insulin replacement paradigms, but then also, using real-world clinical experience backed by some evidence-based guidance, get creative in exploring new ways to approach treatment that might not have been conceived of by the insulin developers in their laboratories.

For people with type 1 diabetes, the current paradigm of treatment design is usually a multiple daily injection program of insulin replacement, usually referred to as "basal/bolus" treatment.[89] These programs seek use exogenous to mimic natural endogenous insulin physiology by providing consistent levels of basal insulin as well as postprandial increases in insulin action to cover mealtime needs. Studies, such as the DCCT, demonstrated that physiologically based treatments that can mimic these patterns using multiple daily injections or continuous subcutaneous insulin infusion ("insulin pumps") decrease the risk of developing some complications.[90,91] However, since that trial, we have many new insulins and devices now available, and we are seeing how those tools are facilitating the evolution of physiologic insulin replacement design that was first confirmed by the DCCT as the recommended treatment approach.

The approach to insulin therapy for type 2 diabetes, owing to the heterogeneity of this condition, has required more individualization and has shown considerable evolutionary change over recent years.[89,92] The differing perspectives and variability in recommendations starts with defining the therapeutic target itself. The American Diabetes Association suggests a hemoglobin A1C level of less than 7%[87] and the American Association of Clinical Endocrinologists suggests less than 6.5%.[88] However, both groups also cite glucose targets before and after meals, reflecting the need to consider glycemic patterns as a treatment target as well. Using those patterns requires self-monitoring of blood glucose, which is strongly recommended for all people with diabetes using insulin,[87] and even those who do not use insulin.[93,94] However, there is firmer supportive data in those with type 1 diabetes.[95] Modification of those ideal targets is also recommended in clinical situations where aggressive treatment may be harmful to the patient or the use of treatments necessary to achieve them may be difficult or pose risks for the patient, such as those with coronary artery disease and older individuals.[87,89,96] Many diabetes experts recommend the engagement of patients in the assessment of their own glycemic patterns, which provides key direction to the design and implementation of insulin treatment programs.[67,97] After considering the A1C to provide a perspective on how close to target the control may be, start by considering the fasting glucose level as the starting point of the day, reflecting basal insulin effect overnight. Next, look at the premeal and bedtime trends during the day—are they upward, downward, or even? Finally, look at postprandial glycemia, both the absolute height of a 2-hour postprandial glycemic level and the increase relative to the preprandial level. Throughout, consider the level of nocturnal glycemia, particularly watching for hypoglycemia.

Insulin is typically indicated for people with type 2 diabetes[88,89,98] who are newly diagnosed and have marked hyperglycemia or when they fail to meet their individualized treatment goals using multiple antidiabetic medications. Insulin is also indicated when there are contraindications or intolerance to the medications, and certainly in the setting of other significant medical conditions, which are promoting increases in glucose, often the case in hospitalized patients. There has been some suggestion that early initiation of insulin therapy for type 2 diabetes may help preserve beta-cell function over time.[99–101] These data can be compelling, but keep in mind that some of these studies were done in China where hospitalizing individuals for aggressive early initiation of such therapy is easier and less expensive.

Typical initiation and treatment advancement plans have been recommended in national guidelines and standards.[88,89] Typically, initial insulin dosing may be basal insulin given once daily at bedtime. It can be started at a dose of 0.1 to 0.2 U/kg body weight, depending on the degree of hyperglycemia, and usually is given along with other noninsulin agents.[98] Patient self-titration methods have been demonstrated to be effective and safe when compared with clinician-driven programs, and can be considered with capable, engaged patients when adequate educational support is available.[5,102] As we think about the newer insulins, it is important to remember that many studies have demonstrated that both NPH and the basal insulin analogs can achieve comparable lowering of hemoglobin A1C, but the ultra-long basal insulin analogs have the advantage of resulting in less hypoglycemia and weight gain, and provide basal coverage for a full 24 hours or longer with a single injection.[5,6,103,104]

When Is Basal Insulin Not Enough?

Titration of a program using basal insulin only will likely help improve the overall control as reflected by the hemoglobin A1C level, but there are limits to how far this type of insulin can be increased before some other approach is needed. The usual recommendations as found in treatment guidelines[88,89,98] suggest certain key findings that suggest the limit of basal insulin titration may have been reached. Key among them is the overarching consideration where the hemoglobin A1C is not at target but unacceptable levels of hypoglycemia occur with further basal insulin titration. However, it is often postprandial hyperglycemia that is a key finding; again, the usefulness of pattern examination is underscored. When the postprandial glucose level is greater than 180 mg/dL, or greater than 50 mg/dL higher than preprandial glycemic levels, further therapeutic advancement is often needed. If a patient is not adequately checking all postprandial glucose levels, then the typical pattern is increasing glucose levels between breakfast and lunch, lunch and supper, and then on to bedtime. What is likely happening is that postprandial glucose levels increase but never adequately return to baseline by the next meal. Bedtime glucose levels are high, but then decrease overnight as the excessive basal insulin quantity is working, only to start that pattern over again the next day. Nocturnal hypoglycemia is often seen in these situations.

Next Steps Beyond Basal Insulin Only

When basal insulin alone is deemed to be insufficient to provide glycemic control, there are a number of options to consider as next steps (**Fig. 5**).[88,89,98]

- Basal plus GLP-1 agonist.
- Switch to a premixed analog (1, 2, or 3 daily injections).
- "Basal plus" program: Add an injection of rapid-acting insulin before 1 or possibly 2 meals.
- Use a full basal/bolus program with balanced doses of basal insulin and bolus doses of rapid-acting insulin before each meal.

The key is that we are advancing to provide more prandial coverage, either through boosted endogenous insulin responses using a GLP-1 receptor agonist, the rapid-acting portion of the premixed insulin, or a rapid-acting insulin before 1, 2, or 3 daily meals. The various options are reviewed.

Adding a glucagonlike protein-1 receptor agonist to basal insulin

Adding a GLP-1 RA to basal insulin is one option that has been suggested, and has been demonstrated effective in multiple studies.[105–107] Although it is beyond the scope of this review to delve into all of the data on this class of medications, there are some important aspects of this treatment design to consider when advancing beyond treatment with basal insulin.[108] This treatment design is becoming more popular because it is less cumbersome for many people than adding mealtime rapid-acting insulin, and promotes glucose-dependent insulin release, which has advantages. Key among them are the efficacy of treatment without an increase in the incidence of hypoglycemia and weight gain.[109] Interestingly, in looking at various study protocols, when the study is designed to minimize the amount of insulin used, the glycemic improvements were less but the weight reduction was greater.[110,111]

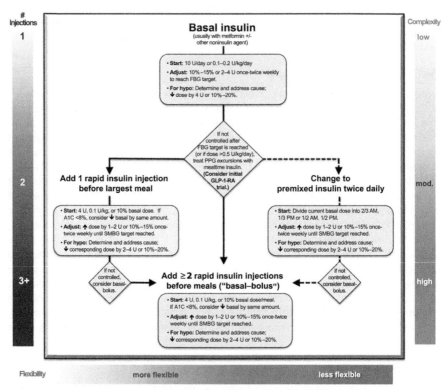

Fig. 5. American Diabetes Association and European Association for the Study of Diabetes schematic algorithm for the advancement of therapy beyond basal-only treatment. Major options include consideration of adding a glucagonlike peptide-1 receptor agonist (GLP-1-RA), change to premixed insulin twice daily, adding rapid-acting insulin before the largest meal of the day and then advancing to a second and then a third premeal injection, the "basal-bolus" treatment design. With advancing therapies along this algorithm comes increased complexity of the self-care program. FBG, fasting blood glucose; PPG, postprandial glucose; SMBG, self-monitoring of blood glucose. (*From* Inzucchi SE, Bergenstal RM, Buse JB, et al. Management of hyperglycemia in type 2 diabetes, 2015: a patient-centred approach. Update to a Position Statement of the American Diabetes Association and the European Association for the Study of Diabetes. Diabetologia 2015;58(3):429–42; with permission.)

However, when more aggressive insulin use was part of the protocol, the improvement in A1C hemoglobin was more pronounced but weight loss was minimal.[112]

Several studies have been done to compare the GLP-1 RA versus rapid acting insulins. Some examples are the 4B Trial (Safety, Tolerability, Pharmacokinetics and Pharmacodynamic Effects of Multiple Escalating Oral Doses of LY2393910 in Patients With Type 2 Diabetes Mellitus), a 30-week randomized noninferiority trial, that compared the addition of exenatide twice daily or thrice daily mealtime insulin lispro to glargine and metformin,[113] and the Harmony 6 (A Long Term, Randomised, Double Blind, Placebo-controlled Study to Determine the Effect of Albiglutide, When Added to Standard Blood Glucose Lowering Therapies, on Major Cardiovascular Events in Patients With Type 2 Diabetes Mellitus) trial, a randomized trial that compared the addition of once-weekly albiglutide versus thrice-daily mealtime insulin lispro to insulin glargine.[114] Both studies demonstrated comparable glycemic control with either less weight gain or weight loss and lower rates of hypoglycemia with the addition of the GLP-1 RA.[113,114]

Thus, thinking about the barriers to insulin therapy emanating from both patients and providers, treatment designs that offer efficacy of treatment but with lower hypoglycemia and weight gain can address some of the issues of concern. What about the newer insulins? The combination of insulin degludec and liraglutide (Xultophy, Novo Nordisk, Bagsvaerd, Denmark) has been discussed in detail and likely will provide some further benefit[57–61] in the context of the improved action pattern of the ultra-long acting basal insulin versus the earlier basal analogs. The fixed combination of dosing and potential limitation on the flexibility of dosing, unlike with premixed insulin, does not seem to impact efficacy, as has been demonstrated in a number of studies, and may improve adherence with both treatments administered via a single injection.[57,115]

Changing to premixed insulin

Another advancement pathway to take is to change from basal insulin only to the use of a premixed insulin. Traditionally, these programs have used twice daily administration as an initial regimen, but potentially 1 or 3 daily injections can be used. A number of studies have looked at this treatment design in comparison with other options, particularly the basal-only option. Typically, there is a trade off when using premixed insulin programs. Either you go for more aggressive hemoglobin A1C lowering, and there is more hypoglycemia, or you try to avoid hypoglycemia, and do not do as well with hemoglobin A1C lowering as the comparator. In the INITIATE (INITiation of Insulin to Reach A1c TargEt) trial, subjects treated with twice daily premixed insulin showed better hemoglobin A1C control, although experienced more hypoglycemic events, than those treated with once daily glargine, particularly when the pretreatment hemoglobin A1C was greater than 8.5%.[116] Another study compared initial treatment with basal only versus twice daily premix and found that the basal was safer and more effective.[117]

Another question about using premixed insulin is the number of times per day it should be administered. Many feel that the ideal frequency for biphasic insulin dosing is twice daily, but they actually can be given 1, 2, or 3 times daily. A trial looking at stepwise addition of premeal injections of biphasic insulin showed that there was some improvement with the first premeal injection, but the greatest improvement was when the second premeal injection was added.[118] Slightly greater improvement was seen when the third injection was added. There are limitations as to how aggressively you can adjust the fixed mixture insulin doses owing to the potential for hypoglycemia at certain times and inadequate coverage at others.[119]

Combined inulin degludec and aspart (IDegAsp), one of the newer formulations discussed previously, was compared in a number of studies with biphasic aspart 70/30. The investigators showed comparable glycemic control, but with significantly reduced rates of hypoglycemia.[120] As noted in this discussion, this is likely a reflection of the lower rates of hypoglycemia with insulin degludec compared with NPH, which provides the basal insulin effect in the older premixed insulin formulation. Thus, in clinical use, the effects of IDegAsp is likely to be similar to the "basal plus" treatment design— basal insulin plus 1 injection of rapid-acting insulin at 1 meal. At this writing, it is too soon to see how the usage of this biphasic insulin plays out in actual clinical practice, but, for a population where simplicity of treatment is key, it may be useful. Often these are people for whom safety is also a major concern and the improved safety profile compared with the previous premixed insulins could be a benefit. Still, the reduced flexibility of dosing and the upper limits to both the basal and prandial components in a single injection of this treatment may limit the aggressiveness of regimens that include this formulation.

Concentrated regular insulin (500 U/mL, regular U-500)

It is important to mention regular U-500 insulin. This concentrated form of the U-100 regular insulin that first came to market in 1952 in an animal formulation, has been available as a human recombinant insulin since 1994.[121,122] The increasing rates of obesity leading to extreme insulin resistance have created a therapeutic challenge that has been addressed by this more concentrated insulin.[70,71] Regular U-500 is recommended for use in patients requiring more than 200 U of insulin in a day.[121]

A clear advantage of regular U-500 over regular U-100 for severely insulin-resistant patients is the ability to deliver large doses with a single injection of a smaller volume, which will lead to needing fewer injections in a day improving patient adherence. Other proposed benefits are better absorption and longer duration of action compared with regular U-100.[123]

Recent euglycemic clamp studies evaluated pharmacokinetics and pharmacodynamics of the human form of this insulin. This randomized study of healthy subjects showed that both U-100 and U-500 regular insulins have a comparable action profile in terms of onset and bioavailability, but with a delayed, blunted, and prolonged peak and extended duration of the U-500 compared with U-100 formulation.[124]

Studies, including a pharmacodynamic modeling study and a randomized controlled trial, have attempted to clarify dosing titration and frequency.[124,125] Dose conversion to regular U-500 may be calculated as 80% or 100% of the total daily dose of basal and prandial insulins depending on the hemoglobin A1C and self-monitoring glucose levels.[123,125,126] It may be divided into either 2 or 3 premeal doses, using the prolonged duration of action to provide a basal insulin effect.[121,124,125] The distribution of the dose is frequently recommended to have a greater proportion of the dose administered as the first injection or within the first two-thirds of the day likely to decrease the risk of nocturnal hypoglycemia. Dosage adjustment algorithms based on self-monitoring glucose levels are readily available.[125,127]

For many years, regular U-500 was only available in a 20 mL vial containing 10,000 U of insulin without a syringe calibrated for its higher concentration. This lack of a designated administration device required dose conversion to be made by prescribers and patients to administer the insulin via either a tuberculin syringe or a U-100 insulin syringe. The potential for dangerous dosing errors was significant, and education and communication about syringe use was crucial.[21,121,128] However, recently this insulin has become available in a prefilled insulin pen dosed in actual units, thus requires no dose conversion for use.[122] This may ease fears and confusion allowing more patients who require it to use this insulin.

Basal insulin plus rapid-acting insulin at 1 or 2 meals: "basal plus"

Another option for advancement beyond the basal insulin only approach is the "basal plus" regimen.[89] With this approach, an injection of rapid-acting insulin is added to a basal-only program before one of the meals. This concept was been demonstrated effective a number of years ago. In 1 noncontrolled study, insulin glulisine was added before breakfast or before the main meal to insulin glargine and oral antidiabetes medications.[129] There was improvement in hemoglobin A1C, with no difference between breakfast and main meal injection times. Despite the lack of a control group in this study, the key point is that the concept of basal plus injection before 1 meal is a more convenient approach than basal/bolus with injections before all meals, and would be an appropriate consideration for people with type 2 diabetes inadequately controlled with basal insulin only. Subsequent studies have borne this out.[130]

The question of which meal to start with is an important one, but it does not seem to matter. The "Step-Wise" study (Comparison of the Efficacy and Safety of Two Different Dose Adjustment Regimens for Insulin Degludec/Insulin Aspart in Subjects With Type 2 Diabetes Mellitus Previously Treated With Insulin Glargine) compared the simpler addition of the first injection of rapid-acting insulin to the largest meal of the day with titration based on premeal values to a step requiring extra checking, adding the injection to the meal with the largest incremental glucose rise after eating, with titration based on those postmeal values.[131] Titration was conducted aiming for a hemoglobin A1C value of less than 7%, and injections at additional meals were added if that goal was not reached. Both groups showed comparable improvements. Thus, the simpler approach is a reasonable method of advancing therapy. Further, the greatest improvement in the hemoglobinA1C was seen with the addition of the first and second injections.

Full basal/bolus treatment programs

When adequate glycemic control cannot be safely achieved with any of the above programs, the advancement to full basal/bolus treatment is often needed.[88,89] Most guidelines have some variation on the same basic approach to designing these treatments:

- Use 50% of the total daily dose as the basal insulin;
- Use the other 50% given as premeal rapid-acting insulin before meals[132,133]; and
- The total daily dose is estimated as 0.3 to 0.5 U/kg; however this may be modified based on experience with previous insulin dosing.

A common mistake is to add a 3rd injection to a "basal plus" program using a large basal dose and 1 to 2 relatively small premeal rapid-acting insulin doses. The third mealtime dose quantity is often small and tentative, and the balance of basal to bolus is heavily weighted to the basal. Owing to the predominance of the basal insulin, hypoglycemic events have occurred and continued hypoglycemia can further the tentativeness of dose advancement. It is therefore often best to just convert to the 50/50 ratio, and then adjust further based on that as a starting point.

There are 2 ways to calculate the premeal rapid-acting insulin dosages.[132] One uses an insulin algorithm, which indicates an insulin dose based on the premeal glucose level. The other is the more sophisticated carbohydrate counting program, which determines the dose based on an estimate of the carbohydrate intake for that meal, adjusted for the level of the premeal glucose level, and may be further adjusted for activity and other confounding factors. The method of dosing of the premeal insulins is often determined the patient's individual lifestyle, day-to-day variability, intellectual levels, and self-care abilities.[134]

When calculating an algorithm, of the 50% of the daily dose allocated to the mealtime injections for use with an algorithm, it is often initially distributed as 40% before breakfast, 30% before lunch, and 30% before supper, based on a premeal glucose reading of about 100 to 150 mg/dL. Typically, the dose is increased by 1 to 2 U for each 50 mg/dL premeal glucose increment above that range, and similarly decreased below that range. However, determination of individual eating and glucose patterns often leads to modifications of this initial dosing formula. Once in use, additional adjustments can be made based on actual usage experience.

Carbohydrate counting has been increasingly the recommended system for determining the premeal rapid-acting insulin dose based on carbohydrate intake.

Carbohydrate is the food component that most affects blood glucose. As with the use of algorithms, such programs take into consideration the premeal glucose level by using a correction or sensitivity factor for dose adjustments to compensate for a high or low blood premeal glucose level. However, they also factor in the anticipated carbohydrate intake for that meal and use an insulin to carbohydrate ratio: 1 U of insulin for every x grams of carbohydrate to be consumed. Training patients to perform carbohydrate counting for dose determination usually requires an experienced registered dietitian. Some patients have functional barriers to successfully learning to use carbohydrate counting.[67]

A study conducted a few years ago compared the 2 approaches.[132] One group used an adjustment algorithm to determine premeal insulin doses based on glucose levels and the other group used carbohydrate counting. At the end of the 24-week study, both approaches achieved a hemoglobin A1C reduction of about 1.5%, with a trend toward less insulin use and less weight gain in the carbohydrate counting group. However, patients may become more involved in their care when using carbohydrate counting, and with significant variability in eating, this can be a useful approach owing to its added flexibility.

There are a number of calculations used to determine the dosing for carbohydrate counting.[135–137] Currently, a reasonable and simple, but not the only, formula is:

- To calculate the mealtime ratio's divide 450 (some prefer to use 500) by the total daily dose of insulin. Rounding to the nearest integer, call it x, that gives you the ratio, 1 U of rapid-acting insulin before the meal for every x grams of carbohydrate to be consumed.
- To calculate the sensitivity factor (some call it a correction factor), divide 1500 by the total daily dose of insulin and round to an easily worked with integer y. Then, determine a reasonable target glucose for that patient. Often 120 is used initially, but may be adjusted based on risk or fear of hypoglycemia or differing premeal glucose targets. Thus, for every y mg/dL a premeal glucose level is above the target {120}, add 1 U of rapid-acting insulin to the premeal quantity already determined by the carbohydrate estimate.
- Some people use a negative sensitivity factor as well: subtract 1 U of rapid-acting insulin for every y mg/dL below the target {120} that glucose value is.

There are many variations on this basic approach and, once initiated, most people need considerable adjustment based on actual usage date. Help from a dietitian experienced in the use of carbohydrate counting and training people to use it can be an important component of the treatment initiation phase of this treatment, and lack of such support can reflect one of the "systems barriers" that we discussed earlier.

How May Our New Insulins Impact These Treatment Regimens?

First, for any of the bolus insulin selections, the inhaled insulin (Afrezza) is an alternative to subcutaneous rapid-acting insulin injections for prandial mealtime coverage. However, it is important to note that it has a very rapid action with an onset of about 12 to 15 minutes, peaking at 60 minutes with a shorter duration of action of 2.5 to 3 hours.[68,79] The rapidity with which it acts is touted as its most notable feature; however, it may not provide a long enough duration of activity for a meal containing a higher fat content so a second postprandial dose may be necessary. The ability to inhale the insulin also provides an administration option that does not require giving an injection while out in public, but may require and toting around different cartridge sizes and multiple inhalations for a single dose.

The concentrated form of insulin lispro is another alternative for prandial coverage. Determination of the ideal candidate for this insulin may be less clear, because it is dosed in the same dosing increments and same maximal dose for a single injection as the standard concentration. However, it may allow a patient to use fewer insulin pens each month (accounting for less garbage for our environmentally conscious patients) and, anecdotally, may provide better absorption at higher individual doses allowing for better glucose coverage at similar dosing. An important note is that administration of lispro U-200 does not require any dosage conversion, unlike the concentrated version of regular insulin (Humulin R U-500), owing to the limited availability to adjust the appropriately calibrated prefilled insulin pen.[3] In mid 2016, a calibrated prefilled insulin pen of the concentrated U-500 regular insulin was also made available.[122] If used for administration, this insulin pen will also allow patients to avoid dosing conversions, because it is dosed in actual units. However, vials of this insulin are also still available without an appropriately calibrated unit-based administration device.

Will the newer basal insulins have a significant clinical impact? It is certainly possible based on the considerations discussed earlier. Key issues for people using basal/bolus regimens, particularly when carbohydrate counting and focused on daily variability in food consumption and activity levels, is the variability in the glycemic patterns from one day to the next. Some of that variability is likely lifestyle related, but some may reflect the day-to-day variability in insulin action noted. People tend to focus on insulin dose adjustments, but clinical experience often demonstrates that only increases the pattern variability and patient's frustration. If even a small amount of the day-to-day variability is reduced by using a basal insulin with more consistent action, then the ability to be more aggressive with insulin dose advancement while maintaining safety, and more precise with rapid-acting insulin adjustments could be more successful.

Another advantage of the newer basal insulins are a longer durations of action. Many of our patients have an inconsistent schedule and struggle administering their basal insulin at the exact frequency required to maintain the basal activity. Both glargine U-300 and insulin degludec have been studied in dosing intervals of longer than every 24 hours.[39,138] Thus, these options may offer more flexibility in dosing interval, with or without minimal impact on glycemic control, for our patients who struggle with schedules owing to shift work or have differing daily schedules.

The potential impact of these benefits, however, must be considered in the context of the potential increased cost of the new insulins. Many have decried the issue of costs, coverage, and copayments in pharmaceuticals in general, and insulin, in particular.[139] It is beyond the scope of this article to delve into the rationale for any pharmaceutical pricing policies; however, the adage that individualized decisions of cost effectiveness must be made, and having a sense for how to gauge the benefits may help with this task.

One important note of caution with the addition of more insulins, administration devices, and formulations to our armamentarium is the potential for prescribing or dispensing errors. As we have noted, 3 insulins are currently marketed in 2 different concentrations under the same proprietary name. As also mentioned, 1 concentrated insulin formulation is available in both a vial and a prefilled insulin pen. Ensuring that the correct formulation or product is selected for individual patients is of utmost importance, so care should be taken to avoid these errors both by prescribers and dispensers of these therapies.

SUMMARY

Insulin today as we know it has come a long way since its discovery in 1921. There have been many incremental steps since then, none of which individually may be considered monumental. However, taken in the aggregate, there has been a giant leap for people who require this therapy for their diabetes in the last 95 years. We have evolved from the antigen-laden impure animal extracts given in the early decades of the insulin era using cumbersome reusable syringes and needles, to the modern insulins with reduced antigenicity and increased purity, more precise in their ability to mimic natural insulin patterns and delivered using devices that are approaching painless, and having reached that milestone with the inhaled formulation. Yet with these advances come challenges for patients to accept and learn the self-administration of these insulins, and cost barriers that can prevent access for many people who might otherwise benefit from the improved pharmacology. Further, as we learn more about the impact of newer antidiabetes medications on the indication for insulin and how these medications, when used in combination with basal insulin, can impact treatment design,[105–111,140–143] the advancement protocols beyond treatment with basal insulin alone may evolve further.

Insulin treatment design decisions must therefore be made based on an individualized assessment all of these considerations so as to select the program and insulin(s) that are the optimal balance of all. That is where the art of medicine comes into play. We can pull data and assess the evidence, but ultimately, it is human beings talking to other human beings, guided by that evidence and data, making that personalized decision on how to design an insulin replacement program that makes treatment of diabetes challenging, and extremely interesting.

REFERENCES

1. Karamanou M, Protogerou A, Tsoucalas G, et al. Milestones in the history of diabetes mellitus: the main contributors. World J Diabetes 2016;7:1–7.
2. White Junod S. Celebrating a milestone: FDA's approval of first genetically-engineered product. Update Magazine, FDA Originally September-October 2007, Updated 2009. Available at: http://www.fda.gov/AboutFDA/WhatWeDo/History/ProductRegulation/SelectionsFromFDLIUpdateSeriesonFDAHistory/ucm081964.htm. Accessed March 22, 2016.
3. Humalog [package insert]. Indianapolis, IN: Eli Lilly & Co.; 2015.
4. Lantus [package insert]. Bridgewater, NJ: Sanofi-Aventis US LLC; 2015.
5. Riddle MC, Rosenstock J, Gerich J, et al. The treat-to-target trial: randomized addition of glargine or human NPH insulin to oral therapy of type 2 diabetic patients. Diabetes Care 2003;26:3080–6.
6. Hermansen K, Davies M, Derezinski T, et al. A 26-week, randomized, parallel, treat-to-target trial comparing insulin detemir with NPH insulin as add-on therapy to oral glucose-lowering drugs in insulin-naive people with type 2 diabetes. Diabetes Care 2006;29:1269–74.
7. Grunberger G. The need for better insulin therapy. Diabetes Obes Metab 2013; 15(Suppl 1):1–5.
8. Nathan DM, for the DCCT/EDIC Research Group. The diabetes control and complications trial/epidemiology of diabetes interventions and complications study at 30 years: overview. Diabetes Care 2014;37(1):9–16.
9. Garber AJ. Will the next generation of basal insulins offer clinical advantages? Diabetes Obes Metab 2014;16:483–91.
10. Eliaschewitz FG, Barreto T. Concepts and clinical use of ultra-long basal insulin. Diabetol Metab Syndr 2016;8:2.
11. DeVries JH, Nattrass M, Pieber TR. Refining basal insulin therapy: what have we learned in the age of analogues? Diabetes Metab Res Rev 2007;23:441–54.

12. de la Pena A, Riddle M, Morrow LA, et al. Pharmacokinetics and pharmacody-namics of high-dose human regular u-500 insulin versus human regular u-100 insulin in healthy obese subjects. Diabetes Care 2011;34:2496–501.

13. Dailey G, Lavernia F. A review of the safety and efficacy data for insulin glargine 300 units/ml, a new formulation of insulin glargine. Diabetes Obes Metab 2015; 17(12):1107–14.

14. Becker RA, Nowotny I, Teichert L, et al. Low within- and between-day variability in exposure to new insulin glargine 300u/mL. Diabetes Obes Metab 2015;17(3): 261–7.

15. Riddle MC, Bolli GB, Ziemen M, et al. New insulin glargine 300 units/ml versus glargine 100 units/ml in people with type 2 diabetes using basal and mealtime insulin: glucose control and hypoglycemia in a 6-month randomized controlled trial (EDITION 1). Diabetes Care 2014;37:2755–62.

16. Yki-Jarvinen H, Bergenstal R, Ziemen M, et al. New insulin glargine 300 units/ml versus glargine 100 units/ml in people with type 2 diabetes using oral agents and basal insulin: glucose control and hypoglycemia in a 6-month randomized controlled trial (EDITION 2). Diabetes Care 2014;37:3235–43.

17. Yki-Jarvinen H, Bergenstal RM, Bolli GB, et al. Glycaemic control and hypogly-caemia with new insulin glargine 300 u/ml versus insulin glargine 100 u/ml in people with type 2 diabetes using basal insulin and oral antihyperglycaemic drugs: the EDITION 2 randomized 12-month trial including 6-month extension. Diabetes Obes Metab 2015;17:1142–9.

18. Bolli GB, Riddle MC, Bergenstal RM, et al. New insulin glargine 300 U/ml compared with glargine 100 U/ml in insulin-naïve people with type 2 diabetes on oral glucose-lowering drugs: a randomized controlled trial (EDITION 3). Dia-betes Obes Metab 2015;17(4):386–94.

19. Home PD, Bergenstal RM, Bolli GB, et al. New insulin glargine 300 units/ml versus glargine 100 units/ml in people with type 1 diabetes: A randomized, phase 3a, open-label clinical trial (EDITION 4). Diabetes Care 2015;38:2217–25.

20. Ritzel R, Roussel R, Bolli GB, et al. Patient-level meta-analysis of the EDITION 1, 2 and 3 studies: glycaemic control and hypoglycaemia with new insulin glargine 300 U/ml versus glargine 100 U/ml in people with type 2 diabetes. Diabetes Obes Metab 2015;17(9):859–67.

21. Segal AR, El Sayed N. Are you ready for more insulin concentrations? J Diabetes Sci Technol 2015;9:331–8.

22. Toujeo [package insert]. Bridgewater, NJ: Sanofi-Aventis US LLC; 2015.

23. Heinemann L, Hompesch M. Biosimilar insulins: basic considerations. J Diabetes Sci Technol 2014;8(1):6–13.

24. Peters AL, Pollom RD, Zielonka JS, et al. Biosimilars and new insulin versions. Endocr Pract 2015;21(12):1387–94.

25. FDA: FDA approves basaglar, the first "follow-on" insulin glargine product to treat diabetes. FDA News Release, U.S. Food and Drug Administration, December 16, 2015. Available at: http://www.fda.gov/NewsEvents/Newsroom/ PressAnnouncements/ucm477734.htm. Accessed March 22, 2016.

26. Linnebjerg H, Lam EC, Seger ME, et al. Comparison of the pharmacokinetics and pharmacodynamics of ly2963016 insulin glargine and EU- and US-approved versions of lantus insulin glargine in healthy subjects: three random-ized euglycemic clamp studies. Diabetes Care 2015;38:2226–33.

27. Heise T, Zhang X, Quin Lam EC, et al. Duration of action of 2 insulin glargine products, LY2963016 and Lantus®, in subjects with type I diabetes mellitus (T1DM). Diabetes 2014;63(Suppl 1):891-P.

28. Blevins TC, Dahl D, Rosenstock J, et al. Efficacy and safety of LY2963016 insulin glargine compared with insulin glargine (Lantus®) in patients with type 1 diabetes in a randomized controlled trial: the ELEMENT 1 study. Diabetes Obes Metab 2015;17:726–33.

29. Rosenstock J, Hollander P, Bhargava A, et al. Similar efficacy and safety of LY2963016 insulin glargine and insulin glargine (Lantus®) in patients with type 2 diabetes who were insulin-naive or previously treated with insulin glargine: a randomized, double-blind controlled trial (the ELEMENT 2 study). Diabetes Obes Metab 2015;17:734–41.

30. Basaglar [package insert]. Indianapolis, IN: Lilly USA, LLC; 2015.

31. Mulcahy AW, Predmore Z, Mattke S. The cost savings potential of biosimilar drugs in the United States. Available at: https://www.rand.org/content/dam/rand/pubs/perspectives/PE100/PE127/RAND_PE127.pdf. Accessed March 22, 2016.

32. Heinemann L, Home PD, Hompesch M. Biosimilar insulins: guidance for data interpretation by clinicians and users. Diabetes Obes Metab 2015;17:911–8.

33. Tresiba [package insert]. Plainsboro, NJ: Novo Nordisk, Inc; 2015.

34. Ryzodeg [package insert]. Plainsboro, NJ: Novo Nordisk, Inc; 2015.

35. Jonassen I, Havelund S, Hoeg-Jensen T, et al. Design of the novel protraction mechanism of insulin degludec, an ultra-long-acting basal insulin. Pharm Res 2012;29:2104–14.

36. Heise T, Nosek L, Bøttcher, et al. Ultra-long-acting insulin degludec has a flat and stable glucose-lowering effect in type 2 diabetes. Diabetes Obes Metab 2012;14:944–50.

37. Haahr H, Heise T. A review of the pharmacological properties of insulin degludec and their clinical relevance. Clin Pharmacokinet 2014;53:787–800.

38. Heise T, Hermanski L, Nosek L, et al. Insulin degludec: four times lower pharmacodynamic variability than insulin glargine under steady-state conditions in type 1 diabetes. Diabetes Obes Metab 2012;14:859–64.

39. Mathieu C, Hollander P, Miranda-Palma B, et al. Efficacy and safety of insulin degludec in a flexible dosing regimen vs insulin glargine in patients with type 1 diabetes (BEGIN: Flex T1): a 26-week randomized, treat-to-target trial with a 26-week extension. J Clin Endocrinol Metab 2013;98(3):1154–62.

40. Ratner RE, Gough SC, Mathieu C, et al. Hypoglycaemia risk with insulin degludec compared with insulin glargine in type 2 and type 1 diabetes: a pre-planned meta-analysis of phase 3 trials. Diabetes Obes Metab 2013;15:175–84.

41. Vora J, Christensen T, Rana A, et al. Insulin degludec versus insulin glargine in type 1 and type 2 diabetes mellitus: a meta-analysis of endpoints in phase 3a trials. Diabetes Ther 2014;5:435–46.

42. Thuillier P, Alavi Z, Kerlan V. Long-term safety and efficacy of insulin degludec in the management of type 2 diabetes. Diabetes Metab Syndr Obes 2015;8: 483–93.

43. Gough SC, Harris S, Woo V, et al. Insulin degludec: overview of a novel ultra long-acting basal insulin. Diabetes Obes Metab 2013;15:301–9.

44. Vora J, Cariou B, Evans M, et al. Clinical use of insulin degludec. Diabetes Res Clin Pract 2015;109:19–31.

45. Novo Nordisk A/S: A trial comparing cardiovascular safety of insulin degludec versus insulin glargine in subjects with type 2 diabetes at high risk of cardiovascular events (DEVOTE), Available at: https://clinicaltrials.gov/ct2/show/NCT01959529. Accessed March 22, 2016.

46. Novo Nordisk A/S: Novo Nordisk receives US FDA approval for Tresiba® and Ryzodeg®, September, 25, 2015. Available at: https://globenewswire.com/news-release/2015/09/25/771147/0/en/Novo-Nordisk-receives-US-FDA-approval-for-Tresiba-and-Ryzodeg-70-30.html. Accessed March 22, 2016.

47. Korsatko S, Deller S, Koehler G, et al. A comparison of the steady-state pharmacokinetic and pharmacodynamic profiles of 100 and 200 u/ml formulations of ultra-long-acting insulin degludec. Clin Drug Investig 2013;33:515–21.

48. Bode BW, Chaykin LB, Sussman AM, et al. Efficacy and safety of insulin degludec 200 u/ml and insulin degludec 100 u/ml in patients with type 2 diabetes (BEGIN: COMPARE). Endocr Pract 2014;20:785–91.

49. Gough SC, Bhargava A, Jain R, et al. Low-volume insulin degludec 200 units/ml once daily improves glycemic control similarly to insulin glargine with a low risk of hypoglycemia in insulin-naive patients with type 2 diabetes: a 26-week, randomized, controlled, multinational, treat-to-target trial: the BEGIN LOW VOLUME trial. Diabetes Care 2013;36:2536–42.

50. Warren M, Chaykin LB, Jabbour S, et al. Efficacy, patient-reported outcomes (PRO), and safety of insulin degludec U200 vs. insulin glargine in patients with type 2 diabetes (T2D) requiring high-dose insulin [Abstract]. Diabetes 2015;64(Suppl 1):A266.

51. Dardano A, Bianchi C, Del Prato S, et al. Insulin degludec/insulin aspart combination for the treatment of type 1 and type 2 diabetes. Vasc Health Risk Manag 2014;10:465–75.

52. Heise T, Tack CJ, Cuddihy R, et al. A new-generation ultra-long-acting basal insulin with a bolus boost compared with insulin glargine in insulin-naive people with type 2 diabetes: A randomized, controlled trial. Diabetes Care 2011;34:669–74.

53. Niskanen L, Leiter LA, Franek E, et al. Comparison of a soluble co-formulation of insulin degludec/insulin aspart vs biphasic insulin aspart 30 in type 2 diabetes: a randomised trial. Eur J Endocrinol 2012;167:287–94.

54. Onishi Y, Ono Y, Rabol R, et al. Superior glycaemic control with once-daily insulin degludec/insulin aspart versus insulin glargine in Japanese adults with type 2 diabetes inadequately controlled with oral drugs: a randomized, controlled phase 3 trial. Diabetes Obes Metab 2013;15:826–32.

55. Hirsch IB, Bode B, Courreges JP, et al. Insulin degludec/insulin aspart administered once daily at any meal, with insulin aspart at other meals versus a standard basal-bolus regimen in patients with type 1 diabetes: a 26-week, phase 3, randomized, open-label, treat-to-target trial. Diabetes Care 2012;35:2174–81.

56. Xultophy [package insert]. Bagsvaerd, Denmark: Novo Nordisk A/S; 2014.

57. Gough SC, Bode B, Woo V, et al. Efficacy and safety of a fixed-ratio combination of insulin degludec and liraglutide (IDegLira) compared with its components given alone: results of a phase 3, open-label, randomised, 26-week, treat-to-target trial in insulin-naive patients with type 2 diabetes. Lancet Diabetes Endocrinol 2014;2:885–93.

58. Linjawi S, Bode BW, Chaykin LB, et al. Efficacy and safety of IDegLira (combination of insulin degludec + liraglutide), in insulin naïve patients with T2D uncontrolled on GLP-1 receptor agonist (GLP-1 RA) therapy. Diabetes 2015;64(Suppl 1):A255.

59. Rodbard HW, Bode BW, Harris SB, et al. IDegLira in insulin-naïve patients with type 2 diabetes (T2D) inadequately controlled on sulfonylureas (SU) alone or in combination with metformin: the DUAL IV study. Diabetes 2015;64(Suppl 1):A255–6.

60. Buse JB, Vilsboll T, Thurman J, et al. Contribution of liraglutide in the fixed-ratio combination of insulin degludec and liraglutide (IDegLira). Diabetes Care 2014; 37:2926–33.

61. Buse JB, Pérez Manghi FC, Garcia-Hernandez PA, et al. Insulin degludec/liraglutide (IDegLira) is superior to insulin glargine (IG) in A1C reduction, risk of hypoglycemia and weight change: DUAL V study [Abstract]. Diabetes 2015; 64(Suppl 1):A43.

62. Curry D, Bennett L, Grodsky G. Dynamics of insulin secretion by the perfused rat pancreas. Endocrinology 1968;83:572–84.

63. Heinemann L, Muchmore DB. Ultrafast-acting insulins: state of the art. J Diabetes Sci Technol 2012;6:728–42.

64. Polonsky KS, Given BD, Van Cauter E. Twenty-four-hour profiles and pulsatile patterns of insulin secretion in normal and obese subjects. J Clin Investig 1988;81(2):442–8.

65. Gerich JE. Is reduced first-phase insulin release the earliest detectable abnormality in individuals destined to develop type 2 diabetes? Diabetes 2002; 51(Suppl 1):S117–21.

66. Monnier L, Lapinski H, Colette C. Contributions of fasting and postprandial plasma glucose increments to the overall diurnal hyperglycemia of type 2 diabetic patients: variations with increasing levels of HbA1c. Diabetes Care 2003;26(3):881–5.

67. Beaser RS. Designing and managing insulin replacement programs. In: Beaser RS, Staff of Joslin Diabetes Center, editors. Joslin's Diabetes Deskbook: a guide for primary care providers. 3rd edition. Boston: Joslin Diabetes Center; 2014. p. 349–456.

68. Boss AH, Petrucci R, Lorber D. Coverage of prandial insulin requirements by means of an ultra-rapid-acting inhaled insulin. J Diabetes Sci Technol 2012; 6(4):773–9.

69. Wilde MI, McTavish D. Insulin lispro: a review of its pharmacological properties and therapeutic use in the management of diabetes mellitus. Drugs 1997;54: 597–614.

70. Ng M, Fleming T, Robinson M, et al. Global, regional, and national prevalence of overweight and obesity in children and adults during 1980-2013: a systematic analysis for the global burden of disease study 2013. Lancet 2014;384:766–81.

71. Kahn BB, Flier JS. Obesity and insulin resistance. J Clin Invest 2000;106: 473–81.

72. Danne T, Heinemann L, Bolinder J. New insulins, biosimilars, and insulin therapy. Diabetes Technol Ther 2016;18(Suppl 1):S43–55.

73. de la Peña A, Seger M, Soon D, et al. Bioequivalence and comparative pharmacodynamics of insulin lispro 200 U/mL relative to insulin lispro (Humalog®) 100 U/mL. Clin Pharmacol Drug Dev 2016;5(1):69–75.

74. Mack GS. Pfizer dumps exubera. Nat Biotechnol 2007;25:1331–2.

75. Inhaled human insulin. new drug. no short-term advantages, too many unknowns in the long term. Prescrire Int 2006;15:203–9.

76. Inhaled insulin no longer marketed. discontinuation. welcome news. Prescrire Int 2008;17:139.

77. Afrezza [package insert]. Danbury, CT: MannKind Corporation; 2014.

78. Potocka E, Cassidy JP, Haworth P, et al. Pharmacokinetic characterization of the novel pulmonary delivery excipient fumaryl diketopiperazine. J Diabetes Sci Technol 2010;4:1164–73.

79. Rave K, Heise T, Heinemann L, et al. Inhaled technosphere® insulin in comparison to subcutaneous regular human insulin: time action profile and variability in subjects with type 2 diabetes. J Diabetes Sci Technol 2008;2(2):205–12.

80. Bode BW, McGill JB, Lorber DL, et al. Affinity 1 study G: inhaled technosphere insulin compared with injected prandial insulin in type 1 diabetes: a randomized 24-week trial. Diabetes Care 2015;38:2266–73.

81. Rosenstock J, Franco D, Korpachev V, et al. Affinity 2 Study G: Inhaled technosphere insulin versus inhaled technosphere placebo in insulin-naive subjects with type 2 diabetes inadequately controlled on oral antidiabetes agents. Diabetes Care 2015;38:2274–81.

82. Afrezza FL. (insulin human) inhalation powder approved for the treatment of patients with type 1 or type 2 diabetes. Am Health Drug Benefits 2015;8:40–3.

83. Nelson LS, Loh M, Perrone J. Assuring safety of inherently unsafe medications: the FDA risk evaluation and mitigation strategies. J Med Toxicol 2014;10(2): 165–72.

84. FDA: Nda 022472 afrezza® (insulin human) inhalation powder - risk evaluation and mitigation strategy (REMS), U.S. Food and Drug Administration, 2015. Available at: http://www.accessdata.fda.gov/drugsatfda_docs/rems/Afrezza_2015.04. 20_REMS%20Factsheet.pdf. Accessed March 22, 2016.

85. Funnell MM. Overcoming barriers to the initiation of insulin therapy. Clin Diabetes 2007;25:36–8.

86. Funnell MM, Kruger DF, Spencer M. Self-management support for insulin therapy in type 2 diabetes. Diabetes Educ 2004;30:274–80.

87. American Diabetes Association. 5. Glycemic targets in 2016 Standards of Care. Diabetes Care 2016;39(Suppl 1):S39–46.

88. Garber AJ, Abrahamson MJ, Barzilay JI, et al. Consensus statement by the American Association of Clinical Endocrinologists and American College of Endocrinology on the comprehensive type 2 diabetes management algorithm –2016 executive summary. Endocr Pract 2016;22(1):84–113.

89. American Diabetes Association. Approaches to glycemia treatment in 2016 Standards of Care. Diabetes Care 2016;39(Suppl 1):S52–9.

90. The Diabetes Control and Complications Trial Research Group. The effect of intensive treatment of diabetes on the development and progression of long-term complications in insulin dependent diabetes mellitus. N Engl J Med 1993;329:977–86.

91. Nathan DM, Cleary PA, Backlund J-YC, et al. Intensive diabetes treatment and cardiovascular disease in patients with type 1 diabetes. N Engl J Med 2005;353: 2643–53.

92. Wallia A, Molitch ME. Insulin therapy for type 2 diabetes mellitus. JAMA 2014; 311:2315–25.

93. Bosi E, Scavini M, Ceriello A, et al. Intensive structured self-monitoring of blood glucose and glycemic control in noninsulin-treated type 2 diabetes: the PRISMA randomized trial. Diabetes Care 2013;36(10):2887–94.

94. Polonsky WH, Fisher L, Schikman C, et al. Structured self-monitoring of blood glucose significantly reduces A1C levels in poorly controlled, noninsulin-treated type 2 diabetes. Diabetes Care 2011;34:262–7.

95. Miller KM, Beck RW, Bergenstal RM, et al. Evidence of a strong association between frequency of self-monitoring of blood glucose and hemoglobin A1C levels in T1D Exchange clinic registry participants. Diabetes Care 2013;36:2009–14.

96. Ismail-Beigi F, Moghissi E, Tiktin M, et al. Individualizing glycemic targets in type 2 diabetes mellitus: implications of recent clinical trials. Ann Intern Med 2011; 154(8):554–9.

97. Powers MA, Davidson J, Bergenstal RM. Glucose pattern management teaches glycemia-related problem-solving skills in a diabetes self-management education program. Diabetes Spectr 2013;26:91–7.

98. Inzucchi SE, Bergenstal RM, Buse JB, et al. Management of hyperglycemia in type 2 diabetes, 2015: a patient-centered approach. update to a position statement of the American Diabetes Association and the European Association for the Study of Diabetes. Diabetes Care 2015;38:140–9.

99. Weng J, Li Y, Xu W, et al. Effect of intensive insulin therapy on beta-cell function and glycaemic control in patients with newly diagnosed type 2 diabetes: A multicentre randomised parallel-group trial. Lancet 2008;371:1753–60.

100. Hu Y, Li L, Xu Y, et al. Short-term intensive therapy in newly diagnosed type 2 diabetes partially restores both insulin sensitivity and β-cell function in subjects with long-term remission. Diabetes Care 2011;34(8):1848–53.

101. Alvarsson M, Berntorp K, Fernqvist-Forbes E, et al. Effects of insulin versus sulphonylurea on beta-cell secretion in recently diagnosed type 2 diabetes patients: a 6-year follow-up study. Rev Diabet Stud 2010;7(3):225–32.

102. Blonde L, Merilainen M, Karwe V, et al. Patient-directed titration for achieving glycaemic goals using a once-daily basal insulin analogue: an assessment of two different fasting plasma glucose targets - the TITRATE study. Diabetes Obes Metab 2009;11:623–31.

103. Rosenstock J, Dailey G, Massi-Benedetti M, et al. Reduced hypoglycemia risk with insulin glargine: a meta-analysis comparing insulin glargine with human NPH insulin in type 2 diabetes. Diabetes Care 2005;28:950–5.

104. Home PD, Fritsche A, Schinzel A, et al. Meta-analysis of individual patient data to assess the risk of hypoglycaemia in people with type 2 diabetes using NPH insulin or insulin glargine. Diabetes Obes Metab 2010;12:772–9.

105. Balena R, Hensley IE, Miller S, et al. Combination therapy with GLP-1 receptor agonists and basal insulin: a systematic review of the literature. Diabetes Obes Metab 2013;15:485–502.

106. Thong KY, Jose B, Sukumar N, et al. Safety, efficacy and tolerability of exenatide in combination with insulin in the Association of British Clinical Diabetologists nationwide exenatide audit. Diabetes Obes Metab 2011;13:703–10.

107. Levin PA, Mersey JH, Zhou S, et al. Clinical outcomes using long-term combination therapy with insulin glargine and exenatide in patients with type 2 diabetes. Endocr Pract 2012;18:17–25.

108. Eng C, Kramer CK, Xinman B, et al. Glucagon-like peptide-1 receptor agonist and basal insulin combination treatment for the management of type 2 diabetes: a systematic review and meta-analysis. Lancet 2014;384:2228–34.

109. Holst JJ, Visboll T. Combining GLP-1 receptor agonists with insulin: therapeutic rationales and clinical findings. Diabetes Obes Metab 2013;15:3–14.

110. Viswanathan P, Chaudhuri A, Bhatia R, et al. Exenatide therapy in obese patients with type 2 diabetes mellitus treated with insulin. Endocr Pract 2007;13: 444–50.

111. Nayak UA, Govindan J, Baskar V, et al. Exenatide therapy in insulin-treated type 2 diabetes and obesity. QJM 2010;103:687–94.

112. Phillips S, Gulbranson N, Kabadi U. Marked improvement in glycemic control with exenatide (Byetta®) on addition to metformin, sulfonylurea and insulin glargine in type 2 diabetes mellitus [Abstract]. Diabetes 2011;60(Suppl 1):A614.

113. Diamant M, Nauck MA, Shaginian R, et al. Glucagon-like peptide 1 receptor agonist or bolus insulin with optimized basal insulin in type 2 diabetes. Diabetes Care 2014;37(10):2763–73.

114. Rosenstock J, Fonseca VA, Gross JL, et al. Advancing basal insulin replacement in type 2 diabetes inadequately controlled with insulin glargine plus oral agents: a comparison of adding albiglutide, a weekly GLP-1 receptor agonist, versus thrice-daily prandial insulin lispro. Diabetes Care 2014;37(8):2317–25.

115. Rosenstock J, Diamant M, Silvestre L, et al. Benefits of a fixed-ratio formulation of once-daily insulin glargine/lixisenatide (LixiLan) vs glargine in type 2 diabetes inadequately controlled on metformin [Abstract]. Diabetologia 2014;57(Suppl 1):A241.

116. Raskin P, Allen E, Hollander P, et al. Initiating insulin therapy in type 2 diabetes: a comparison of biphasic and basal insulin analogs. Diabetes Care 2005;28(2): 260–5.

117. Janka HU, Plewe G, Riddle MC, et al. Comparison of basal insulin added to oral agents versus twice-daily premixed insulin as initial insulin therapy for type 2 diabetes. Diabetes Care 2005;28:254–9.

118. Garber AJ, Wahlen J, Wahl T, et al. Attainment of glycaemic goals in type 2 diabetes with once-, twice-, or thrice-daily dosing with biphasic insulin aspart 70/30 (The 1-2-3 study). Diabetes Obes Metab 2006;8:58–66.

119. Fritsche A, Larbig M, Owens D, et al. Comparison between a basal-bolus and a premixed insulin regimen in individuals with type 2 diabetes–results of the GINGER study. Diabetes Obes Metab 2010;12:115–23.

120. Fulcher GR, Christiansen JS, Gantwal G, et al. Comparison of insulin degludec/insulin aspart and biphasic insulin aspart 30 in uncontrolled, insulin-treated type 2 diabetes: a phase 3a, randomized, treat-to-target trial. Diabetes Care 2014; 37:2084–90.

121. Segal AR, Brunner JE, Burch FT, et al. Use of concentrated insulin human regular (U-500) for patients with diabetes. Am J Health Syst Pharm 2010;67: 1526–35.

122. Humulin R U-500 [package insert]. Indianapolis, IN: Lilly USA, LLC; 2016.

123. Lane W, Cochran E, Jackson J, et al. High-dose insulin therapy: is it time for U-500 insulin? Endocr Pract 2009;15(1):71–9.

124. de la Peña A, Ma X, Reddy S, et al. Application of PK/PD modeling and simulation to dosing regimen optimization of high-dose human regular U-500 insulin. J Diabetes Sci Technol 2014;8:821–9.

125. Hood RC, Arakaki RF, Wysham C, et al. Two treatment approaches for human regular U-500 insulin in patients with type 2 diabetes not achieving adequate glycemic control on high-dose U-100 insulin therapy with or without oral agents: a randomized, titration-to-target clinical trial. Endocr Pract 2015;21(7):782–93.

126. Reutrakul S, Wroblewski K, Brown RL. Clinical use of U-500 regular insulin: review and meta-analysis. J Diabetes Sci Technol 2012;6(2):412–20.

127. Ballani P, Tran MT, Navar MD, et al. Clinical experience with U-500 regular insulin in obese, markedly insulin-resistant type 2 diabetic patients. Diabetes Care 2006;29:2504–5 [Erratum appears in Diabetes Care 2007;30:455].

128. Shastay A. As U-500 insulin safety concerns mount, it's time to rethink safe use of strengths above u-100. Home Healthc Now 2015;33:501–2.

129. Lankisch MR, Ferlinz KC, Leahy JL, et al. Introducing a simplified approach to insulin therapy in type 2 diabetes: a comparison of two single-dose regimens of insulin glulisine plus insulin glargine and oral antidiabetic drugs. Diabetes Obes Metab 2008;10:1178–85.

130. Owens DR, Luzio SD, Sert-Langeron C, et al. Effects of initiation and titration of a single pre-prandial dose of insulin glulisine while continuing titrated insulin glargine in type 2 diabetes: a 6-month 'proof-of-concept' study. Diabetes Obes Metab 2011;13:1020–7.

131. Meneghini L, Mersebach H, Kumar S, et al. Comparison of 2 intensification regimens with rapid-acting insulin aspart in type 2 diabetes mellitus inadequately controlled by once-daily insulin detemir and oral antidiabetes drugs: the Step-Wise randomized study. Endocr Pract 2011;17:727–36.

132. Bergenstal RM, Johnson M, Powers MA, et al. Adjust to target in type 2 diabetes: comparison of a simple algorithm with carbohydrate counting for adjustment of mealtime insulin glulisine. Diabetes Care 2008;31(7):1305–10.

133. De Leeuw I, Vague P, Selam JL, et al. Insulin detemir used in basal-bolus therapy in people with type 1 diabetes is associated with a lower risk of nocturnal hypoglycaemia and less weight gain over 12 months in comparison to NPH insulin. Diabetes Obes Metab 2005;7:73–82.

134. American Diabetes Association. 3 Foundations of Care and Comprehensive Medical Evaluation in 2016 Standards of Care. Diabetes Care 2016;39(Suppl 1):S23–35.

135. Davidson PC, Hebblewhite HR, Steed RD, et al. Analysis of guidelines for basal-bolus insulin dosing: basal insulin, correction factor, and carbohydrate-to-insulin ratio. Endocr Pract 2008;14:1095–101.

136. Walsh J, Roberts R, Bailey T. Guidelines for insulin dosing in continuous subcutaneous insulin infusion using new formulas from a retrospective study of individuals with optimal glucose levels. J Diabetes Sci Technol 2010;4:1174–81.

137. Walsh J, Roberts R, Varma C, et al. Using insulin. San Diego (CA): Torrey Pines Press; 2003.

138. Riddle MC, Bolli GB, Home PD, et al. New insulin glargine 300 U/mL: efficacy and safety of adaptable vs. fixed dosing intervals in people with T2DM. [Abstract] American Diabetes Association. Available at: http://ada.scientificposters.com/epsAbstrasctADA.cfm?id=6. Accessed March 22, 2016.

139. Hirsch IB. Diabetes care entering 2015: ineffective ranting. Diabetes Technol Ther 2015;17:69–71.

140. Inzucchi SE, Tunceli K, Qui Y, et al. Progression to insulin therapy among patients with type 2 diabetes treated with sitagliptin or sulphonylurea plus metformin dual therapy. Diabetes Obes Metab 2015;17:956–64.

141. Neal B, Perkovic V, de Zeeuw D, et al, CANVAS Trial Collaborative Group. Efficacy and safety of canagliflozin, an inhibitor of sodium-glucose cotransporter 2, when used in conjunction with insulin therapy in patients with type 2 diabetes. Diabetes Care 2015;38:403–11.

142. Rosenstock J, Jelaska A, Zeller C, et al. Impact of empagliflozin added on to basal insulin in type 2 diabetes inadequately controlled on basal insulin: a 78-week randomized, double-blind, placebo-controlled trial. Diabetes Obes Metab 2015;17:936–48.

143. Munshi MN, Slyne C, Segal AR, et al. Simplification of insulin regimen in older adults improved risk of hypoglycemia without compromising glycemic control. JAMA Intern Med 2016;176:1023–5.

Inpatient Diabetes Management in the Twenty-First Century

Natasha B. Khazai, MD*, Osama Hamdy, MD, PhD

KEYWORDS

- Inpatient diabetes management • Inpatient insulin management • Hospital
- Diabetes • Hyperglycemia • Corticosteroids • Enteral and parenteral nutrition
- Insulin pump

KEY POINTS

- In hospitalized critically ill and noncritically ill patients both hyperglycemia and hypoglycemia are associated with poor outcomes.
- Insulin in the form of long-acting, basal insulin and fast but short-acting nutritional and corrective insulin should be used in hospitalized patients with diabetes.
- The total daily insulin dose for each patient depends on their outpatient diabetes regimen, their hemoglobin A1c level before admission, current mode and state of nutrition, and presence or absence of corticosteroids.
- Computerized provider insulin order entry and the live availability of patients' glucose levels can greatly aid in optimizing glycemic management in the hospital.

RATIONALE

In hospitalized patients, both hyperglycemia and hypoglycemia have been associated with poor outcomes. During the inpatient period, hyperglycemia has been associated with increased risk of infection,[1,2] cardiovascular events,[3–5] and mortality.[6,7] It is also associated with longer length of hospital stay.[3,8,9] Hypoglycemia has also been associated with an increased risk of mortality.[10] Therefore, current evidence supports avoidance of both conditions among hospitalized patients whether they are admitted to critical care units or noncritical care units.[5,9,11]

GLUCOSE TARGETS IN NONCRITICALLY ILL PATIENTS

Unfortunately, because of the limited number of trials, optimal blood glucose (BG) targets are still debated.[12] Glucose targets recommended by the consensus guidelines

The authors have nothing to disclose.
Joslin Diabetes Center, Boston, MA, USA
* Corresponding author. Joslin Diabetes Center, One Joslin Place, Boston, MA 02215.
E-mail address: natasha.khazai@joslin.harvard.edu

Endocrinol Metab Clin N Am 45 (2016) 875–894
http://dx.doi.org/10.1016/j.ecl.2016.06.013
0889-8529/16/© 2016 Elsevier Inc. All rights reserved.

endo.theclinics.com

issued jointly by the American Diabetes Association (ADA) and the American Association of Clinical Endocrinologists (AACE)[9] and separately by the Endocrine Society[5] are shown in **Table 1**. Higher BG targets can be set for those who are prone to hypoglycemia, have severe comorbidities, or are terminally ill.[11] However, even then, it is recommended that BG be kept less than 200 mg/dL in order to avoid symptomatic hyperglycemia.[11] The basal-bolus insulin doses should be reduced if BG decreases to less than 100 mg/dL, unless patients are clinically stable and had tight control before admission.[11]

DIABETES MANAGEMENT FOR NONCRITICALLY ILL HOSPITALIZED PATIENTS

In all patients with diabetes, hemoglobin A1c (A1C) should be checked on admission unless patients have a value within the past 3 months.[5,9,11] For patients without diabetes, who have random BG level exceeding 140 mg/dL whether in the emergency department or during hospitalization, A1C should be checked. If A1C is 6.5% or greater, it strongly suggests that diabetes preceded hospitalization.[11] If random BG is greater than 140 mg/dL but A1C is 6.4 or less, diabetes diagnosis cannot be totally excluded and an oral glucose tolerance test should be ordered after discharge.

Involvement of a diabetes educator early in the course of admission will help newly diagnosed patients learn essential skills such as glucose monitoring, prevention and management of hypoglycemia, and proper intake of oral antihyperglycemic medications.[9,11] The same is true for patients starting insulin for the first time, whereby involvement of a diabetes educator not only ensures they receive instructions and have hands-on practice on proper insulin injection technique but also may identify barriers to self-management, such as poor patient dexterity that precludes insulin self-administration. Knowledge of such barriers will allow for early involvement and teaching of the patients' caregiver or, if needed, a change in the patients' diabetes discharge plan to one that either the patients or their caregivers are able to execute. Early identification and management of these issues ensure safe and timely discharge.[13]

Medical Nutrition Therapy

Medical nutrition therapy is important for both outpatient and inpatient diabetes management. All patients with diabetes should be on a balanced, hypocaloric, and carbohydrate-consistent diet. If enteral nutrition is used, a diabetes-specific formula is preferred over standard formula. Carbohydrate consistency helps in proper matching of prandial insulin with carbohydrate content of the meals.[8] Carbohydrates should be from whole grains, vegetables, fruits, and low-fat dairy with restricted amounts of added sugar and sucrose-containing foods.[14]

Oral Antihyperglycemic Medications and Glucagon Like Peptide-1 Receptor Agonists

The most recent guidelines from the ADA, AACE, and Endocrine Society recommend against the inpatient use of oral antihyperglycemic medications or

Table 1		
Blood glucose targets in inpatient setting for noncritically ill patients		
Random or Bedtime	**Fasting and Premeal**	**Hypoglycemia**
<180 mg/dL	100–140 mg/dL	<70 mg/dL

Data from Moghissi ES, Korytkowski MT, DiNardo M, et al. American Association of Clinical Endocrinologists and American Diabetes Association consensus statement on inpatient glycemic control. Diabetes Care 2009;32(6):1119–31.

glucagonlike peptide-1 receptor agonists (GLP-1 RA) because of the lack of efficacy studies and because of safety issues.[5,9,11] Metformin use in hospitalized patients may potentially lead to lactic acidosis, in the event of continued use during renal insufficiency, sepsis, hypotension, or a hypoxic state, such as heart failure. Sulfonylureas are associated with an increased risk of hypoglycemia, especially on unpredicted discontinuation of patients' diet oral feeding (nothing by mouth). In case of declining renal function, hypoglycemia due to sulfonylureas may become severe and protracted. A few studies investigating the use of among hospitalized patients with type 2 diabetes showed noninferior glycemic control and hypoglycemic event rates, when compared basal-bolus insulin.[15] However, these therapies often need additional basal insulin therapy to maintain optimal glycemic control. GLP-1 RA therapies are associated with early gastrointestinal side effects, such as nausea and vomiting, in up to 66% of patients. These side effects are specifically undesirable in already anorexic patients or in patients who are sedated, as they put them at higher risk for aspiration pneumonia.[16] Hospitalized patients may continue their oral medications and/or GLP-1 RA only if they meet all the criteria listed in **Box 1**, while taking into consideration all the precautions listed in **Box 2**. All other patients should be treated with insulin. It needs to be noted that if oral agents are held, the treating physician should have a plan to resume them 1 to 2 days before discharge to ensure their efficacy and safety.[11]

Insulin

Patients with established or newly diagnosed diabetes and a good nutrition plan should be started on long-acting basal insulin plus rapid-acting bolus insulin for meals and correction of hyperglycemia while in the hospital.[5,9] Those who have poor nutritional intake or who are taking nothing by mouth should receive basal insulin along with corrective doses of rapid-acting insulin.[9,15] Once they resume nutritional intake, a safe step can be administering nutritional (bolus) insulin right after patients eat in order to allow for better matching of insulin with actual carbohydrate intake.[11] Patients who are well trained and use carbohydrate counting should have the option to continue using the same outpatient insulin to carbohydrate ratio to calculate their nutritional insulin needs for each meal. The use of sliding-scale (corrective) insulin alone without basal and nutritional insulin is strongly discouraged (except in select cases, **Table 2**), with strong evidence showing its inferior performance compared

---

Box 1
Criteria for continuing oral antihyperglycemic medications and glucagonlike peptide-1 receptor agonists during hospital admission

- Low risk, stable patient
- A1C <8%
- Eating greater than 50% of diet
- Expected discharge within 24 to 48 hours
- No plans for contrast studies
- No acute renal failure
- No steroid therapy
- No infection

Box 2
Cautions for use of oral antihyperglycemic medications and glucagonlike peptide-1 receptor agonists during hospital admission

Metformin

- Discontinue if Cr is greater than 1.4 mg/dL and/or eGFR is less than 60 mL/min per 1.73 m^2
- Hold for 48 hours after IV contrast study and check renal function daily for 2 days[17]
- Discontinue in hypoxic states (CHF, COPD exacerbation, sepsis)
- Discontinue if patients have liver disease

Sulfonylurea

- Discontinue if patients have renal acute or chronic insufficiency
- Discontinue if patients are made NPO

Pioglitazone

- Discontinue if patients have CHF or lower extremity edema

GLP-1 RA

- Discontinue if patients develop pancreatitis, nausea, or vomiting

Abbreviations: CHF, congestive heart failure; Cr, creatinine; COPD, chronic obstructive pulmonary disease; eGFR, estimated glomerular filtration rate; IV, intravenous.

---

with a basal-nutritional-corrective regimen.[18] The basal, bolus, and corrective insulin dose for each patient depends on several factors. These factors include the presence or absence of diabetes, type of diabetes, admission A1C level, and how diabetes was managed before admission. It is expected that patients with type 2 diabetes who are well controlled on oral medications as outpatients will need a smaller total daily dose (TDD) of insulin compared with patients with type 2 diabetes who are poorly controlled on insulin as outpatients. Suggested guidelines for calculating TDD of insulin are summarized in **Table 2**.[5,9,19,20] It needs to be stressed that similar to an outpatient setting, inpatient diabetes management also needs individualization for each patient and that the suggested calculations should only serve as starting points. Of note, for patients who are inadequately controlled (A1C >10%) on oral antihyperglycemic medications with or without GLP-1 RA as outpatients, basal insulin will likely be added to their

Table 2
Calculation of total daily dose of insulin

Patient and Glycemic Profile	TDD U/kg of Body Weight
Oral agents or lifestyle therapy as outpatient, A1C <7% Newly diagnosed patients, A1C <7%	Consider corrective insulin only If BG is consistently >140 mg/dL, add basal insulin (0.1 U/kg body weight)
Oral agents as outpatient, A1C 7.0%–7.9% Any treatment and aged ≥70 y and/or eGFR <60 mL/min per 1.73 m^{2}[21]	0.2–0.3 U/kg body weight
Any DM with BG 140–200 mg/dL or admission A1C <10%	0.4 U/kg body weight
Any DM with BG 200–400 mg/dL or admission A1C ≥10%	0.5 U/kg body weight

outpatient diabetes regimen on discharge. Early involvement of a diabetes educator for insulin teaching is strongly advised for those patients. Patients who were well controlled on basal and nutritional insulin as outpatients can continue on their home dose of basal insulin. It is recommended to reduce home doses of their nutritional insulin by 25% to 50% initially to avoid hypoglycemia in case the carbohydrate content in their hospital meals is significantly less than their diet at home. On the other hand, patients who were adherent to their insulin regimen at home but were poorly controlled (A1C >10%) should have their TDD calculated based on **Table 2**. If the calculated TDD is lower than what they were using at home, they should be started on their outpatient regimen with daily up-titration of their TDD based on BG response in the hospital. Frequently, poor outpatient control among those patients is related to poor dietary adherence. This poor dietary adherence is mostly eliminated in the hospital with institution of a calorie-restricted, carbohydrate-consistent diet. Calculation of basal, nutritional, and corrective insulin doses based on TDD is outlined in **Table 3**. It was shown that patients with renal insufficiency (estimated glomerular filtration rate <60 mL/min/1.73 m^2) who started on glargine or detemir insulin using a lower multiplier of 0.2 (instead of 0.5) multiplied by the patients' body weight had reduced incidence of hypoglycemia by around 50%.[21]

Adjusting Basal and Bolus (Nutritional) Insulin

When adjusting insulin doses, one has to take into account the patients' clinical status, concomitant medications (see Glucocorticoid section), BG values, individualized glucose targets, and nutritional status (see Enteral and Parenteral section) among other factors.[9] Insulin adjustment, therefore, is a highly individualized process. Some guidelines that are commonly used for adjusting basal and nutritional insulin, along with examples to help highlight these guidelines, are shown in **Table 4**.

Computerized Provider Insulin Order Entry

Computerized provider order entry (CPOE) for insulin has shown to significantly improve percent times of patients' BG within target range and lower mean BG without an increase in hypoglycemic events.[22,23] Institution of a CPOE is a core requirement of the Health Information Technology and Clinical Health Act (HITECH) and is also recommended by the Institute of Medicine.[11] Routine structured order sets for basal, nutritional, and corrective insulin should be made part of CPOE. Ordering individualized corrective insulin scales, using the patients' calculated correction factor, can be made possible in such computerized order sets.

Glucose Monitoring

BG should be checked before meals and at bedtime. For patients who are taking nothing by mouth, frequency may be increased to every 4 hours while awake. For patients who are at risk of hypoglycemia, a 3-AM BG check is recommended.[11] Glucometers that connect wirelessly to the hospital's electronic health record system can greatly facilitate and expedite needed changes in patients' insulin orders and prevent recurrent hypoglycemia or hyperglycemia. Continuous glucose monitoring (CGM) promises to reduce incidence of severe hypoglycemia, but more research is needed to establish its accuracy and reliability in the hospital setting.[11] Therefore, CGM is not currently recommended for routine hospital use except for patients who are already using them as outpatients and wish to cautiously continue using them in hospital.

Table 3	
Basal-bolus (nutritional) and corrective insulin dose calculation	
Basal insulin	Starting dose = TDD[a] × 0.5 • Glargine insulin: one dose at bedtime or • Detemir insulin: one dose at bedtime (type 2) or split to 2 equal doses AM and bedtime (type 1) or • NPH insulin: two-thirds AM and one-third bedtime • Premixed insulin 70/30, 75/25, or 50/50 not generally recommended in the hospital unless patients need to be discharged on this regimen Note 1: Glargine and detemir are preferred over NPH in the hospital setting (lower risk of hypoglycemia as NPH peak may seriously decrease BG when patients are fasting for a procedure or any other reason). Note 2: Use NPH if short hospital stay is anticipated and patients are unable to afford/switch to glargine/detemir as outpatient. NPH is also preferred in patients on oral steroid therapy.
Nutritional (bolus) insulin	Starting dose = TDD[a] × 0.5 divided equally before each meal • Lispro, aspart, and glulisine are preferred over regular insulin for hospitalized patients (less risk of hypoglycemia). Note 3: Inject 50% or less of calculated nutritional insulin if patients have reduced intake. Note 4: Hold nutritional insulin if patients are not able to eat.

Corrective insulin	CF = 1700 ÷ TDD[a]
	The correction factor is the amount of BG in mg/dl that 1 unit of insulin will lower, therefore
	Corrective insulin dose = (current BG − 100) ÷ CF
	• Build the scale by increasing insulin dose by 1 U for every CF
	• Give nutritional and correction doses as 1 injection with meals
	Example: An 80-kg patient with type 2 diabetes and A1C of 11% needs
	TDD = 60 kg × 0.5 = 40 U
	Basal insulin = TDD × 50% = 20 U of glargine or detemir insulin q h
	Nutritional insulin = 20 ÷ 3 = ~7 units rapid-acting insulin with each meal
	Correction factor = 1700 ÷ 40 = 42 mg/dL
	This means that 1 U of insulin is expected to lower BG by ~ 40 mg/dL
	corrective insulin dose = (BG −100)/CF
	A scale can be made as follows:
	Premeal corrective insulin scale (BG goal <140 mg/dL)
	  Scale
	    140–180 mg/dL = 1 U
	    181–220 mg/dL = 2 U
	    221–260 mg/dL = 3 U and so forth
	Bedtime corrective insulin scale (BG goal <180 mg/dL)
	  Scale
	    141–180 mg/dL = 0 U
	    181–220 mg/dL = 1 U
	    221–260 mg/dL = 2 U and so forth

Abbreviation: CF, correction factor.
[a] TDD is calculated using instructions in **Table 2**.

Corticosteroids

Glucocorticoid-induced hyperglycemia, defined as BG levels greater than 180 mg/dL after initiation of glucocorticoids, has been reported in 32%[24] to 52%[25] of inpatients. Of these, 18%[24] to 25%[25] were diagnosed with diabetes. Hyperglycemia in these patients has been shown to be associated with an increased risk of mortality,[26] infections,[27] and length of stay.[28] Despite the importance of controlling hyperglycemia in these patients,

Table 4 General guidelines for adjusting basal and nutritional insulin	

Fasting BG >140 mg/dL	• Increase bedtime long-acting insulin; if NPH or detemir are used q 12 h, increase bedtime dose:
	  ○ 10% if fasting BG is 140–199 mg/dL
	  ○ 20% if fasting BG is 200–299 mg/dL
	  ○ 30% if fasting BG is 300–399 mg/dL
	Example: Fasting BG: 190 mg/dL, prelunch: 135 mg/dL, predinner: 120 mg/dL, bedtime: 140 mg/dL; patient on 40 U of glargine insulin at bedtime
	Increase basal glargine insulin by 10% from 40 U to 44 U

Premeal BG >140 mg/dL or bedtime BG >180 mg/dL and fasting BG <140 mg/dL	• Increase nutritional rapid-acting insulin:
	  ○ 10% if BG is 140–199 mg/dL
	  ○ 20% if BG is 200–299 mg/dL
	  ○ 30% if BG is 300–399 mg/dL
	Example: Fasting BG: 120 mg/dL, prelunch: 200 mg/dL, predinner: 230 mg/dL, bedtime: 280 mg/dL; total nutritional insulin is 20 U
	Increase nutritional insulin by 20% from 20 U to 24 U

Fasting and premeal BG >140 mg/dL and bedtime BG >180 mg/dL	• Sum up total amount of basal, nutritional and corrective insulin from day prior and calculate new TDD by increasing this sum as follows:
	  ○ 10% if BGs 140–199
	  ○ 20% if BGs 200–299
	  ○ 30% if BGs 300–399
	  ○ 40% if BGs 400–499
	Calculate new basal, bolus and corrective insulin using the new TDD.

not enough head-to-head randomized controlled trials (RCTs) exist to recommend a specific type or a starting dose of insulin for a certain type of steroid. Because hyperglycemia in response to morning oral steroid is predominately seen from noontime until evening, an additional single dose of neutral protamine hagedorn (NPH) insulin given in the morning should be most effective[11] compared with adjusting basal-bolus (even when the noon and presupper bolus doses are increased).[29] In the only single RCT done to date,[19] when NPH was added onto the patient's basal-bolus-corrective regimen, there was a trend toward improved glycemic control without increased risk of hypoglycemia, compared with adjusting patients' basal-bolus-corrective insulin alone. This finding seems intuitive because NPH insulin peaks 4 to 10 hours after injection, around the same time prednisone exerts its hyperglycemic effects (4–8 hours). In addition, NPH has a duration of action of approximately 12 to 18 hours, similar to the duration of hyperglycemic effects of prednisone.[30] A slightly simplified version of an insulin protocol for patients on glucocorticoids by Grommesh and colleagues[19] is shown in **Table 5**. In this protocol, the starting dose of NPH depends on the patients' prednisone dose and absence or presence of diabetes. It needs to be emphasized that the NPH dose has to be added on to the patients' existing basal-bolus and corrective dose. Instead of using a fixed NPH dose, the NPH dose can be calculated as 0.27 units per kilogram.[31]

Multiple daily doses of glucocorticoids, such as hydrocortisone and methylprednisolone, and longer-acting glucocorticoids, such as dexamethasone, may be better

Table 5
NPH insulin dose administered at the time of glucocorticoid administration

	Prednisone <40 mg/d as Single Morning Dose	Prednisone ≥40 mg/d as Single Morning Dose
Hyperglycemia but no history of diabetes	5 U	10 U
Established diabetes	10 U	20 U

- Increase NPH by 25% if BG >180 mg/dL and increase by 50% if BG >300 mg/dL
- Taper NPH by same percentage as prednisone is tapered
- NPH can be stopped when prednisone dose is reduced to <10 mg/d

It is recommended that a mechanism be implemented in the CPOE that links the prednisone order to the NPH order, such that it is given at the same time, and signals a need for change or hold in NPH if glucocorticoids are changed or held.

controlled with longer-acting insulin like glargine and detemir insulin.[11] A retrospective study by Gosmanov and colleagues[32] assessing the glycemic control of patients with diabetes and hematologic malignancies who were receiving dexamethasone found that a daily-adjusted basal-bolus regimen achieved lower average BG levels compared with fixed sliding-scale insulin. For patients starting dexamethasone therapy, a TDD is somewhere between 0.66 units per kilogram and 1.2 units per kilogram.

In those patients who remain uncontrolled with BG levels greater than 400 mg/dL on a subcutaneous regimen, an intravenous (IV) insulin infusion should be considered.

Enteral and Parenteral Nutrition

It is recommended that patients be started on nutritional support within 24 to 48 hours if they are critically ill or after 7 to 14 days if they are not critically ill[33] but unable to meet greater than 60% of nutritional needs by mouth. The recommended glycemic goal is less than 180 mg/dL (see **Table 1**); however, observational studies suggest that a lower BG target of less than 150 mg/dL improves clinical outcomes for those receiving nutritional support without increasing hypoglycemia risk.[34]

Enteral nutrition

Multiple RCTs support the use of lower-carbohydrate-content (diabetes specific) enteral formulas because of their association with reduced hyperglycemia.[35–39] In standard enteral formulas, 55% to 60% of the calories are provided by carbohydrates, whereas diabetic-specific formulas reduce carbohydrate contribution by a maximum of 40% of the total caloric content. This reduction is made possible by substituting some of the carbohydrate content with monounsaturated fatty acids and dietary fiber.[40,41] A variety of insulin regimens are used to manage hyperglycemia for patients on parenteral nutrition. The superiority of one regimen over the other remains to be established. To date there have been several retrospective study[42] and only one RCT examining this question.[40] This RCT[43] showed that one dose of glargine insulin with corrective regular insulin performed just as well as NPH twice daily with corrective regular insulin, with no difference in target BG achieved or hypoglycemic events[44] (see Method 1, **Table 6**).[45]

Total parenteral nutrition

Administering insulin directly into the total parenteral nutrition (TPN) solution is associated with lower hypoglycemia risk in the event of abrupt TPN discontinuation. For patients with diabetes, start with 0.1 unit or regular insulin per 1 g of dextrose with daily

Table 6
Diabetes management for patients on enteral and parenteral nutrition

Continuous enteral nutrition	Method 1 Initial TDD = 0.3–0.6 U/kg body weight • One-half TDD as basal: glargine insulin q 24 h • One-half TDD as prandial: NPH q 8–12[1] or regular q 6 h • Corrective insulin: regular q 6 h[2] • BG checked q 6 h • Prandial insulin to be held if parenteral nutrition stopped • Prandial insulin adjusted by adding 80% of previous day's correctional insulin to current prandial dose[3] Method 2 TDD given as just basal: 2 doses of NPH or detemir 1 dose of glargine[4] Corrective insulin: regular insulin q 6 h[2] • Basal insulin adjusted by adding 50% of previous day's correctional insulin to current basal dose[3] • If parenteral nutrition stopped, give only 0.3 U/kg basal insulin along with corrective insulin
Cyclic enteral nutrition	• Continue existing basal, bolus, and corrective insulin • In addition, give extra insulin dose for cyclic EN = 60% of (0.3–0.6) unit per kilogram of body weight • Given as NPH/regular or premixed 70/30 (or 75/25) at the time of TF initiation • Titrate based on midnight, 3 AM, and 6 AM BG
Bolus enteral nutrition	• Continue existing basal, bolus, and corrective insulin • Add additional rapid-acting insulin for each bolus feeding • BG checked before meals and bedtime
TPN	• Continue existing basal, bolus, and corrective insulin • Add insulin to TPN bag (0.1 U/1 g of dextrose) • Titrate 0.05 U/1g of dextrose daily if BG >150 mg/dL • BG checked q 6 h
Interruption of enteral feedings	• Adjust insulin appropriately with planned withholding of enteral nutrition • Standing orders for prandial insulin held and MD notified if enteral feeds are to be stopped at any point • If unexpected and abrupt interruption of enteral feedings exceeding 2 h, start D10W IV at the same rate as enteral feedings were given to prevent hypoglycemia and dehydration

Abbreviations: EN, enteral nutrition; TF, tube feeding; TPN, total parenteral nutrition.

titration by 0.05 units per 1 g dextrose if BG remains greater than 150 mg/dL.[46] For patients without diabetes the unit per dextrose grams ratio has been shown to be lower at 0.1 unit per 2.0 g of dextrose.[47]

1. This decreases injection frequency while still remaining a good option for lowering the risk of hypoglycemia if enteral nutrition is abruptly stopped.
2. Please see **Table 3** for how to calculate this dose.
3. If the previous day correctional insulin is added to the basal insulin, a higher risk of hypoglycemia ensues on abrupt or planned discontinuation of enteral nutrition. In the former case, providers might overestimate the true basal insulin needs.
4. There is a higher risk of hypoglycemia with this regimen if enteral nutrition is abruptly stopped.

INSULIN PUMP MANAGEMENT IN THE HOSPITAL

Approximately 30% to 40% of patients with type 1 diabetes and an increasing number of insulin requiring patients with type 2 diabetes are using insulin pumps.[48] Most insulin pump users are well trained on diabetes self-management and frequently get frustrated when they are asked to stop using their insulin pump during hospitalization. Adding to this frustration is the nonintentional delay in administering their bolus or corrective insulin by hospital staff. It is recommended that insulin pump users be allowed to self-manage their diabetes during hospitalization provided they are able to demonstrate adequate skill and ability to manage their pumps and are able to procure their pump supplies.[11,49] An insulin pump agreement helps outline expectations that patients need to collaborate and communicate with the hospital team by reporting BG and basal levels and any boluses given for meals or correction. These values need to be documented on a special insulin pump record sheet. A hospital-wide insulin pump policy can help in smoothing transition to subcutaneous (SC) insulin in the event of pump failure or change in patients' cognition that prevents continued self-management. This policy should delineate responsibilities for hospital team members and ensure ultimate patient safety. Involvement of a diabetologist, either on site or by phone, is highly recommended to assist in recommending changes in basal, bolus, or corrective settings while patients are in the hospital.[48,50]

In the Event of Surgery

Patients who are on an insulin pump can continue their usual basal rate during minor surgeries and major noncardiac surgeries lasting less than 6 hours, providing that their ongoing basal rate is not causing hypoglycemia. If there is any concern about possible fasting hypoglycemia, a temporary basal rate should be set at 80% of patients' usual basal rate. The infusion set should be changed 24 hours before surgery, and the insertion site should be selected away from the surgical site. The chosen site can be anywhere on the upper outer thighs, upper arms, or abdomen 2 in away from the umbilicus. BG should be checked every hour during surgery. Transition to insulin infusion should be considered if BG exceeds and remains greater than 180 mg/dL.

Critical Illness

Patients on insulin pumps need to be transitioned to an IV insulin infusion in critical illness.[48]

PERIOPERATIVE DIABETES MANAGEMENT

Patients with diabetes should be given preference for early morning surgery. Doing so may decrease the risk of hyperglycemia and hypoglycemia resulting from disruption in typical medication and food schedules. On the day before surgery, patients with diabetes should continue their usual hospital-ordered, calorie-restricted, carbohydrate-consistent diabetic diet along with their ordered insulin and/or oral antihyperglycemic medications. Changes that need to be made to patients' diabetes medication regimen are listed in **Box 3**. The patients' health care team needs to ensure that patients are not sent to the preanesthesia unit without receiving their adjusted scheduled dose of long-acting or intermediate-acting insulin. This point is especially important in patients with type 1 diabetes who are traditionally at higher risk of diabetic ketoacidosis if their insulin regimen is disrupted.

Intraoperative

On arrival to the preanesthesia unit, diabetes management depends largely on the patients' type of diabetes, BG on arrival, and the type of surgery. The target BG range in

---

Box 3
Preoperative diabetes management night before or morning of surgery

Diabetes medication management

- *Long-acting (glargine or detemir) insulin:* Inject 80% of the scheduled dose at bedtime or in the morning before surgery depending on the patients' usual administration time.

- *Intermediate acting (NPH) insulin:* Inject one-half of the usual dose.

- *Rapid (aspart, lispro, glulisine) or short-acting (regular) insulin:* Omit the morning dose (including inhaled insulin).

- *Premixed insulin (70/30, 75/25, 50/50):* Inject one-half of the NPH component of the usual premixed insulin and no rapid or short-acting insulin on the morning of surgery.

- *Oral and noninsulin injectable diabetes medications:* Discontinue it on the morning of surgery.[9]

BG monitoring

- Check BG at bedtime and on the morning of surgery, and every 4 to 6 h thereafter.

- If hypoglycemic at bedtime or overnight, patients should be treated with glucose gel and not by juice.

---

the perioperative period is 80 to 180 mg/dL.[11] Tighter perioperative glycemic control does not improve outcomes and has been associated with hypoglycemia.[51]

Minor Surgeries

Patients' BG on arrival to the preanesthesia unit can determine treatment and BG monitoring frequency as outlined in **Table 3**. Patients who have a BG level greater than 180 mg/dL and are not responding to SC insulin within an hour can be started on IV insulin infusion. On the other hand, patients with a BG less than 100 mg/dL should be started on IV dextrose infusion as outlined in **Table 7**. All other patients should receive maintenance IV fluids that do not contain dextrose, such as lactated ringers, normal saline, or 0.45% normal saline.

Major Surgeries

It is recommended that IV insulin infusion be started for patients undergoing chest, abdominal cavity, vascular bypass, transplant, spinal or brain surgery, total hip or knee replacement surgeries, or a surgery anticipated to last longer than 4 hours. For patients who are started on IV insulin infusion, a dextrose containing IV fluid is necessary. Dextrose 5% in water (D5W) at 40 mL/h or Dextrose 10% in water (D10W) at 20 mL/h should be started to provide approximately 50 g of glucose over 24 hours.

Postoperative

While patients are in the postanesthesia unit, management and frequency of BG monitoring remains similar to during surgery (see **Table 7**). If the patients' BG is greater than

---

Table 7
Intraoperative diabetes management for non-major surgery

BG <80 mg/dL	BG 80–100 mg/dL	BG 101–180 mg/dL	BG >180 mg/dL
Give at least 100 mL D10W IV or 25–50 mL (0.5–1.0 amp) of D50, check BG in 15–30 min	Begin D5W at 40 mL/h or D10W at 20 mL/h, check BG in 1 h	Continue to monitor BG every 2 h	Give corrective rapid-acting insulin q 4 h (see **Table 3**) or start insulin infusion, check BG every hour

180 mg/dL, BG should be checked hourly. A corrective dose of rapid-acting insulin should be administered every 4 hours. On arrival to the regular floor, it is recommended to start basal plus nutritional or basal plus corrective rapid-acting insulin regimen.[52,53] If patients are not eating, nutritional insulin should be held. It may start later at reduced doses based oral nutrition intake.[9,53] Patients who have undergone cardiac surgery should continue on IV insulin infusion.

HYPERGLYCEMIA MANAGEMENT OF CRITICALLY ILL INPATIENTS

It is well established that mortality, morbidity, and length of stay increases when BG levels increase greater than 180 to 200 mg/dL in critically ill patients.[5,9] More recently it has been established that hypoglycemia in these patients is also associated with increased mortality. It is, therefore, important to have a form of insulin that both acts as well as clears rapidly in order to quickly correct and prevent hyperglycemia and hypoglycemia. When regular insulin is injected by IV versus SC routes, peak serum levels are reached within 2 minutes by IV route versus 60 minutes by SC route resulting in peak glucose lowering at 15 minutes by IV route versus 180 minutes by SC route. Rapid glucose lowering by IV insulin coupled with rapid insulin clearance allows BG levels to return to baseline 30 minutes after injection if the insulin infusion is stopped.[54–56] The slower performance of SC-administered regular insulin is because regular insulin is crystalized around a zinc molecule in the shape of a hexamer. It takes time for this hexamer to dissociate into first dimers; then monomers form, which rapidly crosses the capillary membrane and binds to insulin receptors. Thus, IV insulin infusions are the standard of care in critically ill patients. Exceptions are patients who are predicted to be discharged from the intensive care unit (ICU) in less than 24 hours. Those patients may start or continue SC insulin as previously discussed.

Target Blood Glucose Range

The current BG recommendations for critically ill patients by the ADA in conjunction with the AACE[9] and separately by the Society of Critical Care Medicine[57] are listed in **Table 8**. In order to understand the rationale behind these recommendations, the authors briefly review the landmark RCTs leading to them. The Leuven trial in 2001[58] was a single-center trial that compared the BG target of 80 to 110 mg/dL versus 180 to 200 mg/dL in the surgical ICU. It showed 42% reduction in mortality and 34% reduction in length of stay. The Leuven group repeated their study in the medical ICU but were not able to show similar reduction in mortality. In fact, there was a trend toward increase mortality that was found to be strongly associated with hypoglycemia.[59] The efficacy of volume substitution and insulin therapy in severe sepsis (VISEP) study[60] compared the 2 target BG range groups defined by the Leuven trials[58,59] but in patients with septic shock. The study reported a significant increase in adverse events (11% vs 5%) in the 80 to 110 mg/dL group versus the 180 to 200 mg/dL group, and the study was stopped early because of the significantly increased rate of hypoglycemia (17% vs 4%) in the tightly controlled group. The normoglycemia in

Table 8	
Glucose targets in critically ill patients with and without diabetes	
Established diabetes	No diabetes • After cardiac surgery or • After ischemic cardiac or neurological event
140–180 mg/dL	100–150 mg/dL

intensive care evaluation-survival using glucose algorithm regulation (NICE-SUGAR) study,[61] a large, multinational study, compared a target range of 81 to 108 mg/dL with 140 to 180 mg/dL in both surgical and medical ICUs. The trial showed significant increase in 90-day mortality. This increased mortality was shown to be associated with hypoglycemia, although no causal relationship was established.[62] Of note, this was the only study that had a comparison group with BG levels less than 180 mg/dL, which is well below the 200 mg/dL threshold that prior studies had shown to increase morbidity and mortality. It is worth noting that the safety of BG levels between 110 mg/dL and 140 mg/dL is still unanswered. The ADA/AACE's recommendations[9] aim to keep the lower end of their target higher enough (140 mg/dL) to preemptively prevent less experienced ICU teams from entering their patients to the danger BG zone of less than 110 mg/dL, which was associated with higher mortality as shown in the NICE-SUGAR study,[61] and an upper end of the range less than 180 mg/dL to avoid falling into the greater than 200 mg/dL danger zone. It is recommended that BG should be kept in the lower end of this range.[9] However, certain hospitals with lower hypoglycemia rates have chosen tighter target ranges, such as 120 to 160 mg/dL, presuming the unexamined 110 to 140 mg/dL to be safe, and trying to keep their upper target range away from 200 mg/dL.

For patients who have had cardiac surgery, the Society of Critical Care Medicine recommends a target range of 100 to 150 mg/dL[57] (see **Table 8**). However, tight control (100–140 mg/dL) on IV insulin infusion in patients who have had cardiac surgery has shown to lower adverse outcomes for patients without diabetes. Patients with diabetes have no increased complications in the 140 to 180 mg/dL target group when compared with the 100 to 140 mg/dL target group.[63,64] Other patients without diabetes who may benefit from tighter glycemic control are those who are admitted for an acute ischemic cardiac[65] or neurologic event, provided these targets can be achieved without significant hypoglycemia.[57]

Effective insulin infusion protocols must use dynamic as opposed to static algorithms that use both the last BG, the rate of change in BG, as well as the current insulin infusion rate when recommending the new insulin infusion rate.[11] This practice will help prevent hyperglycemia if the rate of correction is too slow and prevent hypoglycemia if the rate of correction is too fast. Many different paper-based and computer-based dynamic algorithms are available, and no single protocol or algorithm has been established as the most effective for achieving and maintaining glucose targets or achieving lowest hypoglycemia rates.[66,67] It is important that the hospital's chosen protocol is validated and has demonstrated safety and efficacy.[67] Key elements of an IV insulin infusion protocol are listed in **Box 4**.[66–68] In general, a potential hypoglycemic or hyperglycemic scenario should be anticipated and proactively addressed with clear guidelines in the protocol. For example, in the event of abrupt TPN/peripheral parenteral nutrition (PPN) or steroid or vasopressor discontinuation, the infusion rate should be reduced by 50%, with resumption of BG checks once every hour until BGs are stable. It needs to be noted that patients with diabetic ketoacidosis and hyperglycemic hyperosmolar syndrome will need modified insulin infusion protocols that prevent rapid correction of hyperglycemia.

Transitioning off insulin drip
Once critically ill patients become clinically stable and ready for transfer out of the ICU, and are tolerating at least 50% of their diet, or are on a stable regimen of TPN or PPN, they are ready to come off the insulin infusion. Not all patients who were on an insulin infusion in the critical care unit will need to transition to SC insulin. Patients who need to be transitioned are those with type 1 diabetes, type 2 diabetes, or those without

---

Box 4

Key elements of an intravenous insulin infusion protocol

1. Clear instructions on the criteria for initiation of IV insulin infusion

2. Clearly stated target BG

3. Clear instructions on how to calculate initial IV insulin infusion rate

4. Instructions on frequency of BG monitoring

5. Clear instructions on management of hypoglycemia

6. Guidance for handling situations whereby peripheral parenteral nutrition (TPN), steroids, or vasopressors are added or removed

7. Guidance for transitioning from IV insulin to SC insulin

8. Instructions on how to change insulin infusion rate

---

diabetes requiring more than 1 to 2 units per hour of insulin.[69] The Joslin Diabetes Center's guidelines for transitioning patient from IV to SC insulin are listed in **Box 5**.[69,70]

HYPOGLYCEMIA

Early recognition and treatment of hypoglycemia, using a hospital-wide nurse-led protocol, significantly reduces adverse outcomes.[73,74] Treatment depends on severity of hypoglycemic episode and whether or not patients are conscious. The hypoglycemia management guidelines by the Joslin Diabetes Center are listed in **Table 9**.[75] Recurrence of hypoglycemia is common. In one study, 84% of patients with severe hypoglycemia had had one prior episode of hypoglycemia.[11] Failing to adjust the insulin regimen after a hypoglycemic event is common[11] and is a strong predictor of recurrence of hypoglycemia and declining renal function.[9] Therefore, it is important for the treating provider to review the patients' insulin regimen and adjust basal or corrective bedtime insulin doses in the event of fasting hypoglycemia or bolus and/or corrective insulin doses in the event of postprandial hypoglycemia.[5] The Joslin Diabetes Center's guidelines on insulin adjustments for hypoglycemia are detailed in **Box 6**.[75] In about 20% of cases, rebound hyperglycemia is experienced after a hypoglycemic

---

Box 5

Guidance for transitioning from intravenous to subcutaneous insulin

1. Determine the average hourly rate of insulin over the past 8 hours.

2. Multiply this number by 24 to determine the total IV insulin requirements in past 24 hours (TDD-IV).

3. Use 60% to 80%[71,72] of the total TDD-IV to derive your TDD of SC insulin (TDD-SC).

4. If patients were taking nothing by mouth, the TDD-SC number is equivalent to the patients' basal insulin.

5. If patients were eating over the past 24 hours, then one-half of the TDD-SC is bolus and the other half basal.

6. Overlap IV insulin infusion for a minimum of 4 hours if SC insulin glargine is given without SC fast-acting insulin or only 2 hours if SC fast-acting insulin is given along with glargine.

Table 9
Hypoglycemia management (noncritically ill patients)

		Treatment
Conscious on oral feeding	BG: 50–69 mg/dL BG <50 mg/dL	15–20 g of simple carbohydrates 20–30 g of simple carbohydrates
Conscious but NPO	On IV insulin	• Stop insulin infusion • Inject bolus dose D50W IV; dose in milliliters = (100 − BG) × 0.4 • Start D10W IV at 25 mL/h • Once BG is back to >100 mg/dL, stop D10W and resume insulin infusion at 50% of the previous rate
	On SC insulin	• Inject bolus dose D50W dose in milliliters = (100 − BG) × 0.4 • Start D10W IV at 25 mL/h • Once BG is back to >100 mg/dL, stop D10W and resume insulin regimen after appropriate adjustments are made
Unconscious	No IV access	• Give 1 mg glucagon intramuscularly or 0.5 mg for patients <50 kg body weight • Once IV access is established, proceed with steps outlined for conscious patients
		Insulin Adjustment
Fasting hypoglycemia		• Reduce long-acting basal insulin by 20% if BG is 50–70 mg/dL. • Reduce long-acting basal insulin by 30% if BG is <50 mg/dL. • If patients received corrective insulin before the event, consider increasing sensitivity factor of corrective insulin.
Postprandial hypoglycemia		• Reduce bolus (nutritional) insulin by 20%–50% for the duration that patients' oral food intake is below baseline. • If patients had received corrective insulin before the event, consider increasing sensitivity factor of corrective insulin.

event. Close communication between physicians and nursing staff before making any changes to patients' insulin regimen is quite important. Overcorrection with carbohydrates is frequently the main cause of rebound hyperglycemia. For example, giving no more than 20 g of carbohydrate for correction of BG between 50 and 70 mg/dL and calculating the D50 dose based on BG reading at the time of a hypoglycemic episode instead of injecting full ampule are good practice. It needs to be noted that patients with gastroparesis should receive treatment with glucose gel because of their delayed gastrointestinal absorption. BG should be checked 15 minutes later; if BG remains less than 70 mg/dL, another 15 g of simple carbohydrates should be given. As discussed in a previous section, for critically ill patients the consensus bar for hypoglycemia is considered 100 mg/dL.

Box 6
Examples of 15 g of carbohydrate

- 4 glucose tablets
- 1 tube glucose gel
- 4 oz (0.5 c) of juice or regular soda
- 4 tsp of sugar

SUMMARY

During hospital admission, proactive glycemic control for critically ill and noncritically ill patients with diabetes is important to prevent hospital complications and mortality whether patients are managed in surgical or medical units. Hyperglycemia needs to be avoided with institution of long-acting basal plus nutritional and corrective rapid-acting bolus insulin and not only by corrective regular insulin doses before the sliding scale. Timely detection of hypoglycemia and nurse-led management protocols have become a standard of care. Timely changes in treatment are greatly facilitated by glucose meters that are wirelessly connected to the hospitals electronic health record system as well as by using computerized physician insulin order entry systems. This combination allows physicians to rapidly access patients' BG readings from anywhere in the hospital and immediately intervene. Good communication between the hospital team and availability of a certified diabetes educator are shown to improve diabetes control during hospital admission and ensure patient safety after discharge. As tight glycemic control may be associated with increased hypoglycemia risk, further studies are still needed to determine ideal BG targets for both critically ill and noncritically ill patients. With increasing attention to medication errors and iatrogenic complications in the hospital setting, safely achieving euglycemia will be of paramount importance.

REFERENCES

1. Pomposelli JJ, Baxter JK 3rd, Babineau TJ, et al. Early postoperative glucose control predicts nosocomial infection rate in diabetic patients. JPEN J Parenter Enteral Nutr 1998;22(2):77–81.
2. Baker EH, Janaway CH, Philips BJ, et al. Hyperglycaemia is associated with poor outcomes in patients admitted to hospital with acute exacerbations of chronic obstructive pulmonary disease. Thorax 2006;61(4):284–9.
3. McAlister FA, Majumdar SR, Blitz S, et al. The relation between hyperglycemia and outcomes in 2,471 patients admitted to the hospital with community-acquired pneumonia. Diabetes Care 2005;28(4):810–5.
4. McAlister FA, Man J, Bistritz L, et al. Diabetes and coronary artery bypass surgery: an examination of perioperative glycemic control and outcomes. Diabetes Care 2003;26(5):1518–24.
5. Umpierrez GE, Hellman R, Korytkowski MT, et al. Management of hyperglycemia in hospitalized patients in non-critical care setting: an Endocrine Society clinical practice guideline. J Clin Endocrinol Metab 2012;97(1):16–38.
6. Umpierrez GE, Isaacs SD, Bazargan N, et al. Hyperglycemia: an independent marker of in-hospital mortality in patients with undiagnosed diabetes. J Clin Endocrinol Metab 2002;87(3):978–82.
7. Ainla T, Baburin A, Teesalu R, et al. The association between hyperglycaemia on admission and 180-day mortality in acute myocardial infarction patients with and without diabetes. Diabet Med 2005;22(10):1321–5.
8. Clement S, Braithwaite SS, Magee MF, et al. Management of diabetes and hyperglycemia in hospitals. Diabetes Care 2004;27(2):553–91.
9. Moghissi ES, Korytkowski MT, DiNardo M, et al. American Association of Clinical Endocrinologists and American Diabetes Association consensus statement on inpatient glycemic control. Diabetes Care 2009;32(6):1119–31.
10. Seaquist ER, Anderson J, Childs B, et al. Hypoglycemia and diabetes: a report of a workgroup of the American Diabetes Association and the Endocrine Society. Diabetes Care 2013;36(5):1384–95.

11. American Diabetes Association. Standards of medical care in diabetes-2016 abridged for primary care providers. Clin Diabetes 2016;34(1):3–21.

12. Draznin B, Gilden J, Golden SH, et al. Pathways to quality inpatient management of hyperglycemia and diabetes: a call to action. Diabetes Care 2013;36(7):1807–14.

13. Healy SJ, Black D, Harris C, et al. Inpatient diabetes education is associated with less frequent hospital readmission among patients with poor glycemic control. Diabetes Care 2013;36(10):2960–7.

14. Curll M, Dinardo M, Noschese M, et al. Menu selection, glycaemic control and satisfaction with standard and patient-controlled consistent carbohydrate meal plans in hospitalised patients with diabetes. Qual Saf Health Care 2010;19(4):355–9.

15. Umpierrez GE, Gianchandani R, Smiley D, et al. Safety and efficacy of sitagliptin therapy for the inpatient management of general medicine and surgery patients with type 2 diabetes: a pilot, randomized, controlled study. Diabetes Care 2013;36(11):3430–5.

16. Umpierrez GE, Korytkowski M. Is incretin-based therapy ready for the care of hospitalized patients with type 2 diabetes?: Insulin therapy has proven itself and is considered the mainstay of treatment. Diabetes Care 2013;36(7):2112–7.

17. Thomsen HS, European Society of Urogenital Radiology. European Society of Urogenital Radiology guidelines on contrast media application. Curr Opin Urol 2007;17(1):70–6.

18. McDonnell ME, Umpierrez GE. Insulin therapy for the management of hyperglycemia in hospitalized patients. Endocrinol Metab Clin North Am 2012;41(1):175–201.

19. Grommesh B, Lausch MJ, Vannelli AJ, et al. Hospital insulin protocol aims for glucose control in glucocorticoid-induced hyperglycemia. Endocr Pract 2016;22(2):180–9.

20. Joslin Diabetes Center Inpatient Hyperglycemia Protocol. 2016.

21. Baldwin D, Zander J, Munoz C, et al. A randomized trial of two weight-based doses of insulin glargine and glulisine in hospitalized subjects with type 2 diabetes and renal insufficiency. Diabetes Care 2012;35(10):1970–4.

22. Gillaizeau F, Chan E, Trinquart L, et al. Computerized advice on drug dosage to improve prescribing practice. Cochrane Database Syst Rev 2013;(11):CD002894.

23. Kennihan M, Zohra T, Devi R, et al. Individualization through standardization: electronic orders for subcutaneous insulin in the hospital. Endocr Pract 2012;18(6):976–87.

24. Liu XX, Zhu XM, Miao Q, et al. Hyperglycemia induced by glucocorticoids in nondiabetic patients: a meta-analysis. Ann Nutr Metab 2014;65(4):324–32.

25. Donihi AC, Raval D, Saul M, et al. Prevalence and predictors of corticosteroid-related hyperglycemia in hospitalized patients. Endocr Pract 2006;12(4):358–62.

26. Ali NA, O'Brien JM Jr, Blum W, et al. Hyperglycemia in patients with acute myeloid leukemia is associated with increased hospital mortality. Cancer 2007;110(1):96–102.

27. Derr RL, Hsiao VC, Saudek CD. Antecedent hyperglycemia is associated with an increased risk of neutropenic infections during bone marrow transplantation. Diabetes Care 2008;31(10):1972–7.

28. Garg R, Bhutani H, Alyea E, et al. Hyperglycemia and length of stay in patients hospitalized for bone marrow transplantation. Diabetes Care 2007;30(4):993–4.

29. Burt MG, Drake SM, Aguilar-Loza NR, et al. Efficacy of a basal bolus insulin protocol to treat prednisolone-induced hyperglycaemia in hospitalised patients. Intern Med J 2015;45(3):261–6.

30. Low Wang CC, Draznin B. Use of Nph insulin for glucocorticoid-induced hyperglycemia. Endocr Pract 2016;22(2):271–3.

31. Dhital SM, Shenker Y, Meredith M, et al. A retrospective study comparing neutral protamine Hagedorn insulin with glargine as basal therapy in prednisone-associated diabetes mellitus in hospitalized patients. Endocr Pract 2012;18(5):712–9.

32. Gosmanov AR, Goorha S, Stelts S, et al. Management of hyperglycemia in diabetic patients with hematologic malignancies during dexamethasone therapy. Endocr Pract 2013;19(2):231–5.

33. Dhaliwal R, Cahill N, Lemieux M, et al. The Canadian critical care nutrition guidelines in 2013: an update on current recommendations and implementation strategies. Nutr Clin Pract 2014;29(1):29–43.

34. Marik PE, Preiser JC. Toward understanding tight glycemic control in the ICU: a systematic review and meta-analysis. Chest 2010;137(3):544–51.

35. Leon-Sanz M, Garcia-Luna PP, Sanz-Paris A, et al. Glycemic and lipid control in hospitalized type 2 diabetic patients: evaluation of 2 enteral nutrition formulas (low carbohydrate-high monounsaturated fat vs high carbohydrate). JPEN J Parenter Enteral Nutr 2005;29(1):21–9.

36. Elia M, Ceriello A, Laube H, et al. Enteral nutritional support and use of diabetes-specific formulas for patients with diabetes: a systematic review and meta-analysis. Diabetes Care 2005;28(9):2267–79.

37. Alish CJ, Garvey WT, Maki KC, et al. A diabetes-specific enteral formula improves glycemic variability in patients with type 2 diabetes. Diabetes Technol Ther 2010;12(6):419–25.

38. Vaisman N, Lansink M, Rouws CH, et al. Tube feeding with a diabetes-specific feed for 12 weeks improves glycaemic control in type 2 diabetes patients. Clin Nutr 2009;28(5):549–55.

39. Pohl M, Mayr P, Mertl-Roetzer M, et al. Glycemic control in patients with type 2 diabetes mellitus with a disease-specific enteral formula: stage II of a randomized, controlled multicenter trial. JPEN J Parenter Enteral Nutr 2009;33(1):37–49.

40. Gosmanov AR, Umpierrez GE. Management of hyperglycemia during enteral and parenteral nutrition therapy. Curr Diab Rep 2013;13(1):155–62.

41. Malone A. Enteral formula selection: a review of selected product categories. Practical Gastroenterol 2005;28:44–74.

42. Hsia E, Seggelke SA, Gibbs J, et al. Comparison of 70/30 biphasic insulin with glargine/lispro regimen in non-critically ill diabetic patients on continuous enteral nutrition therapy. Nutr Clin Pract 2011;26(6):714–7.

43. Dickerson RN, Wilson VC, Maish GO 3rd, et al. Transitional NPH insulin therapy for critically ill patients receiving continuous enteral nutrition and intravenous regular human insulin. JPEN J Parenter Enteral Nutr 2013;37(4):506–16.

44. Korytkowski MT, Salata RJ, Koerbel GL, et al. Insulin therapy and glycemic control in hospitalized patients with diabetes during enteral nutrition therapy: a randomized controlled clinical trial. Diabetes Care 2009;32(4):594–6.

45. Joslin Diabetes Center Enteral and Parenteral Nutrition Protocol. 2015.

46. Hongsermeier T, Bistrian BR. Evaluation of a practical technique for determining insulin requirements in diabetic patients receiving total parenteral nutrition. JPEN J Parenter Enteral Nutr 1993;17(1):16–9.

47. Jakoby MG, Nannapaneni N. An insulin protocol for management of hyperglycemia in patients receiving parenteral nutrition is superior to ad hoc management. JPEN J Parenter Enteral Nutr 2012;36(2):183–8.

48. Grunberger G, Abelseth JM, Bailey TS, et al. Consensus statement by the American Association of Clinical Endocrinologists/American College of Endocrinology insulin pump management task force. Endocr Pract 2014;20(5):463–89.

49. Houlden RL, Moore S. In-hospital management of adults using insulin pump therapy. Can J Diabetes 2014;38(2):126–33.

50. Bhatt D, Reynolds LR. Keep your hands off my insulin pump! The dilemma of the hospitalized insulin pump patient. Am J Med 2015;128(9):936–7.

51. Buchleitner AM, Martinez-Alonso M, Hernandez M, et al. Perioperative glycaemic control for diabetic patients undergoing surgery. Cochrane Database Syst Rev 2012;(9):CD007315.

52. Umpierrez GE, Smiley D, Jacobs S, et al. Randomized study of basal-bolus insulin therapy in the inpatient management of patients with type 2 diabetes undergoing general surgery (RABBIT 2 surgery). Diabetes Care 2011;34(2):256–61.

53. Umpierrez GE, Smiley D, Hermayer K, et al. Randomized study comparing a basal-bolus with a basal plus correction insulin regimen for the hospital management of medical and surgical patients with type 2 diabetes: basal plus trial. Diabetes Care 2013;36(8):2169–74.

54. Guerra SM, Kitabchi AE. Comparison of the effectiveness of various routes of insulin injection: insulin levels and glucose response in normal subjects. J Clin Endocrinol Metab 1976;42(5):869–74.

55. Shahshahani MN, Kitabchi A. Glucose-lowering effect of insulin by different routes in obese and lean nonketotic diabetic patients. J Clin Endocrinol Metab 1978;47(1):34–40.

56. Skjaervold NK, Lyng O, Spigset O, et al. Pharmacology of intravenous insulin administration: implications for future closed-loop glycemic control by the intravenous/intravenous route. Diabetes Technol Ther 2012;14(1):23–9.

57. Jacobi J, Bircher N, Krinsley J, et al. Guidelines for the use of an insulin infusion for the management of hyperglycemia in critically ill patients. Crit Care Med 2012; 40(12):3251–76.

58. van den Berghe G, Wouters P, Weekers F, et al. Intensive insulin therapy in critically ill patients. N Engl J Med 2001;345(19):1359–67.

59. Van den Berghe G, Wilmer A, Hermans G, et al. Intensive insulin therapy in the medical ICU. N Engl J Med 2006;354(5):449–61.

60. Brunkhorst FM, Engel C, Bloos F, et al. Intensive insulin therapy and pentastarch resuscitation in severe sepsis. N Engl J Med 2008;358(2):125–39.

61. Investigators N-SS, Finfer S, Chittock DR, et al. Intensive versus conventional glucose control in critically ill patients. N Engl J Med 2009;360(13):1283–97.

62. Investigators N-SS, Finfer S, Liu B, et al. Hypoglycemia and risk of death in critically ill patients. N Engl J Med 2012;367(12):1108–18.

63. Vellanki P, Bean R, Oyedokun FA, et al. Randomized controlled trial of insulin supplementation for correction of bedtime hyperglycemia in hospitalized patients with type 2 diabetes. Diabetes Care 2015;38(4):568–74.

64. Umpierrez G, Cardona S, Pasquel F, et al. Randomized controlled trial of intensive versus conservative glucose control in patients undergoing coronary artery bypass graft surgery: GLUCO-CABG Trial. Diabetes Care 2015;38(9):1665–72.

65. Task Force on the management of ST-segment elevation acute myocardial infarction of the European Society of Cardiology (ESC), Steg PG, James SK, et al. ESC

guidelines for the management of acute myocardial infarction in patients presenting with ST-segment elevation. Eur Heart J 2012;33(20):2569–619.

66. Krikorian A, Ismail-Beigi F, Moghissi ES. Comparisons of different insulin infusion protocols: a review of recent literature. Curr Opin Clin Nutr Metab Care 2010; 13(2):198–204.

67. Steil GM, Deiss D, Shih J, et al. Intensive care unit insulin delivery algorithms: why so many? How to choose? J Diabetes Sci Technol 2009;3(1):125–40.

68. Boutin JM, Gauthier L. Insulin infusion therapy in critically ill patients. Can J Diabetes 2014;38(2):144–50.

69. Joslin Diabetes Center Medical Intensive Care Unit Protocol. 2015.

70. Joslin Diabetes Center Surgical Intensive Care Unit Protocol. 2015.

71. Schmeltz LR, DeSantis AJ, Thiyagarajan V, et al. Reduction of surgical mortality and morbidity in diabetic patients undergoing cardiac surgery with a combined intravenous and subcutaneous insulin glucose management strategy. Diabetes Care 2007;30(4):823–8.

72. Shomali ME, Herr DL, Hill PC, et al. Conversion from intravenous insulin to subcutaneous insulin after cardiovascular surgery: transition to target study. Diabetes Technol Ther 2011;13(2):121–6.

73. DiNardo M, Noschese M, Korytkowski M, et al. The medical emergency team and rapid response system: finding, treating, and preventing hypoglycemia. Jt Comm J Qual Patient Saf 2006;32(10):591–5.

74. Siminerio LM, Piatt G, Zgibor JC. Implementing the chronic care model for improvements in diabetes care and education in a rural primary care practice. Diabetes Educ 2005;31(2):225–34.

75. Joslin Diabetes Center Hypoglycemia Protocol. 2015.

Utility of Continuous Glucose Monitoring in Type 1 and Type 2 Diabetes

Elena Toschi, MD*, Howard Wolpert, MD

KEYWORDS

- Technology • Type 1 diabetes mellitus • Type 2 diabetes mellitus
- Continuous glucose monitoring

KEY POINTS

- Continuous glucose monitoring (CGM) improves glycemic control in adults with type 1 diabetes and reduces the risk of hypoglycemia.
- Short-term, intermittent use of CGM has been shown to be effective in adults with type 2 diabetes (not on prandial insulin) who have a hemoglobin A1c of 7% or greater.
- The use of technological devices in clinical practice is time intensive and requires a substantial investment in education of both practitioners and patients.
- Cost-effectiveness studies are needed to further document health care cost reduction associated with CGM.
- Sensor-augmented insulin pump therapy and closed-loop "artificial pancreas" systems are currently in development and show great promise to automate insulin delivery with minimal patient intervention.

INTRODUCTION

Results from the Diabetes Control and Complication Trial have underlined the importance of glucose control in prevention of microvascular and macrovascular disease, and over the last 4 decades the use of self-monitoring blood glucose (SMBG) has become the standard of care.[1]

However, striving toward near-normal glycemia is difficult to achieve without substantial patient and health care provider effort, and leads to an increase in episodes of hypoglycemia. Moreover, although SMBG is a widely used and important component of therapy for type 1 diabetes mellitus (T1DM), it is challenging in day-to-day practice: patients' monitoring may be infrequent or intermittent, and overnight glucose

The authors have nothing to disclose.
Joslin Diabetes Center, Adult Section, One Joslin Place, Boston, MA 02215, USA
* Corresponding author.
E-mail address: elena.toschi@joslin.harvard.edu

Endocrinol Metab Clin N Am 45 (2016) 895–904
http://dx.doi.org/10.1016/j.ecl.2016.06.003
0889-8529/16/© 2016 Elsevier Inc. All rights reserved.

levels are seldom measured. Given these limitations, episodes of hypoglycemia and hyperglycemia may be missed and not factored into treatment decisions.[2,3]

Real-time (RT) continuous glucose monitoring (CGM)—the newest diabetes technological device—has been commercially available since the mid 2000s. The potential clinical benefit of this technology as a tool to assist with optimization of glucose control for both T1DM and types 2 diabetes mellitus (T2DM) adult populations is reviewed in this article.

CONTINUOUS GLUCOSE MONITORING TECHNOLOGY

Current models of CGM measure the glucose concentration in the interstitial fluid every 1 to 5 minutes for up to 7 days via a short subcutaneous probe (glucose sensor). There is a lag of several minutes between plasma and interstitial fluid concentrations, which also depends on the glucose rate of change at any given time; this can lead to inconsistencies between SMBG and CGM values in excess of 20 mg/dL. SMBG values are still required to calibrate CGM devices—the best time to calibrate is during glucose steady state—and SMBG is required to confirm glucose levels before an insulin bolus is administered and to confirm hypoglycemia before treatment. At this time, CGM devices cannot substitute SMBG, but they are valuable in providing detailed information on blood glucose trends in between SMBG, especially after meals and overnight. Moreover, whereas SMBG is a static value, CGM shows current glucose levels along with trend arrows, providing a dynamic tracing, which is likely much more helpful in decision making throughout the day. It also provides threshold alerts for low and high blood glucose values. Currently, we do not have guidelines on how to choose and adjust alert settings, and it is up to the clinician along with the patient to decide what works best to tighten glucose control, reduce hypoglycemic risk, and avoid alert fatigue. This technology is evolving steadily in terms of accuracy and ease of use. Factory-calibrated devices are in development that could reduce common calibration errors.

Recent enhancements have also made it possible to project data to other devices such as smartphones, smart wrist-watches, and computers with the possibility of sharing data safely with clinicians, spouses, and others remotely. In 2015, the US Food and Drug Administration approved 3 such systems: the Dexcom Share (Dexcom, Inc., San Diego, CA),[4] Dexcom G5 with Bluetooth (Dexcom, Inc.),[5] and MiniMed Connect (Medtronic, North Haven, CT).[6] An open-source system (not US Food and Drug Administration approved) called Nightscout is also available.

USE OF CONTINUOUS GLUCOSE MONITORING IN TYPE 1 DIABETES MELLITUS
Impact of Continuous Glucose Monitoring on Glycemic Control

Several major studies have evaluated the use of CGM in adults with T1DM (**Table 1**): the Juvenile Diabetes Research Foundation (JDRF) CGM randomized controlled trial,[7] the GuardControl Study,[8] and O'Connell and colleagues,[9] and they all demonstrated that adults with T1DM with a hemoglobin A1c of at least 7.0% had a greater reduction in hemoglobin A1c with the use of RT-CGM than with intermittent SMBG (0.5%, 0.6% and 0.43%, respectively). Furthermore, unlike findings with SMBG, the improvement in hemoglobin A1c with CGM is not accompanied by an increase in biochemical hypoglycemia.[8,10] Interestingly, in the JDRF 6-month trial, the improvement in hemoglobin A1c in the subjects using CGM was sustained over the 6-month observational period that followed completion of the trial.[11] This ongoing benefit occurred despite reduction in office visit frequency during this observational period to levels (2.7 ± 1.2 visits over 6 months), similar to routine care.

| Table 1 |
| Results for type 1 diabetes mellitus reduction in hemoglobin A1c and hypoglycemia |

			Baseline		Outcome		
			Hemoglobin	Δ Hemoglobin	Hemoglobin	Severe	
Study	n	Length	A1c	A1c	A1c <7.0%	Hypoglycemia	
JDRF-CGM	52	6 mo	7.6	−0.5	30%	21.8	
JDRF-CGM 6 mo	51	1 y	7.6	−0.5	29%	7.1	
Deiss	81	3 mo	8.1	−0.6	27%	NA	
O'Connell	15	3 mo	7.3	−0.4	56%	NA	

Abbreviations: JDRF-CGM, Juvenile Diabetes Research Foundation Continuous Glucose Monitoring; NA, not applicable.

To date, there are no trials focusing on evaluation of benefit of use of CGM in T1DM on multiple daily injections (MDI). In the JDRF CGM trial,[7] the patients using continuous subcutaneous insulin infusion (CSII) and MDI had similar reductions in hemoglobin A1c. However, because MDI users comprised only 20% of the total study population, the improvement in this subgroup did not attain significance. The ongoing Diamond study (Multiple Daily Injections and Continuous Glucose Monitoring in Diabetes),[12] which is examining the use of RT-CGM in adults with T1DM and T2DM on MDI, should provide conclusive data about the benefit of this technology in individuals using insulin injections for diabetes self-management.

Impact of Continuous Glucose Monitoring on Frequency of Hypoglycemia

The JDRF CGM Study Group has also demonstrated that in patients with T1DM who have achieved hemoglobin A1c levels of less than 7.0%, RT-CGM use can reduce the frequency of biochemical hypoglycemia measured by CGM and maintain hemoglobin A1c levels of less than 7.0% compared with standard blood glucose monitoring over a 6-month study period. The median time per day with a glucose level of 70 mg/dL or less as measured by CGM was less in the CGM group than in the control group; however, the difference was not significant. In this study, almost all the other analyses (including the time per day at ≤60 mg/dL, time per day between 71 and 180 mg/dL, and combined outcomes involving hemoglobin A1c coupled with hypoglycemia) statically favored the CGM group compared with the control group. Furthermore, the incidence rate of severe hypoglycemia declined from 20.5 events per 100 patient-years during the initial 6-month randomized trial to 12.1 events per 100 patient-years during the 6-month observational follow-up.[11]

These data clearly support the efficacy of CGM in reducing the incidence rate of hypoglycemic events and could be beneficial in high-risk groups, such as long-standing T1DM subjects and pregnant women with T1DM. Hypoglycemia unawareness and episodes of severe hypoglycemia are challenges that people with long-standing T1DM face. These patients are at higher risk of severe hypoglycemia partly owing to age, longer duration of diabetes, and associated hypoglycemic unawareness. Very little attention has been given to these high-risk patients, and more work needs to be done in this area.[13]

Although the JDRF CGM trial included some subjects over 65 years old who derived benefit from CGM, there have been no trials exclusively enrolling older patients, and thus far Medicare does not cover this technology.

Hypoglycemia, in particular asymptomatic hypoglycemia, is a key safety concern during pregnancy. However, the potential benefit of CGM in pregnant women with preexisting diabetes is unclear based on current available data.[14] An ongoing study (CONCEPTT; Continuous Glucose Monitoring in Women with Type 1 Diabetes in Pregnancy Trial) is evaluating if CGM can safely improve glycemic control in patients with T1DM who are pregnant or planning pregnancy.[15]

Factors Predicting Successful Use of Continuous Glucose Monitoring

A post hoc analysis of the JDRF-CGM study data was conducted to determine what factors, if any, predicted successful CGM use in month 6 of the trial and reduction in hemoglobin A1c.[16] In the sixth month of the trial, 50% of subjects were using the CGM 6 or more days per week. The only baseline factors associated with CGM use in month 6 were age greater than 25 and reported number of home glucose meter checks per day. Additional factors predictive of CGM use were frequency of CGM use in the first month and the percentage of values in the target range of 71 to 180 mg/dL during the first month. For subjects with a baseline hemoglobin A1c of greater than 7.0%, use of CGM for more than 6 days per week was associated with a greater than 0.5% reduction in hemoglobin A1c[17] (**Box 1**).

Interestingly, none of the psychosocial surveys used in the trial, including the Hypoglycemia Fear Survey,[18] the Blood Glucose Monitoring System Rating Questionnaire,[19] and the Problem Areas in Diabetes Questionnaire,[7] were predictive of improvement in glycemic control.[20] A small subset of subjects (n = 20) participating in the JDRF trial participated in semistructured interviews focusing on their psychosocial experiences with CGM. Subjects that had either (A) improvement in glucose control with baseline hemoglobin A1c of greater than 7.0% and/or (B) demonstrated decreased time of blood glucose at less than 70 mg/dL while remaining within target hemoglobin A1c were able to cope with frustrations. They used self-control rather than emotions-based coping when faced with CGM frustrations; were able to use retrospective pattern analysis, not just minute-by-minute data analysis, in glycemic management; and had "significant other" involvement—interest, encouragement, and participation by their loved ones. However, all subjects expressed body image concerns when wearing CGM devices.[21]

There is an ongoing learning curve while using CGM. In the JDRF study, CGM users whose hemoglobin A1c levels was already at target (<7.0%) had a decrease in the incidence of episodes of hypoglycemia from 23.6 events per 100 person-years during the 6-month randomized controlled trial and 0 per 100 patient-years during the 6 months of continued CGM use after the conclusion of the randomized clinical trial.[11]

In a survey performed in 300 individuals with T1DM (n = 222) and insulin-treated T2DM (n = 78) using CGM data and responding to their glucose information in real-world settings, it was found that respondents use the CGM data to alter multiple aspects of their diabetes care, including insulin dose timing, dose adjustments, and in hypoglycemia prevention. Moreover, the insulin adjustments reported by respondents

---

Box 1
Potential advantages of continuous glucose monitoring used in type 1 diabetes mellitus

Better glucose control reflected by hemoglobin A1c

Reduced risk of hypoglycemia episodes

Reduced glycemic variability

Improved quality of life

were much greater than the 10% to 20% recommended.[19,22,23] A subsequent study that evaluated the use of the rate of change arrows again reported that the majority of respondents make multiple and more significant changes in their insulin dosages than the 10% to 20% recommended. There is no standardization on how to use this information for bolusing/correction.[24]

Furthermore, CGM data highlight the complexity of postprandial glucose patterns present in T1DM. A systematic review of studies that evaluated the effects of dietary fat, protein, and glycemic index on acute postprandial glucose control in T1DM indicated that all these dietary factors modify postprandial glycemia. Specifically high-fat/protein meals require more insulin than lower fat/protein meals with identical carbohydrate content.[25] Currently, a carbohydrate-based approach to bolus dose calculation is used, but this clearly has limitations and there is a need for alternative insulin dosing algorithms for high-fat/high-protein meals.

Still, little is known about how patients use CGM data around their behavior toward exercise and food choices, and how they adjust their insulin therapy on a day-to-day basis and if there are differences between individuals who use MDI therapy and those who use CSII.

CONTINUOUS GLUCOSE MONITORING IN TYPE 2 DIABETES MELLITUS
Impact of Continuous Glucose Monitoring on Glycemic Control

There are even fewer data available on T2DM and the use of CGM. In the following, the results of 2 studies using the most up-to-date devices are discussed. One well-performed large-scale randomized controlled trial[26] involving 100 adults with T2DM on therapies including diet and exercise alone and various combinations of antidiabetes medications, including basal but not prandial insulin, showed that intermittent use of CGM for 12 weeks (4 cycles of 2 weeks use/1 week off) resulted in significant improvement in hemoglobin A1c, sustained during a 40-week follow-up period (hemoglobin A1c at 12 weeks and 52 weeks were $1.0 \pm 1.1\%$ and $0.8 \pm 1.5\%$ in the CGM group vs $0.5 \pm 0.8\%$ and $0.2 \pm 1.3\%$ in the SMBG control group; $P = .04$). This improvement in the CGM group occurred without greater intensification of medication than the control group, indicating that it probably reflected changes in self-care prompted by use of CGM.[26,27] A follow-up analysis showed that patients with T2DM with higher starting A1Cs benefit the most of using short-term CGM, and clinicians should closely monitor for worsening glycemia that might be the result of burnout.[28]

In a less rigorous study, Yoo and colleagues[29] randomized patients with T2DM and hemoglobin A1c levels of 8% to 10% on oral agents or insulin to use of CGM for 3 days per month for 12 weeks versus SMBG 6 times per week in the control group. Both the CGM and SMBG groups had significant reductions in the hemoglobin A1c at the 12-week follow-up (CGM: $9.1\% \pm 1.0\%$ to $8.0 \pm 1.2\%$ [$P < .001$]; SMBG: $8.7 \pm 0.7\%$ to $8.3 \pm 1.1\%$ [$P = .01$]), with a significant difference in the improvement between the 2 groups ($P = .004$). Reduction in hemoglobin A1c in the control group occurred despite a very modest increase in SMBG frequency from 3.9 times per week at baseline to 6.1 times per week in the trial, suggesting that study effect and increased intensity of follow-up and guidance in this trial may have added to the apparent benefit seen in the CGM group.

Consistent data from additional well-performed randomized, controlled trials in patients with different health literacy and sociodemographic characteristics to those studied in these 2 trials are needed to confirm that these findings are generalizable to the broader T2DM population. At present, no data exist for use of RT-CGM in patients with T2DM on prandial insulin. The ongoing Diamond study[12] should provide conclusive data about the potential benefits of this technology in this population.

An analysis projected that lifetime clinical and economic outcomes for CGM versus SMBG only showed that CGM, as a self-care tool, is a cost-effective disease management option in the United States for people with T2DM not on prandial insulin. Repeated use of CGM may result in additional cost effectiveness.[30]

Education and Training on Use of Real-Time Continuous Glucose Monitoring

There are few data about how best to train individuals on the use of CGM to optimize glycemic control, reduce risk of hypoglycemic events, and all the while minimize alert fatigue. A review of the literature revealed no evidence of randomized trials that have evaluated the effectiveness of educational strategies and protocols on how to best use CGM. A recent consensus statement and guidelines from American Association of Clinical Endocrinologists recommend education regarding the interpretation and use of CGM data to help modify patient behaviors, enhance ability to self-adjust therapy, and help decide when to seek medical assistance.[14]

At this point in time, reports of CGM are not standardized and use of how to analyze the data, how to set alarms, and how to use trend arrows have not been standardized. This makes the use of this technology still challenging especially, for physicians who do not use CGM technology on a daily basis. The development of standardized metrics and reporting among available CGM devices would facilitate better interpretation of the data. Downloading CGM should become faster and easier, and should be accessible remotely by physicians, health care providers, and significant others. Moreover, development of pattern recognition software that identifies risk patterns would help clinicians to interpret data and educate patients in a meaningful way.

Even without this standardization, experiences reported in the literature were overwhelmingly positive, with improved glycemic control, diet and exercise management, quality of life, and physical and psychological well-being, as well as reduced frequency of SMBG.[31]

In the near future, tools should be developed to integrate data gathered from common mobile device apps, such as step counters, heart rate monitors, meals/calorie counters, exercise trackers, and so on. This will minimize patient data entry and will ease physicians' evaluation of CGM data in the context of other variables influencing glucose levels. Further studies are needed to determine how to develop tools to train subjects on how to best use their CGM data.

THE FUTURE
Continuous Glucose Monitoring Along with Continuous Subcutaneous Insulin Infusion

Continuous subcutaneous insulin infusion with stand-alone real-time continuous glucose monitoring

CGM has been used both as a stand-alone along with CSII or through integration with pump technology in so-called "sensor-augmented insulin pumps" (SIP). Studies have shown that the use of SIP technology in T1DM can improve both glucose control and, if using a low glucose threshold suspend, can reduce hypoglycemic events.[32,33] Successful use of SIP or CSII with stand-alone CGM is determined by the amount of time a patient has spent using this technology, whether the patient feels he or she can rely on the accuracy of data, and whether the patient understands how to use the information for daily diabetes self-management. In a small ambulatory study, 38 subjects with T1DM used the Dexcom G4 and Medtronic Enlite sensors simultaneously for 4 to

6 days. The results showed that the Dexcom G4 sensor was associated with greater accuracy, especially in the hypoglycemic range, than the Enlite sensor. Moreover, patients reported a significantly more positive experience using the Dexcom G4 and were more willing to use the system in daily life.[34] These data call for a randomized controlled trial evaluating head-to-head the different CGM devices rather than an evaluation of SIP technology versus CSII. By the same token, no official recommendations currently exist for selecting a particular CGM system, and individual diabetes centers generally base the selection on local experience and preferences.

Closed-Loop Insulin Delivery Systems

Improvements in CGM accuracy have allowed scientists and researchers to close the loop—creating an "artificial pancreas."[35,36] Closed-loop systems feature CGM and automated insulin delivery with minimal patient intervention. In a randomized controlled trial in adults, overnight closed-loop insulin delivery improved glucose control and reduced hypoglycemia, even after a large carbohydrate meal with alcohol.[37] Recent trials show near-normal glucose levels in adults with T1DM using a bihormonal (insulin and glucagon) closed-loop system, even in outpatient-monitored settings.[38–40] Additional studies are in progress to refine closed-loop algorithms and further evaluate their performance in adult home settings. Several companies and investigators are taking different approaches to make an artificial pancreas.

SUMMARY

The studies performed so far suggest that CGM is beneficial to improve glycemic control and prevent hypoglycemic episodes in T1DM and improve glycemic control in T2DM. The Endocrine Society Clinical Practice Guidelines[41] recommended that CGM devices should be used by all adults with T1DM, as long they can demonstrate use of these devices on a nearly daily basis, to achieve or maintain hemoglobin A1c levels less than 7.0%, and to reduce the frequency of biochemical hypoglycemia. Similarly, the benefit of using CGM has been also shown for T2DM and short-term, intermittent use of CGM should be considered in adult patients with T2DM (not on prandial insulin) who have a hemoglobin A1c of 7% or greater.[41]

Adults with T1DM and T2DM using CGM should receive education, training, and ongoing support to help achieve and maintain individualized glycemic goals. Development of pattern recognition software could facilitate interpretation and utilization of the data by both patients and physicians. Encouragingly, the ongoing Diamond study[12] should provide conclusive data about the benefit of this technology in individuals using MDI, and the REPLACE-BG[42] will do the same regarding the safety of using only a CGM for insulin bolusing.

A consensus conference of the American Association of Clinical Endocrinologists and American College of Endocrinology held in February 2016 advocated expanding the use of CGM in the management of diabetes. Based on the data described in this paper, CGM use is shown to improve glucose control and reduce hypoglycemic events, and therefore has the potential to reduce the risk of acute and chronic complications of diabetes. Likely, all of the above would not only improve the quality of life and life expectancy of people with diabetes, but would also have a positive impact on health-related cost.[43]

We expect some time in the next decade CGM will replace SMBG and be considered as a stand-alone entity.[44]

REFERENCES

1. The Diabetes Control and Complications Trial Research Group. The effect of intensive treatment diabetes on the development and progression of long-term complications in insulin-dependent diabetes mellitus. N Engl J Med 1993;329: 977–86.
2. Kaufman FR, Gibson LC, Halvorson M, et al. A pilot study of the continuous glucose monitoring system: clinical decisions and glycemic control after its use in pediatric type 1 diabetic subjects. Diabetes Care 2001;24:2030–4.
3. Chitayat L, Zisser H, Jovanovic L. Continuous glucose monitoring during pregnancy. Diabetes Technol Ther 2009;11(Suppl 1):S105–11.
4. US Food and Drug Administration (FDA). Press announcements: FDA permits marketing of first system of mobile medical apps for continuous glucose monitoring. Available at: http://www.fda.gov/newsevents/newsroom/pressannounce ments/ucm431385.htm. Accessed April 2016.
5. FDA Approves Dexcom G5® Mobile Continuous Glucose Monitoring System | Dexcom. 2015. Available at: http://dexcom.com/news/1257506247-f-da-approves-dexcom-g5®-mobile-continuous-glucose-monitoring-system. Accessed April 2016.
6. Medtronic receives FDA clearance of MiniMed® Connect for more convenient access to personal diabetes data. 2015. Available at: http://newsroom.medtronic. com/phoenix. Accessed April 2016.
7. Juvenile Diabetes Research Foundation Continuous Glucose Monitoring Study Group. Continuous Glucose Monitoring and Intensive Treatment of Type 1 Diabetes. N Engl J Med 2008;359:1464–76.
8. Deiss D, Bolinder J, Riveline JP, et al. Improved Glycemic Control in Poorly Controlled Patients with Type 1 Diabetes Using Real-Time Continuous Glucose Monitoring. Diabetes Care 2006;29(12):2730–2.
9. O'Connell MA, Donath S, O'Neal DN, et al. Glycaemic impact of patient-led use of sensor-guided pump therapy in type 1 diabetes: a randomized controlled trial. Diabetologia 2009;52:1250–7.
10. Diabetes Research in Children Network (DirecNet) Study Group. Continuous glucose monitoring in children with type 1 diabetes. J Pediatr 2007;151(4): 388–93.
11. Juvenile Diabetes Research Foundation Continuous Glucose Monitoring Study Group. Sustained benefit of continuous glucose monitoring on A1C, glucose profiles, and hypoglycemia in adults with type 1 diabetes. Diabetes Care 2009; 32(11):2047–9.
12. Multiple Daily Injections and Continuous Glucose Monitoring in Diabetes (DIaMonD). ClinicalTrials.gov: NCT02282397. Available at: https://www.clinicaltrials.gov/ct2/ show/NCT02282397?term=NCT02282397&rank=1. Accessed April 2016.
13. Weinstock RS, DuBose SN, Bergenstal RM, et al. T1D Exchange Severe Hypoglycemia in Older Adults with Type 1 Diabetes Study Groups: risk factors associated with severe hypoglycemia in older adults with type 1 diabetes. Diabetes Care 2016;39(4):603–10.
14. Bailey TS, Grunberger G, Bode BW, et al. American Association of Clinical Endocrinologists and American College of Endocrinology 2016 Outpatient Glucose Monitoring Consensus Statement. Endocr Pract 2016;22(2):231–61.
15. Continuous Glucose Monitoring in Women With Type 1 Diabetes in Pregnancy Trial (CONCEPTT). Available at: http://clinicaltrials.gov/show/NCT01788527. Accessed April 2016.

16. The Juvenile Diabetes Research Foundation Continuous Glucose Monitoring Study Group. Factors predictive of use and of benefit from continuous glucose monitoring in type 1 diabetes. Diabetes Care 2009;32:1947–53.
17. Ruedy K, Tamborlane W. The Landmark JDRF Continuous Glucose Monitoring Randomized Trials: a look back at the accumulated evidence. J Cardiovasc Trans Res 2012;5:380–7.
18. The Juvenile Diabetes Research Foundation Continuous Glucose Monitoring Study Group. Validation of measures of satisfaction with and impact of continuous and conventional glucose monitoring. Diabetes Technol Ther 2010;12(9): 679–84.
19. JDRF CGM Study Group. JDRF randomized clinical trial to assess the efficacy of real-time continuous glucose monitoring in the management of type 1 diabetes: research design and methods. Diabetes Technol Ther 2008;10:310–21.
20. Beck RW, Lawrence JM, Laffel L, et al. Quality-of-life measures in children and adults with type 1 diabetes: Juvenile Diabetes Research Foundation Continuous Glucose Monitoring randomized trial. Diabetes Care 2010;33(10):2175–7.
21. Ritholz MD, Atakov-Castillo A, Beste M, et al. Education and psychological aspects psychosocial factors associated with use of continuous glucose monitoring. Diabetes Med 2010;27:1060–5.
22. Pettus J, Price DA, Edelman SV. How patients with type 1 diabetes translate continuous glucose monitoring data into diabetes management decisions. Endocr Pract 2015;21:613–20.
23. Buckingham B, Xing D, Weinzimer S, et al. Use of the DirecNet Applied Treatment Algorithm (DATA) for diabetes management with a real-time continuous glucose monitor (the FreeStyle Navigator). Pediatr Diabetes 2008;9:142–7.
24. Pettus J, Edelman SV. Use of glucose rate of change arrows to adjust insulin therapy among individuals with type 1 diabetes who use continuous glucose monitoring. Diabetes Technol Ther 2016;18(Suppl 2):S234–42.
25. Bell KJ, Smart CE, Steil GM, et al. Impact of fat, protein, and glycemic index on postprandial glucose control in type 1 diabetes: implications for intensive diabetes management in the continuous glucose monitoring era. Diabetes Care 2015;38:1008–15.
26. Vigersky RA, Fonda SG, Chellappa M, et al. Short- and long-term effects of real-time continuous glucose monitoring in patients with type 2 diabetes. Diabetes Care 2012;35:32–8.
27. Ehrhardt NM, Chellappa M, Walker MS. The effect of real-time continuous glucose monitoring on glycemic control in patients with type 2 diabetes mellitus. J Diabetes Sci Technol 2011;5:668–75.
28. Fonda SJ, Salkind SJ, Walker MS, et al. Heterogeneity of Responses to Real-Time Continuous Glucose Monitoring (RT-CGM) in patients with type 2 diabetes and its implications for application. Diabetes Care 2013;36:786–92.
29. Yoo H, An HG, Park SY, et al. Use of a real time continuous glucose monitoring system as a motivational device for poorly controlled type 2 diabetes. Diabetes Res Clin Pract 2008;82:73–9.
30. Fonda SJ, Graham C, Munakata J, et al. The cost-effectiveness of real-time continuous glucose monitoring (RT-CGM) in type 2 diabetes. J Diabetes Sci Technol 2016;10(4):898–904.
31. Pickup JC, Ford Holloway M. Samsi K Real-time continuous glucose monitoring in type 1 diabetes: a qualitative framework analysis of patient narratives. Diabetes Care 2015;38:544–55.

32. Bergenstal RM, Tamborlane WV, Ahrmann A, et al. Effectiveness of sensor-augmented insulin-pump therapy in type 1 diabetes. N Engl J Med 2010;363:311–20.

33. Bergenstal RM, Klonoff DC, Gard SK, et al. Threshold-based insulin-pump interruption for reduction of hypoglycemia. N Engl J Med 2013;369:224–32.

34. Matuleviciene V, Joseph JI, Andelin M, et al. A Clinical Trial of the Accuracy and Treatment Experience of the Dexcom G4 Sensor (Dexcom G4 System) and Enlite Sensor (Guardian REAL-Time System) Tested Simultaneously in Ambulatory Patients with Type 1 Diabetes. Diabetes Technol Ther 2014;16:759–67.

35. Garg SK, Brazg RL, Bailey TS, et al. Reduction in duration of hypoglycemia by automatic suspension of insulin delivery: the in-clinic ASPIRE study. Diabetes Technol Ther 2012;14:205–9.

36. Klonoff DC, Bergenstal RM, Garg SK, et al. ASPIRE In-Home: rationale, design, and methods of a study to evaluate the safety and efficacy of automatic insulin suspension for nocturnal hypoglycemia. J Diabetes Sci Technol 2013;7:1005–10.

37. Hovorka R, Kumareswaran K, Harris J, et al. Overnight closed loop insulin delivery (artificial pancreas) in adults with type 1 diabetes: crossover randomised controlled studies. BMJ 2011;13:342–52.

38. Russell SJ, El-Khatib FH, Nathan DM, et al. Blood glucose control in type 1 diabetes with a bihormonal bionic endocrine pancreas. Diabetes Care 2012;35:2148–55.

39. Haidar A, Legault L, Dallaire M, et al. Glucose-responsive insulin and glucagon delivery (dual-hormone artificial pancreas) in adults with type 1 diabetes: a randomized crossover controlled trial. CMAJ 2013;185(4):297–305.

40. Russell SJ, El-Khatib FH, Sinha M, et al. Outpatient glycemic control with a bionic pancreas in type 1 diabetes. N Engl J Med 2014;371:313–25.

41. Klonoff DC, Buckingham B, Christiansen JS. Continuous glucose monitoring: an Endocrine Society Clinical Practice Guideline. J Clin Endocrinol Metab 2011;96:2968–79.

42. A Trial Comparing Continuous Glucose Monitoring With and Without Routine Blood Glucose Monitoring in Adults With Type 1 Diabetes (REPLACE-BG). Available at: https://clinicaltrials.gov/ct2/show/NCT02258373. Accessed April 2016.

43. AACE/ACE Consensus Conference on CGM February 20, 2016 Hyatt Regency at Capitol Hill, Washington DC.

44. Garg S. The future of glucose monitoring. Diabetes Technol Ther 2016;18(Suppl 2):1–3.

Bariatric Surgery

Pathophysiology and Outcomes

Sidra Azim, MD, Sangeeta R. Kashyap, MD*

KEYWORDS

- Obesity • Type 2 diabetes • Bariatric surgery • Weight loss • Metabolic effects

KEY POINTS

- Obesity and type 2 diabetes are closely interrelated; excess adiposity leads to inflammation, insulin resistance, and beta cell failure in predisposed individuals.
- Currently, bariatric surgery is the most effective treatment for obesity and results in long-term weight loss and improvement in metabolic profile and obesity-related complications.
- Bariatric surgery leads to significant improvement in glycemic control and metabolic syndrome components through weight loss but benefits for micro/macro vascular complications of diabetes remain unclear.
- Long-term risk for nutritional deficiencies, osteoporosis/bone fractures, and various surgical complications need to be considered for individual patient management.

BACKGROUND

Chronic diseases lead to 7 of 10 deaths every year in the United States and pose a major burden on health care, accounting for 86% of national health care costs.[1,2] Type 2 diabetes mellitus (DM) and obesity are 2 preventable chronic diseases with an approximate prevalence of 9.3% (29.1 million) and 34.9% (78.6 million) in the US population.[3,4] A total of $245 billion were spent on diabetes care in the United States in direct and indirect costs and $147 billion were spent in medical care of obese adults in 2012. Annual medical costs for people with obesity are $1429 higher than those for people of normal weight.[1]

The prevalence of obesity has doubled over the past 40 years, and a similar drift is expected for DM prevalence to double in the next 40 years.[5] This trend illustrates a direct relationship between obesity and DM, which was described in a prior study in which severe obesity with a body mass index (BMI) greater than 35 kg/m² was associated with a 40-fold increased risk of developing DM as compared with normal BMI

Disclosure Statement: The authors have nothing to disclose.
Department of Endocrinology, Diabetes, and Metabolism, Cleveland Clinic, 9500 Euclid Avenue (F-20), Cleveland, OH 44195, USA
* Corresponding author. Department of Endocrinology, Cleveland Clinic Foundation, 9500 Euclid Avenue (F-20), Cleveland, OH 44195.
E-mail address: kashyas@ccf.org

less than 23 kg/m^2.[6] Obesity is an independent risk factor for mortality and increases the risk of developing other comorbidities, such as nonalcoholic fatty liver disease, hypertension, hyperlipidemia, cardiovascular (CV) disease, stroke, degenerative joint disease, obstructive sleep apnea, and cancer.[7,8]

Obesity-related morbidity and mortality risk has been shown to be reversible with modest weight loss.[9] Various weight loss interventions, including lifestyle modifications and weight loss medications, have shown excellent results, with up to 7% to 12% weight loss, but have not been able to show long-term benefits. Weight loss surgeries that were initially introduced in the 1960s have now become standard of care for patients with BMI of 40 kg/m^2 or higher or BMI greater than 35 kg/m^2 with obesity-related comorbidities or obese patients who fail lifestyle and medical management. Bariatric surgery (BS) has shown to be the most effective weight-loss therapy with sustained results with approximated weight loss range of 12% to 39% of presurgical body weight or 40% to 71% excess weight loss (EWL).[10]

We review here the association between obesity and DM, pathophysiology and metabolic benefits of BS on DM and related comorbidities, and clinical implications of BS for DM management.

OBESITY AND TYPE 2 DIABETES

Obesity is a disease state characterized by excess fat accumulation to an extent that is detrimental to health. It is defined as BMI of greater than 30 kg/m^2 by the World Health Organization (WHO). Obesity severity is categorized as class I, BMI 30 to 34.9 kg/m^2; class II, BMI 35 to 39.9 kg/m^2; and class III, BMI greater than 40 kg/m^2.[11] Class III obesity has been further subcategorized to quantify the metabolic disease risk in surgical literature as "severe obesity," BMI greater than or equal to 35 or 40; "morbid obesity," BMI greater than or equal to 35 or 40 to 44.9 or 49.9; and "super obesity," BMI greater than or equal to 45 or 50.

Risk factors that promote obesity include genetics, sedentary lifestyle, excess calorie consumption, and imbalance between peripheral hormones that cause satiety and hunger. Hormones that promote satiety include leptin produced solely in adipose tissue, glucagonlike peptide 1 (GLP-1) produced in the small intestine, cholecystokinin, enterostatin, polypeptide Y 3 to 36, α melanocyte-stimulating hormone, corticotropin-releasing hormone, tumor necrosis factor α (TNF-α), and obestatin.[12] In contrast, ghrelin is a strong appetite stimulant produced in the fundus that also stimulates growth hormone secretion. Other hormones that have a similar effect on appetite include neuropeptide Y, dynorphin, melanin-concentrating hormone, norepinephrine, growth hormone–releasing hormone, orexin-A, and orexin-B. The effect of some of these hormones is discussed in more detail below.

Type 2 diabetes mellitus (DM2) is a complex metabolic disorder triggered by a combination of genetic and environmental factors that leads to development of insulin resistance, progressive pancreatic beta cell insufficiency resulting in hyperglycemia.

There are various hypothesized mechanisms by which obesity may lead to insulin resistance and diabetes. **Fig. 1** describes the possible mechanisms by which obesity may contribute to diabetes and diabetes-related complications.

The lipocentric model suggests that excess caloric intake causes excess lipogenesis, elevation of circulating free fatty acids and ectopic fat deposition in liver and muscle causing insulin resistance and subsequent hyperinsulinemia. This may lead to "lipotoxicity" via activation of inflammatory pathways and production of inflammatory adipocytokines, such as TNF-α, plasminogen activator inhibitor 1, retinol-binding protein 4, and resistin, which disrupt glucose disposal.[12,13] In addition, adiponectin

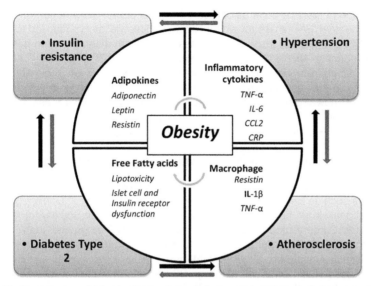

Fig. 1. Mechanisms by which obesity leads to diabetes and diabetes-related complications. C-C motif, chemokine; CCL2, ligand 2; CRP, C-reactive protein; IL-1β, interleukin 1 beta; IL-6, interleukin 6. (*Adapted from* Redinger RN. The pathophysiology of obesity and its clinical manifestations. Gastroenterol Hepatol (NY) 2007;3(11):858.)

(a cytokine released by adipose tissue that decreases insulin resistance) has shown to be deficient in obese patients. It is also suggested that ectopic fat deposition in the pancreas can contribute to impaired insulin secretion and hyperglycemia.

Approximately 75% of patients with DM on insulin have been reported to be overweight.[14] In both men and women, BMI is a major predictor of developing DM. In women, the risk of developing DM is increased 5-fold with BMI greater than 25 kg/m², 28-fold with BMI greater than 30 kg/m², and 93-fold with BMI greater than 35 kg/m².[15] Men are 2.2 times more likely to develop DM if their BMI is greater than 25 kg/m² and 6.7 times more likely if there BMI is greater than 30 kg/m².[6] Westlund and Nicolayson[16] found similar results in their study in which 0.6% of normal weight men developed DM while the incidence of DM was 23.4% in overweight men.

EFFECTS OF WEIGHT LOSS

Various studies have suggested a positive impact of weight loss on DM and other obesity-related complications.

A weight loss of 5 kg has been associated with more than 50% reduction in the risk of developing DM.[15] Similarly, a 9-kg weight loss was associated with 30% to 40% decrease in DM-related death.[17] There is a 15% reduction in fasting blood glucose and a 7% drop in HbA1c seen with weight loss of 5% body weight.[18]

Reisin and colleagues[19] found a 20% reduction in systolic and diastolic blood pressure (BP) with 10-kg weight loss. A similar improvement is seen in the lipid profile of patients, with a decrease in low-density lipoprotein (LDL) by 1%, triglycerides (TG) by 3%, and increase in high-density lipoprotein (HDL) by 1% for every kilogram of weight loss.[20]

The US Diabetes Prevention Program (DPP) study suggested that 5% to 10% of initial body weight loss via lifestyle modifications including diet and exercise reduced the incidence of DM2 by 58% as compared with placebo.[21] The Action for Health in Diabetes (Look AHEAD) trial showed that intensive lifestyle intervention led to a weight loss of 8.6% of initial weight.[22] This was associated with mean glycated hemoglobin (HbA1C) reduction to 6.6%, along with improvement in BP, TG, HDL cholesterol, and urine albumin-to-creatinine ratio. However, no benefits on mortality or CVD (Cardiovascular diseases) events were noted with intensive lifestyle modification.

Obesity is known to be a proinflammatory state, and weight loss is associated with an improvement in obesity-related inflammation via increase in adiponectin and reduction in TNF-α, interleukin-6, leptin, and C-reactive protein.[23]

RESTRICTIVE AND MALABSORPTIVE BARIATRIC SURGERY PROCEDURES

BS procedures are associated with a greater weight loss as compared with other interventions such as lifestyle modification and pharmacotherapy.[24] Current guidelines by the National Heart, Lung, and Blood Institute and American Society for Metabolic and Bariatric Surgery recommend BS for patients with BMI greater than 40 kg/m^2 and patients with BMI greater than 35 kg/m^2 with comorbid diseases that can be alleviated or significantly improved by weight loss.[25]

Obese patients with DM2 who undergo BS have remarkable improvement in their glycemic control, with approximately 78% obtaining DM resolution and close to 85% experiencing improvement in their blood sugar control and reduction in antidiabetic medications.[26]

The effect of BS on weight loss, resolution of diabetes, and cardiometabolic parameters may vary depending on the type of BS procedures.

BS procedures are classified on the proposed mechanism of weight loss[27] and are described in **Table 1**.

Malabsorptive

Malabsorptive procedures comprise partial resection of small intestine, which causes reduction in intestinal mucosal area leading to lesser nutrient absorption. In addition, these procedures also restrict caloric intake by limiting stomach size. Up to 85% of patients with DM2 who undergo this type of surgery achieve diabetes remission.[28]

Roux-en-Y gastric bypass
Roux-en-Y gastric bypass (RYGB), commonly known as gastric bypass surgery, is the most commonly performed procedure and is gold standard for BS.[29] This procedure comprises constructing a small stomach pouch, Roux, and biliary limb, which leads to restricted caloric intake and decreased absorption of nutrients; 95% of the stomach, the entire duodenum, and a portion of the jejunum are bypassed. This surgery is primarily restrictive with some malabsorption.

Biliopancreatic diversion with duodenal switch
The biliopancreatic diversion with duodenal switch (BPD/DS) consists of 2 components: a partial gastrectomy and intestinal bypass. This procedure is thought to preserve physiologic digestive process. This surgery is majorly malabsorptive with some restriction.

Restrictive

Gastric restrictive procedures reduce caloric intake and cause satiety by limiting gastric volume. This can be done by surgically resizing the stomach as done in sleeve gastrostomy (SG) or laparoscopic adjustable gastric banding (LAGB) or vertical gastroplasty (VBG). These procedures are associated with approximately 46.2% of

Table 1
Commonly performed bariatric surgery procedure types, brief description of the procedure, and illustrations of anatomic changes

Procedures	Description	Figures
Malabsorptive		
Roux-en-Y gastric bypass (RYGB)	15–30-mL gastric pouch with gastro-jejunal anastomosis	
Biliopancreatic diversion with duodenal switch (BPD/DS)	Distal gastrectomy with anastomoses to distal ileum; proximal ileum is anastomosed to terminal ileum	
Restrictive		
Laparoscopic adjustable gastric banding (LAGB)	Adjustable silicone band is positioned around the stomach to create a 15-mL pouch	
Sleeve gastrostomy (SG)	Removal of greater curvature to create a tubular stomach	

excess body weight (EBW) loss. These types of surgeries have shown to lead to DM remission in 56.7% of patients.

Laparoscopic adjustable gastric banding
The LAGB is characterized by placement of adjustable band around the proximal stomach below the gastro-esophageal junction, forming a small pouch. This procedure has lower morbidity and mortality as compared with other bariatric procedures, but has shown to be less beneficial than a malabsorptive procedure and is associated with higher risk of reoperations.[30]

Sleeve gastrostomy
The laparoscopic SG comprises partial resection of the greater curvature of the stomach. This procedure is comparable to the malabsorptive procedures but has shown to have a greater effect than that of LAGB.

The efficacy of BS on metabolic pathways and diabetes remission depend on the type of surgery. Malabsorptive procedures lead to diabetes remission within days, whereas this response is not seen with gastric restrictive procedures.[31] Diabetes remission was shown in 98% of patients with DM2 undergoing BPD, 84% with RYGB, 72% with VGB, and 48% with LAGB.[26]

MECHANISMS FOR DIABETES REMISSION

The main processes that lead to weight loss after BS are calorie restriction via anatomic restriction and malabsorption.[10] Thirty percent to 70% of patients undergoing bariatric surgery develop some degree of malnutrition, including protein–calorie deficiency, fat malabsorption, fat-soluble vitamins, vitamins B12 and C, iron, calcium, copper, and zinc. Vagal denervation performed with some bariatric procedures may additionally contribute to weight loss via decreasing ghrelin levels. The role of ghrelin is described later. Another hypothesized modification, which promotes weight loss, is change in intestinal microbiome after bariatric surgery. There is decrease in Firmicutes and increase in Bacteroides/Prevotella and Escherichia coli depicting adaptation to a malnourished state.

There are various hypothesized mechanisms by which BS leads to improvement in glucose homeostasis. Of these, 3 major contributors are weight loss, nutrient malabsorption and rerouting, and gut hormonal changes.[32]

Weight Loss

Weight loss is a key driver for achieving euglycemia in obese patients with DM who undergo BS. Gastric volume restriction leads to early satiety, smaller meal consumption, and reduced caloric intake. This improves hepatic insulin sensitivity and improves insulin clearance in the liver, leading to lowering of fasting glucose levels. Additionally, caloric restriction reduces hyperinsulinemia and provides "rest" for beta-cell, which results in enhanced beta-cell function.[33] The rate of DM remission after BS correlates with the degree of weight loss.[34] Relapse of glycemic control post-BS is linked to inadequate surgical weight loss and weight regain. Patients after BS have an overall decrease in amount of food intake and change in food choices, with a decline in inclination toward calorie-rich, sugary, and fat-rich foods.[10,35] It is interesting that restrictive procedures lead to a lower rate of DM remission as compared with malabsorptive procedures such as RYGB or BPD in which patients become euglycemic within days of surgery and before significant weight loss.[36,37] This suggests that weight loss is not the sole factor contributing to diabetes remission.

Malabsorption of Nutrients

Malabsorptive procedures reduce excess intestinal absorption of glucose and lipids, which are thought to increase inflammation by increasing reactive oxygen species. This leads to improved insulin resistance and pancreatic beta-cell function, which decreases deposition of lipid metabolites in adipose and extra-adipose tissue, such as skeletal muscles and liver and corrects the impaired adipose tissue signaling.[38] This malabsorption of nutrients is more pronounced with BPD and is not as significant with RYGB, suggesting that additional factors may drive improvements in glycemic control.[39,40]

Foregut Versus Hindgut Hypothesis

Another principle to explain the effect of BS on glucose homeostasis is the redirecting of food course via anatomic changes in the gastrointestinal tract as seen with RYGB and BPD. Rubino and colleagues[33] suggested that obesity-related overeating leads to chronic overstimulation of the alimental system causing metabolic and hormonal disruptions that are diabetogenic.

Based on rat studies, they also proposed the theory of the "foregut exclusion hypothesis," which suggests that delivery of nutrients to the proximal small intestine leads to a release of a prodiabetic factor, which is oversecreted in diabetic patients.[32] Bypass of the duodenum and proximal jejunum avoids this effect and improves glycemic control.

Cummings[41] explained this via the "hindgut hypothesis," which indicates that the improved glucose homeostasis after BS is attributable to hormonal responses to the increased nutrient delivery to the distal small intestine. The delivery of incompletely digested food causes overstimulation of specialized entero-endocrine L-cells that cause increased production of incretin hormones GLP-1 and peptide YY (PYY). GLP-1 improves glucose processing by increasing insulin secretion and action and slowing gastric emptying, which also contributes to satiety. PYY regulates appetite, decreases adiposity, and contributes to insulin-induced glucose disposal. Kindel and colleagues[42] suggested GLP-1 as a main component of gluco-regulation after BS.

Entero-Endocrine Hormones

The gastrointestinal tract comprises an intricate neuroendocrine system and produces more than 100 hormonally active peptides.[10] Incretins are neuroendocrine hormones produced by the intestinal mucosa in response to food stimulus that cause increased insulin secretion.[43] Glucose-dependent insulinotropic peptide (GIP) is produced by duodenal K cells and GLP-1 comes from ileal L-cells and together these hormones account for 60% of the nutrient-dependent insulin release. This incretin effect on insulin secretion is impaired in DM2.

Glucagonlike peptide-1

GLP-1 is the best-studied incretin and appears to play an important role in glucose regulation, satiety, and weight loss after BS. GLP-1 suppresses glucagon and ghrelin secretion and delays gastric emptying, which improves postprandial hyperglycemia.[44] In some patients following RYGB, hyperinsulinemic hypoglycemia with neuroglycopenia is observed and attributed to increases in GLP-1. Increases are also observed following SG but not after lap banding.

Laferrère[43] found no difference in GLP-1 levels with diet-induced weight loss but reported an increase in postprandial GLP-1 levels within 4 weeks of RYGB. Samat and colleagues[45] saw similar results in obese patients with DM2 at 1 year after gastric bypass surgery. They found that GLP-1 was significantly elevated and was associated with increased insulin sensitivity and suppressed ghrelin. This increase in GLP-1 and improvement in beta-cell function was more pronounced in the RYGB group as compared with SG or intensive medical therapy group 2 years post-BS in the Surgical Therapy and Medications Potentially Eradicate Diabetes Efficiently (STAMPEDE) trial.[46]

Ghrelin

Ghrelin is an appetite stimulant hormone that is produced by A-like cells in the stomach fundus. This hormone regulates food intake, and has additional effects that lead to impaired insulin sensitivity and reduced glucose-stimulated insulin secretion.[43] Ghrelin levels increase after diet-induced weight loss.[47] On the contrary, low levels of ghrelin have been associated with RYGB and GS and may contribute to weight loss but are not seen with LAGB.[10] Ghrelin levels are affected by type of BS, time from surgery, and vagal nerve involvement.

Glucose-dependent insulinotropic peptide

GIP plays a part in lipid metabolism and is thought to have a direct relation to obesity. The impact of BS on GIP is not well understood but is thought to be related to removal of duodenal K cells during BS, which leads to low GIP levels, less fat deposition, and weight loss.[10]

Additional neuroendocrine hormones, which play a role in BS-induced weight loss and glucose homeostasis, include PYY, GLP-2, and oxyntomodulin. Other gastrointestinal hormones that have been studied in this regard and do not appear to play a major role include obestatin, cholecystokinin, apolipoprotein A4, enterostatin, neurotensin, motilin, and vasoactive intestinal peptide.

METABOLIC EFFECTS OF BARIATRIC SURGERY AND OUTCOMES

The metabolic effects of different types of BS on some of the obesity-related complications and gut neuroendocrine hormones are described in **Fig. 2** and **Table 2**.

Weight Loss

Presently, BS is the most effective approach to obesity in terms of magnitude of weight loss achieved and long-term results. It has been associated with weight loss in the range of 12% to 39% of presurgical body weight or 40% to 71% EWL.[10]

The Swedish Obese Subject (SOS) study was a major prospective study that assessed the effects of intentional weight loss via conventional treatment versus BS in obese patients.[48] The results revealed that the intervention group had a percentage body weight loss of approximately 23% at 2 years, 17% at 10 years, 16% at 15 years, and 18% at 20 years postsurgery.[49] The average weight loss in the control group was 0% to 1% during this time.

Similar results were seen in a meta-analysis by Buchwald and colleagues,[26] and a systematic review by Ribaric and colleagues[50] showed an average EWL of 61.2% and 75.3%, respectively, in patients undergoing BS. Gill and colleagues[51] found a similar trend in obese patients with DM2 who underwent SG with EWL of 47%.

The STAMPEDE trial showed more weight loss in the BS group as compared with the medical-therapy group after 1 year (RYGB −29.4 ± 9.0 kg, SG −25.1 ± 8.5 kg, medical therapy −5.4 ± 8.0 kg, $P<.001$) and 3 years (RYGB −24.5% ± 9.1%, SG −21.1% ± 8.9%, medical-therapy −4.2% ± 8.3%, $P<.001$).[52,53]

Meta-analysis of randomized controlled trials (RCTs) in patients with DM2 and obesity undergoing BS by Gloy and colleagues[54] showed a greater weight loss with

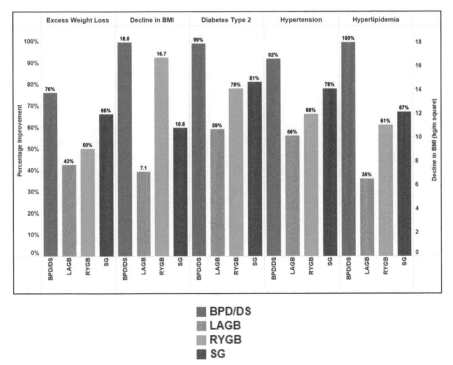

Fig. 2. Bariatric surgery procedures and their effect on metabolic parameters and obesity related complications. (*Data from* Keshishian A. Weight loss procedure surgical I procedures and outcomes. Available at: http://www.dssurgery.com/weight-loss-surgery-poster.php. Accessed March 18, 2016.)

BS (mean difference −26 kg [95% confidence interval −31 to −21], *P*<.001) as compared with conventional treatment.

Glycemic Control in Diabetes (Observational and Randomized Controlled Trials)

BS contributes to improved glycemic control via various mechanisms, as described previously and in **Fig. 3**.

The concept of BS as a potential remedy for DM initially came from observational studies. Pories and colleagues[55] found normalization of glucose tolerance in patients

Table 2				
Effects of bariatric surgery on intestinal neuroendocrine hormones				
Procedures	**GLP-1**	**GIP**	**PYY**	**Ghrelin**
Roux-en-Y gastric bypass (RYGB)	↑↑	↑→↓	↑	↓
Biliopancreatic diversion with duodenal switch (BPD/DS)	↑↑	↓	↑	↓
Laparoscopic adjustable gastric banding (LAGB)	→	→	→	↑→
Sleeve gastrostomy (SG)	↑	→	→	↓

Abbreviations: ↑↑, very increased; ↑, increased; ↓, decreased; →, no change; GIP, glucose-dependent insulinotropic peptide; GLP-1, glucagonlike peptide 1; PYY, peptide YY.

Adapted from Mingrone G. Role of the incretin system in the remission of type 2 diabetes following bariatric surgery. Nutr Metab Cardiovasc Dis 2008;18(8):578.

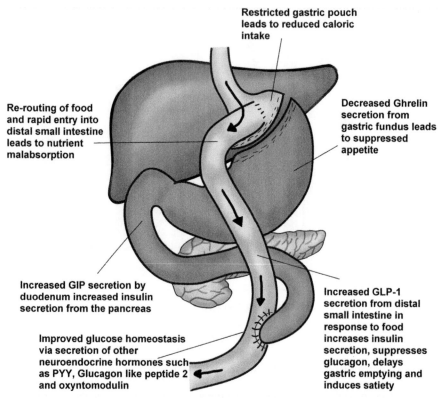

Fig. 3. Role of intestinal hormones in glucose homeostasis following Roux-en-Y surgery. (*Adapted from* Ionut V, Bergman RN. Mechanisms responsible for excess weight loss after bariatric surgery. J Diabetes Sci Technol 2011;5(5):1265.)

with DM undergoing RYGB as early as 10 days after the procedure; 99% of obese patients with DM2 showed an improvement in fasting plasma glucose and 83% of these patients had normalization of HBA1c and did not require any diabetes therapy at 7.6 years post-BS.[56] The SOS study found diabetes remission in 72% of patients with DM2 undergoing BS as compared with 21% in the conventional group.[57] The DM prevalence 8 years after BS in the SOS study remained stable, whereas an increase in incidence of diabetes in the control group was noted from 7.8% to 24.9%.

There is a persistent improvement in glycemia in obese patients with DM2 undergoing BS in RCTs. Schauer and colleagues[52,53] found a reduction in HbA1c in the BS arm (mean HbA1c 6.5%) as compared with the medical therapy group (mean HbA1c 7.5%) at 1 year and 3 years (mean HbA1c RYGB 6.7%, SG 7%, medical therapy 8.4%). In the BS group, the mean HbA1c and fasting serum glucose decreased to the normal range in 83% of patients and the diabetes medication requirements declined in 80%.[58]

Mingrone and colleagues[59] found biochemical remission of DM in obese patients with DM2 undergoing BS at 2 years (RYGB 75% and BPPD 95%). HbA1c was remarkably improved from baseline in the BS group (RYGB −25.18% ± 20.89%, BPD −43.01% ± 9.64%, medical-therapy group −8.39% ± 9.93%). At 5 years of follow-up 50% of the patients in the BS arm maintained DM remission.[60]

In the Diabetes Surgery Study, Ikrammuddin and colleagues[61] found a goal HbA1c of 7% or lower in 75% of patients undergoing BS as compared with 32% in the medical therapy group (odds ratio 6.0; 95% confidence interval 2.6–13.9).

Gloy and colleagues[54] noted a pooled relative risk for diabetes remission with BS of 22.1 (3.2–154.3, $P = .002$) as compared with nonsurgical treatment.

The role of BS in diabetes remission and the magnitude of improvement in glycemia are dependent on various factors. Procedure type (malabsorptive BS [BPD and RYGB]), younger age, higher peak weight loss, shorter duration of diabetes (<5 years 95%, 6–10 years 75%, >10 years 54%), lower diabetes severity (diet controlled), and lower central obesity have been associated with a higher DM remission rate.[26,62,63]

Patients with type 1 DM undergoing BS did had some minor improvement in HbA1c despite similar weight loss to patients with DM2.[62]

Dyslipidemia

Visceral obesity is a key factor in developing insulin resistance and impairment of lipids metabolic pathway. BS plays an important role in correction of impaired lipid processing due to insulin resistance by inducing weight loss and improving insulin-dependent glucose uptake. Hyperlipidemia improved in 70% of patients receiving BS with a decline in Total Cholesterol (TC), LDL, and TG and increase in HDL.[31,64]

The SOS study reported an improvement in lipid profile of patients after BS, with an increase in HDL concentrations by 18.7% and decrease in TG by 29.9% in the surgical versus control group.[49] Garcia-Marirrodriga and colleagues[65] found a positive impact of BS in patients undergoing RYGB with a decline in TC, LDL and TG, and significant increase in HDL levels. There was a direct correlation between the improvement in lipid profile and extent of EWL.

RCTs, including the study by Mingrone and colleagues,[59] the STAMPEDE trial, and the Diabetes Surgery Study found a decrease in TG and increase in HDL but no significant difference in LDL concentrations with BS as compared with medical therapy.[52,61]

A meta-analysis of RCTs for bariatric surgery by Gloy and colleagues[54] found no difference in mean change in TC from pooled data from RCTs between BS and nonsurgical arms (mean difference −0.4 mmol/L [−0.8–0.00], $P = .05$).

The positive effects of BS on lipid profile can be explained by the direct response to weight loss, as well as changes is neuroendocrine hormones, such as GLP1, PYY, and ghrelin.

BARIATRIC SURGERY AND MACROVASCULAR COMPLICATIONS OF DIABETES

Hypertension, CV disease, and peripheral vascular disease are the major macrovascular complications of DM2. Obesity has been related to the development of hypertension and CV disease, which is attributed to metabolic derangement seen with obesity.

Hypertension

Hypertension has a strong association with obesity and approximately 1% body weight loss can improve systolic BP by 1 mm Hg and diastolic BP by 2 mm Hg.[7] Patients with hypertension had improvement in their BP in 79% of the cases and complete resolution in 61% of cases after BS.[27]

The SOS study had mixed results regarding effects of BS on hypertension. Patients receiving BS showed an improvement in BP at 1 year, followed by progressive rise over the consequent years, which was thought to be associated with increasing age and weight gain.[7,66] Meta-analysis by Wilhelm and colleagues[67] showed a significant benefit in obese patients undergoing BS with BP improvement reported in 63% and resolution in 50% of patients.

The study by Mingrone and colleagues,[59] the STAMPEDE trial, and the Diabetes Surgery Study in patients with DM2 undergoing BS versus medical therapy did not show any significant difference in BP between the 2 groups, but there was a notable decrease in the number of antihypertensive medications.[52,61]

There is a complex association between BS and the effects it has on hypertension, which can be confounded by other variables, such as age, degree of weight loss, weight regain, and other comorbidities.

Cardiovascular Disease

Obesity has an association with impaired heart function, which may be due to left ventricular hypertrophy and diastolic dysfunction or early atherosclerosis leading to ischemic heart disease. It is also an independent risk factor for atrial fibrillation. Weight loss has been associated with improvement in CV risk. Benraouane and Litwin[68] estimated a CV risk reduction from 6% to 4% after BS.

The SOS study reported a decrease in CV events and CV mortality in patients undergoing BS as compared with the control group.[49] The STAMPEDE trial showed a significant decrease in the high-sensitivity CRP level and need for cardiovascular medication.[52] The Utah obesity study showed a lower coronary calcium score at 5 years in patients post-BS as compared with the conventional therapy group.[69]

This suggests that BS can over time delay the progression of atherosclerosis. These findings can be attributed to the overall improvement in metabolic profile of these patients and improvement in the obesity-related proinflammatory state and CV risk factors, such as diabetes, hypertension, and dyslipidemia.

BARIATRIC SURGERY AND MICROVASCULAR COMPLICATIONS OF DIABETES

Traditionally, hypertension and glycemic control are key determinants of the development of diabetes-associated microvascular complications that include diabetic nephropathy, neuropathy, and retinopathy. Even though observational studies have shown some association between BS and microvascular complications, the RCTs comparing surgery with medical therapy for DM thus far have not established a significant impact of BS in improving microvascular complications or delaying the progression of microvascular disease with DM.

Diabetic Nephropathy

Diabetic nephropathy affects 40% of patients with DM2 and the conventional therapy for this is aimed at improving BP control, blood sugar control, and hyperlipidemia.[70] Observational studies have shown an improvement in albuminuria with weight loss surgery. RYGB was associated with decrease in proteinuria in prospective studies. The STAMPEDE trial did not show any benefit of BS on development of albuminuria as compared with intensive medical therapy.[53] There was no significant difference in the serum creatinine level and the estimated glomerular filtration rate between the 2 groups.

Diabetic Retinopathy

The effect of BS on diabetic retinopathy was studied in the STAMPEDE trial, which concluded that diabetic retinopathy did not significantly differ between the BS arm and the control arm at 2 years.[63] A recent meta-analysis raised the concern for worsening of diabetic retinopathy post-BS.[71] The study reported that patients without retinopathy before BS did not progress in 92.5% of cases, whereas those with preoperative disease remained stable in 57.4%, progressed in 23.5%, and improved in 19.2%.

Diabetic Neuropathy

Müller-Stich and colleagues[72] evaluated the role of BS in DM2 on diabetic neuropathy in the DiaSurg 1 study. They found a significant improvement in neuropathy symptom score with a 67% reversal in symptomatic neuropathy.[72]

There is a need for multicenter RCTs to better delineate the effect of bariatric procedures on cardiometabolic and microvascular complications of DM2. The Alliance for Randomized Medication versus Metabolic Surgery will aim to do this. The Prevention and Treatment of Diabetes Complications with Gastric Surgery or Intensive Medicines (PRODIGIES) trial is an ongoing trial that may shed light on this issue (ClinicalTrials.gov Identifier: NCT01974544).

BARIATRIC SURGERY–ASSOCIATED ADVERSE EVENTS AND COMPLICATIONS

The mortality associated with bariatric procedures has been reported as 0.28% at 30 days after surgery and 0.35% between 30 days and 2 years after the procedure.[73] The Longitudinal Assessment of Bariatric Surgery showed a similar mortality rate of 0.3% at 30 days.[74] The SOS study reported that bariatric surgery was associated with a lower overall mortality in the BS group (hazard ratio 0.76) as compared with the conventional treatment group (hazard ratio 0.71).[48] There was a need for reoperation due to bleeding, gastric leaks, and small bowel obstruction in 8% of patients undergoing BS in RCTs.[52,59,61]

Major surgical complications (ie, DVTs (Deep vein thrombosis), infection, gastric leaks, fistulas, small bowel obstruction) are seen in 5% to 40% of cases and occur more commonly in smokers and DM.[74,75] Many (30%–70%) patients post-BS suffer from nutritional deficiencies, with anemia being the most common that may necessitate iron infusion therapy.[76] Reactive hypoglycemia is another complication seen with these procedures, hypothesized to be due to exaggerated postprandial insulin response to GLP-1 or from nesidioblastosis.[77] Post-BS hypoglycemia syndrome is rare, but can be debilitating. The exact pathophysiology is variable and management, including reversal of the surgery, can be challenging.

SUMMARY

Diabetes and obesity not only coexist, but promote and exacerbate each other. Weight gain leads to increased insulin resistance, hyperinsulinemia, and a progressive decline in beta-cell function. Insulin analogs and oral hypoglycemic therapies (ie, sulfonylureas and thiazolidinediones) further weight gain and thwart lifestyle modification. BS has shown to be superior to conventional methods for durable weight loss. BS has also shown to have an overall mortality benefit in severe obesity and has favorable effects on metabolic parameters and comorbidities, such as hypertension, hyperlipidemia, metabolic syndrome, cardiovascular risk, and glycemic control in diabetes. Thus far, RCTs of BS versus medical therapy for diabetes have documented superior efficacy of surgical weight loss to produce diabetes remission and improve quality of life. The long-term effects of BS on diabetes complications remain unanswered. Thus, monitoring for glycemic control and serial surveillance remain the treatments of choice for prevention and delaying the progression of diabetes-related vascular complications.

REFERENCES

1. Centers for Disease Control and Prevention. Death and mortality. NCHS FastStats Web site. Available at: http://www.cdc.gov/nchs/fastats/deaths.htm. Accessed March 18, 2016.
2. Gerteis J, Izrael D, Deitz D, et al. Multiple chronic conditions chartbook. AHRQ Publications No, Q14-0038. Rockville (MD): Agency for Healthcare Research and Quality; 2014.
3. National Diabetes Statistics Report, 2014.
4. Ogden C, Carroll M, Kit B, et al. Prevalence of childhood and adult obesity in the United States, 2011-2012. Surv Anesthesiol 2014;58(4):206.
5. Flegal K, Carroll M, Kit B, et al. Prevalence of obesity and trends in the distribution of body mass index among US adults, 1999-2010. JAMA 2012;307(5):491.
6. Chan J, Rimm E, Colditz G, et al. Obesity, fat distribution, and weight gain as risk factors for clinical diabetes in men. Diabetes Care 1994;17(9):961–9.
7. Noria S, Grantcharov T. Biological effects of bariatric surgery on obesity-related comorbidities. Can J Surg 2013;56(1):47–57.
8. Patel A, Hildebrand J, Gapstur S. Body mass index and all-cause mortality in a large prospective cohort of white and black U.S. adults. PLoS One 2014;9(10): e109153.
9. Jensen M, Ryan D, Apovian C, et al. 2013 AHA/ACC/TOS guideline for the management of overweight and obesity in adults. Circulation 2013;129(25 Suppl 2): S102–38.
10. Ionut V, Bergman R. Mechanisms responsible for excess weight loss after bariatric surgery. J Diabetes Sci Technol 2011;5(5):1263–82.
11. Obesity and overweight. Fact sheet no 311. Geneva (Switzerland): World health organization. 2016.
12. McKenney R, Short D. Tipping the balance: the pathophysiology of obesity and type 2 diabetes mellitus. Surg Clin North Am 2011;91(6):1139–48.
13. Mantzoros C. Obesity and diabetes. Totowa (NJ): Humana Press; 2006.
14. Jung R. Obesity as a disease. Br Med Bull 1997;53(2):307–21.
15. Colditz G. Weight gain as a risk factor for clinical diabetes mellitus in women. Ann Intern Med 1995;122(7):481.
16. Westlund K, Nicolayson R. Ten year mortality and morbidity study related to serum cholesterol. A follow-up of 3.751 men aged 40-49. Scand J Lab Invest Suppl 1972;127:1–24.
17. Williamson D, Pamuk E, Thun M, et al. Prospective study of intentional weight loss and mortality in overweight white men aged 40-64 years. Am J Epidemiol 1999; 149(6):491–503.
18. Wing RR, Shoemaker M, Marcus MDM, et al. Variables associated with weight loss and improvements in glycaemic control in type 2 diabetic patients. Arch Intern Med 1990;147:1749–53.
19. Reisin E, Abel R, Modan M, et al. Effect of weight loss without salt restriction on the reduction of blood pressure in overweight hypertensive patients. N Engl J Med 1978;298(1):1–6.
20. Datnlo AM, Kris-Etherton PM. Effects of weight reduction on blood lipids and lipoproteins: a meta analysis. Am J Clin Nutr 1992;56:320–8.
21. Knowler WC, Barrett-Connor E, Fowler SE, et al, Diabetes Prevention Program Research Group. Reduction in the incidence of type 2 diabetes with lifestyle intervention or metformin. N Engl J Med 2002;346(6):393–403.

22. Look AHEAD Research Group, Pi-Sunyer X, Blackburn G, Brancati FL, et al. Reduction in weight and cardiovascular disease risk factors in individuals with type 2 diabetes: one-year results of the look AHEAD trial. Diabetes Care 2007; 30(6):1374–83.

23. Forsythe L, Wallace J, Livingstone M. Obesity and inflammation: the effects of weight loss. Nutr Res Rev 2008;21(02):117.

24. American College of Cardiology/American Heart Association Task Force on Practice Guidelines, Obesity Expert Panel, 2013. Expert panel report: guidelines (2013) for the management of overweight and obesity in adults. Obesity (Silver Spring) 2014;22(S2):S41–410.

25. Sugerman H. The ASBS Consensus Conference on the state of bariatric surgery and morbid obesity: health implications for patients, health professionals and third-party payors. Surg Obes Relat Dis 2005;1(2):105.

26. Buchwald H, Avidor Y, Braunwald E, et al. Bariatric surgery. JAMA 2004;292(14): 1724.

27. Colquitt J, Picot J, Loveman E, et al. Surgery for obesity. Cochrane Database Syst Rev 2009;(2):CD003641.

28. Singh A, Kota S, Singh R. Bariatric surgery and diabetes remission: who would have thought it? Indian J Endocrinol Metab 2015;19(5):563.

29. American Society for Metabolic and Bariatric Surgery. Bariatric surgery procedures. Gainesville (FL): American Society for Metabolic and Bariatric Surgery; 2016. Available at: https://asmbs.org/patients/bariatric-surgery-procedures. Accessed February 13, 2016.

30. Parikh M, Fielding G, Ren C. U.S. experience with 749 laparoscopic adjustable gastric bands: intermediate outcomes. Surg Endosc 2005;19(12):1631–5.

31. Buchwald H, Estok R, Fahrbach K, et al. Weight and type 2 diabetes after bariatric surgery: systematic review and meta-analysis. Am J Med 2009;122(3): 248–56.e5.

32. Karra E, Yousseif A, Batterham RL. Mechanisms facilitating weight loss and resolution of type 2 diabetes following bariatric surgery. Trends Endocrinol Metab 2010;21(6):337–44.

33. Rubino F, R'bibo S, del Genio F, et al. Metabolic surgery: the role of the gastrointestinal tract in diabetes mellitus. Nat Rev Endocrinol 2010;6(2):102–9.

34. Ponce J, Haynes B, Paynter S, et al. Effect of lap-band-induced weight loss on type 2 diabetes mellitus and hypertension. Obes Surg 2004;14(10):1335–42.

35. Halmi KA, Mason E, Falk JR, et al. Appetitive behavior after gastric bypass for obesity. Int J Obes 1981;5:457–64.

36. Isbell J, Tamboli R, Hansen E, et al. The importance of caloric restriction in the early improvements in insulin sensitivity after Roux-en-Y gastric bypass surgery. Diabetes Care 2010;33(7):1438–42.

37. Buchwald H, Oien D. Metabolic/bariatric surgery worldwide 2008. Obes Surg 2009;19(12):1605–11.

38. Evans J, Goldfine I, Maddux B, et al. Are oxidative stress-activated signaling pathways mediators of insulin resistance and -cell dysfunction? Diabetes 2003; 52(1):1–8.

39. Marceau P, Hould FS, Simard S, et al. Biliopancreatic diversion with duodenal switch. World J Surg 1998;22(9):947–54.

40. Brolin R. Malabsorptive gastric bypass in patients with superobesity. J Gastrointest Surg 2002;6(2):195–205.

41. Cummings D. Endocrine mechanisms mediating remission of diabetes after gastric bypass surgery. Int J Obes Relat Metab Disord 2009;33:S33–40.

42. Kindel T, Yoder S, Seeley R, et al. Duodenal-jejunal exclusion improves glucose tolerance in the diabetic, Goto-Kakizaki rat by a GLP-1 receptor-mediated mechanism. J Gastrointest Surg 2009;13(10):1762–72.

43. Laferrère B. Effect of gastric bypass surgery on the incretins. Diabetes Metab 2009;35(6):513–7.

44. Holst J, Vilsboll T, Deacon C. The incretin system and its role in type 2 diabetes mellitus. Mol Cell Endocrinol 2009;297(1–2):127–36.

45. Samat A, Malin S, Huang H, et al. Ghrelin suppression is associated with weight loss and insulin action following gastric bypass surgery at 12 months in obese adults with type 2 diabetes. Diabetes Obes Metab 2013;15(10):963–6.

46. Kashyap S, Bhatt D, Wolski K, et al. Metabolic effects of bariatric surgery in patients with moderate obesity and type 2 diabetes: analysis of a randomized control trial comparing surgery with intensive medical treatment. Diabetes Care 2013; 36(8):2175–82.

47. Cummings D, Weigle D, Frayo R, et al. Plasma ghrelin levels after diet-induced weight loss or gastric bypass surgery. N Engl J Med 2002;346(21):1623–30.

48. Sjöström L, Narbro K, Sjöström C, et al. Effects of bariatric surgery on mortality in Swedish obese subjects. N Engl J Med 2007;357(8):741–52.

49. Sjöström L, Peltonen M, Jacobson P, et al. Bariatric surgery and long-term cardiovascular events. JAMA 2012;307(1):56.

50. Ribaric G, Buchwald J, McGlennon T. Diabetes and weight in comparative studies of bariatric surgery vs conventional medical therapy: a systematic review and meta-analysis. Obes Surg 2013;24(3):437–55.

51. Gill R, Birch D, Shi X, et al. Sleeve gastrectomy and type 2 diabetes mellitus: a systematic review. Surg Obes Relat Dis 2010;6(6):707–13.

52. Schauer P, Kashyap S, Wolski K, et al. Bariatric surgery versus intensive medical therapy in obese patients with diabetes. N Engl J Med 2012;366(17):1567–76.

53. Schauer P, Bhatt D, Kirwan J, et al. Bariatric surgery versus intensive medical therapy for diabetes—3-year outcomes. N Engl J Med 2014;370(21):2002–13.

54. Gloy V, Briel M, Bhatt D, et al. Bariatric surgery versus non-surgical treatment for obesity: a systematic review and meta-analysis of randomised controlled trials. BMJ 2013;347:f5934.

55. Pories W, Card J, Flickinger E, et al. The Control of Diabetes Mellitus (NIDDM) in the morbidly obese with the Greenville gastric bypass. Ann Surg 1987;206(3): 316–23.

56. Pories W, Swanson M, MacDonald K, et al. Who would have thought it? An operation proves to be the most effective therapy for adult-onset diabetes mellitus. Ann Surg 1995;222(3):339–52.

57. Sjostrom C, Peltonen M, Wedel H, et al. Differentiated long-term effects of intentional weight loss on diabetes and hypertension. Hypertension 2000;36(1):20–5.

58. Schauer P, Burguera B, Ikramuddin S, et al. Effect of laparoscopic Roux-en-Y gastric bypass on type 2 diabetes mellitus. Nutr Clin Pract 2004;19(1):60–1.

59. Mingrone G, Panunzi S, De Gaetano A, et al. Bariatric surgery versus conventional medical therapy for type 2 diabetes. N Engl J Med 2012;366(17):1577–85.

60. Mingrone G, Panunzi S, De Gaetano A, et al. Bariatric–metabolic surgery versus conventional medical treatment in obese patients with type 2 diabetes: 5 year follow-up of an open-label, single-centre, randomised controlled trial. Lancet 2015;386(9997):964–73.

61. Ikramuddin S, Korner J, Lee W, et al. Roux-en-Y gastric bypass vs intensive medical management for the control of type 2 diabetes, hypertension, and hyperlipidemia. JAMA 2013;309(21):2240.

62. Maraka S, Kudva Y, Kellogg T, et al. Bariatric surgery and diabetes: implications of type 1 versus insulin-requiring type 2. Obesity (Silver Spring) 2015;23(3): 552–7.
63. Torquati A, Lutfi R, Abumrad N, et al. Is Roux-en-Y gastric bypass surgery the most effective treatment for type 2 diabetes mellitus in morbidly obese patients? J Gastrointest Surg 2005;9(8):1112–8.
64. Bouldin M, Ross L, Sumrall C, et al. The effect of obesity surgery on obesity co-morbidity. Am J Med Sci 2006;331(4):183–93.
65. Garcia-Marirrodriga I, Amaya-Romero C, Ruiz-Diaz G, et al. Evolution of lipid profiles after bariatric surgery. Obes Surg 2011;22(4):609–16.
66. Sjöström C, Peltonen M, Sjöström L. Blood pressure and pulse pressure during long-term weight loss in the obese: the Swedish Obese Subjects (SOS) intervention study. Obes Res 2001;9(3):188–95.
67. Wilhelm S, Young J, Kale-Pradhan P. Effect of bariatric surgery on hypertension: a meta-analysis. Ann Pharmacother 2014;48(6):674–82.
68. Benraouane F, Litwin SE. Reductions in cardiovascular risk after bariatric surgery. Curr Opin Cardiol 2011;26(6):555–61.
69. Priester T, Ault T, Davidson L, et al. Coronary calcium scores 6 years after bariatric surgery. Obes Surg 2014;25(1):90–6.
70. Docherty N, le Roux C. Improvements in the metabolic milieu following Roux-en-Y gastric bypass and the arrest of diabetic kidney disease. Exp Physiol 2014;99(9): 1146–53.
71. Cheung D, Switzer N, Ehmann D, et al. The impact of bariatric surgery on diabetic retinopathy: a systematic review and meta-analysis. Obes Surg 2014;25(9): 1604–9.
72. Müller-Stich B, Fischer L, Kenngott H, et al. Gastric bypass leads to improvement of diabetic neuropathy independent of glucose normalization—results of a prospective cohort study (DiaSurg 1 Study). Ann Surg 2013;258(5):760–6.
73. Buchwald H, Estok R, Fahrbach K, et al. Trends in mortality in bariatric surgery: a systematic review and meta-analysis. Surgery 2007;142(4):621–35.
74. Longitudinal Assessment of Bariatric Surgery (LABS) Consortium, Flum DR, Belle SH, King WC, et al. Perioperative safety in the longitudinal assessment of bariatric surgery. N Engl J Med 2009;361(5):445–54.
75. Encinosa W, Bernard D, Du D, et al. Recent improvements in bariatric surgery outcomes. Med Care 2009;47(5):531–5.
76. Davies D, Baxter J, Baxter J. Nutritional deficiencies after bariatric surgery. Obes Surg 2007;17(9):1150–8.
77. Goldfine A, Mun E, Devine E, et al. Patients with neuroglycopenia after gastric bypass surgery have exaggerated incretin and insulin secretory responses to a mixed meal. J Clin Endocrinol Metab 2007;92(12):4678–85.

Islet Cell Transplantation and Alternative Therapies

Betul Hatipoglu, MD

KEYWORDS

- Pancreas transplantation • Islet transplantation • Type 1 diabetes • Beta cells

KEY POINTS

- Pancreas and islet cell transplantation are therapeutic options for patients with type 1 diabetes suffering severe hypoglycemia or worsening complications despite advanced medical therapy.
- Some countries like Canada have both therapies available as accepted medical treatment, whereas in the United States, islet transplantation remains experimental for type 1 diabetes.
- The advances and improvements achieved, especially since 2000, brought this therapy much closer to the clinical use.

In recent years, as the obesity epidemic plateaued, the new cases of type 2 diabetes also slowed down in United States.[1] Unfortunately, in contrast, a nearly 30% increase in the rates of type 1 diabetes in children aged 14 and younger has been reported.[2] According to the US Centers for Disease Control and Prevention, if current trends continue, we will see 23% of type 1 diabetes by 2050. The United States is not alone in this; studies from Europe, Canada and Australia have reported the same trends, largest increases being observed in children under 5 years old.[3] Even though clinical management of type 1 diabetes has improved beyond imagination with the advances in technology, improvements of insulins, and insulin delivery devices, as well as glucose monitoring systems, prevention and cure are the 2 major challenges for future generations of scientists facing this increase in the numbers. This article reviews the advances we achieved on the way to cure type 1 diabetes.

Currently, pancreas transplant is an option for patients with type 1 diabetes who need more help than medical therapy can offer. This is a common practice for patients undergoing kidney transplantation or less commonly as a therapy alone. Performed first in 1966 by Kelly and colleagues,[4] this replacement therapy has now much improved outcomes; for example, the expected 1-year pancreas graft survivals are

The author has nothing to disclose.
Endocrinology and Metabolism Institute, Cleveland Clinic, 9500 Euclid Avenue, F20, Cleveland, OH 44195, USA
E-mail address: hatipob@ccf.org

90% with simultaneous pancreas and kidney (SPK) transplantation, 83% in pancreas after kidney transplantation, and 80% with pancreas transplantation alone, according to the latest accumulated data from scientific registry of transplant recipient. However, it remains a late therapeutic option in advanced disease because it is a major surgery with complications[5] and patients become lifetime dependent on immunosuppression to prevent rejection.

The need for improvement inspired the clinical and scientific community to find a method to separate endocrine tissue, which is only 1% of the pancreas from the rest of bulky exocrine tissue, to develop islet transplantation therapy.

Islet replacement therapy has 2 arms, allogeneic islet transplantation involving harvested islets from deceased organ donors, used in type 1 diabetes patients, and auto-transplantation, which is performed after total pancreatectomy using extracted islets from the individual's own pancreas to prevent or reduce the severity of diabetes after removal of the gland.

Improvement of the isolation techniques have taken decades, and advances observed today are the result of the collaborative effort of many who spent their career in this field. The earliest recorded attempt is transplantation of sheep pancreas injected under skin in 1893.[6] Around 1965, isolation of islets mainly used for research purpose was reported by Moskalewski.[7] Few years later, in 1972, Ballinger and Lacy[8] isolated normal islets and performed successful transplant to restore euglycemia in diabetic rat models. Almost a decade later, the first results from a series of type 1 diabetes patients receiving islet transplantation, by Sutherland and colleagues,[9] was published from the University of Minnesota. Unfortunately, none became insulin independent at the time. But around 1989, clinically successful islet transplantation was achieved, although lasting only 1 month.[10] The following decade until 2000 witnessed attempts of islet transplantation therapy with less than 10% success of insulin independence.[11]

The Edmonton protocol published around 2000 by Shapiro and colleagues[12] was a landmark study that advanced this field once more. The researchers reported that all 7 patients in this study achieved insulin independence at 1 year. The Edmonton protocol separated itself from its predecessors by 4 main variations. The protocol included a steroid-free immunosuppressive regimen, using combinations of sirolimus, low-dose tacrolimus, and an anti-CD25 antibody daclizumab, which enabled them to eliminate the glucocorticoids that was heavily relied on previously. The second variation included the use of a sufficient number of viable islets from multiple donors, as many as 4 to provide enough islets, 10,000 islet equivalents per kilogram, infused usually several weeks apart, instead of the previously used number of 6000 islet equivalents per kilogram. A third point of difference was seen in their isolation and purification method modified by removing nonhuman medium to minimize exposure to xenoproteins. Last, to optimize islet function, they limited the cold storage time to less than 13 hours, by eliminating previous method of culturing the cells several days before the infusions. In 2001, the group published their observation for a median follow-up of 10 months: 11 of 12 patients were reported to be insulin independent (4 with normal glucose tolerance, 5 with impaired glucose tolerance, and 3 with levels in the diabetic range).[13]

A collaboration was born after this new development, bringing multiple international centers together in a multicenter trial supported by the National Institutes of Health and the immune tolerance network. This consortium initiated series of pilot studies around 2004, the Clinical Islet Transplantation Consortium (CIT) currently has 2 phase III studies, CIT-07 for type 1 diabetes with severe hypoglycemia and glycemic lability and CIT-06, which includes type 1 diabetics with kidney transplantation.[14]

Initial results from the multicenter collaborative effort, including 36 patients who underwent islet transplantation using the Edmonton protocol, were published in 2006. A total of 21 (58%) patients became insulin independent, with varied length of time, and only 5 remained insulin independent at the end of 2 years.[15] Some sites achieved 100% success, whereas others had very limited results, which caused a pause in islet transplantation numbers observed before 2008.

Around 1999, the Collaborative Islet Transplantation Registry (CITR) data was established under the support of Juvenile Diabetes Research Foundation to update information and monitor progress from more than 40 centers including from Canada, the United States, Europe, Australia, and Asia.[16] CITR defines insulin independence as no insulin use for 14 or more consecutive days. The review of this public registry results was reported in July 2012. From total of 677 islet recipients, 575 subjects (85%) underwent transplantation as islet alone (with total 1375 infusions, 44% receiving 2 infusions, and 20% more than 2)[17] Insulin independence was observed 51% at 1 year and 27% at 3 years for patients transplanted between 1999 and 2002, whereas for the 2007 to 2010 era these numbers were 66% and 44%, respectively, with a significant continuous decrease over 5 years of follow-up.[17] Insulin independence being the best definition of success for type 1 diabetes replacement therapies started to be questioned.

Currently, the definition of success for both pancreas and islet transplantation heavily focus on insulin independence rates. As discussed by Gruessner and Gruessner,[18] the 5 current primary endpoints include insulin independence, occurrence of hypoglycemia, a hemoglobin A1c of less than 6.5%, a C-peptide of more than 0.3, and improvements in fasting blood glucose. In their article, these investigators argue that avoiding severe hypoglycemia should be used as a clinical success and this mode of therapies should be included in the algorithms for the treatment of severe hypoglycemia, which is currently not listed in any society guidelines. When CITR data are reviewed for the severe hypoglycemia occurrence, regardless of previous graft loss, 90% patients remain free of severe hypoglycemic events, whereas 90% of all subjects had severe hypoglycemia at the time of enrollment.

Within this perspective, in the last decade, islet transplantation was transformed into a treatment option for type 1 diabetic patients suffering hypoglycemic unawareness, and accepted as a nonexperimental treatment offered and reimbursed by health insurance system in several countries.

The need for long-term immunosuppressive therapy and differences between centers in achieving high-quality islets isolation for successful single infusion, kept islet transplantation therapy as an experimental option in many other countries, including in the United States. Recently, data reported[19] from a phase III trial show improvement of common manufacturing process and reproducibility between multiple sites. Outcomes that were presented from this study were promising as insulin independence was achieved about 55% of recipients at 1 year with 1 or 2 infusions, and even without insulin independence, hypoglycemic unawareness was treated effectively.[20]

As reported, insulin independence rates in a single donor islet transplant[21] reaches 50% for 5 years, with better induction therapy and maintenance immunosuppression therapy, as well as observed positive impact of this therapy on complications of diabetes,[22,23] accepting islet transplantation as a clinical treatment option is becoming a reality.

Selection of the most appropriate treatment option for an individual patient has to be done in the countries where islet transplantation is offered as an option in addition to pancreas transplantation.

PANCREAS VERSUS ISLET FOR ENDOCRINE THERAPY

Pancreas transplantation has been performed since 1966, with significant improvements over time. International Pancreas Registry reports more than 42,000 pancreas transplantation worldwide, most commonly performed as SPK. This is a procedure with survival rates at 1 and 5 years of more than 96% and 84%, respectively.[24] Graft function rates, defined as complete insulin independence, are currently 82% and 58% for 1 and 5 years for pancreas alone, and 89% and 71% for SPK, respectively.[24] The expected 10-year survival rates range from 40% for PTA to 55% for SPK per International Pancreas Registry data.

Currently within Canada, the University of Alberta in Edmonton, the University of British Columbia in Vancouver, and McGill University in Montreal provide fully funded islet transplantation to the patients with type 1 diabetes. This is offered as islet alone or islet after kidney transplantation, as recommended by Canada diabetes association for the patients who have undergone successful kidney transplant but have persistent metabolic instability despite efforts to optimize glycemic control. When a comparison study looked into islet versus pancreas with kidney transplant, results demonstrated similar hemoglobin A1c levels, although islet recipients were less likely to achieve insulin independence, whereas pancreas recipients had higher procedure related morbidity.[25]

For countries where both options are available for patients with type 1 diabetes, consideration is made individually for patients, and these procedures are complementary and not competitive. For example, islet transplantation will be an option in cases with high cardiac risk for major surgery and older age, making them ineligible for pancreas transplantation, as well as kidney recipients who cannot receive a pancreas transplant or who do not wish to undergo another major surgery, will be great candidates, with the understanding of the differences in the outcome of insulin independence between these 2 procedure, at the current time.

Lifelong exposure to immunosuppression and its impact on the overall health contraindicates these procedures in a larger number of diabetics who could benefit from tight blood sugar control.

IMMUNOSUPPRESSION AND NEW DEVELOPING STRATEGIES

The main risk and concern for clinicians is the undesirable effects of immunosuppression, such as susceptibility to infections and cancer.[26] The Edmonton protocol using steroid-free immunosuppressive agents such as low-dose tacrolimus, sirolimus, and daclizumab improved the outcome of the procedure but not the concern about immunosuppressive drug use and their side effects. Clinical trials designed to replicate or improve the Edmonton experience have used alternate protocols for immunosuppression such as T-cell–depleting induction therapy to minimize use of islet toxic agents. Hering and colleagues[27] used initially OKT3 and later polyclonal antilymphocyte antibody thymoglobulin, with this approach and a modified maintenance therapy, the University of Minnesota group achieved long-term insulin independence in 4 out of 6 of their small series.[28] Around the same time addition of etanercept, a tumor necrosis factor-alpha inhibitor, in conjunction with T-cell–depleting regimen was reported to outperform previous protocols and became popular between different centers.[29]

Newer modified protocols used drugs such efalizumab and belatacept, novel monoclonal antibodies against specific T-cell antigens with the goal to improve long-term islet survival.[30] For example, the University of San Francisco reported with such modifications that 8 out of 8 patients became insulin independent[31] and 50% of them remained so at 5 years, a success close to pancreas transplant outcomes.

Unfortunately, the agent efalizumab, which was well-tolerated in islets patients, was later linked to progressive multifocal leukoencephalopathy, and the drug was immediately discontinued in all islet patients, after which most maintained their graft function with very low immunosuppressive maintenance therapy.

Extensive work has been done in the development of new strategies to minimize the need for systemic immunosuppression. Eliminating or minimizing exposure to immunosuppressive drugs will, without a doubt, revolutionize this field and open this treatment option to possibly all diabetics on insulin therapy rather than diabetics suffering with severe hypoglycemia or complications of this disease. Several preclinical approaches are being developed and very few protocols are in early phase clinical trials.

ISLET ENCAPSULATION

The idea of creating an environment protected from immune system but still allowing access to nutrient and product delivery has been considered for more than 40 years. An ideal device would allow selective permeability, keeping larger host immune cells and immunoglobulins outside, but allowing smaller molecules necessary for the survival of the cells such as oxygen, CO_2, nutrients, and products desired such as insulin pass freely.[32] There are 2 forms of encapsulation currently being studied for islet transplantation. Microencapsulation is the encapsulation of 1 or 2 islets in 1 semipermeable microcapsule, whereas multiple islets reside in 1 device in macroencapsulation.

Macrodevices designed to keep total cell volume in 1 device have been tested in animal studies and even in a small number of human trials. Although they are works in progress, so far they continue to be promising.

Some areas of improvements are the issue of islets being crowded within 1 device, resulting in low surface to volume ratio and interference with optimal diffusion of nutrients and oxygen. The islets density in the macrocapsule have to be 5% to 10% of the volume, and this results in the need to implant multiple units to achieve sufficient islets mass. Currently, there are intravascular or extravascular forms. The intravascular devices for macroencapsulation have a high risk of thrombosis and need for major surgery, making them less desirable for clinical use.[33]

Macrodevices implanted in an extravascular space such as skin are more attractive. Original studies dates back to late 1940s; continued efforts resulted in the formation of a sheet device by Baxter Health Care (Deerfield, IL) and later used by ViaCyte Company (San Diego, CA) as a semipermeable encapsulation device called the Encaptra Drug Delivery System. It is designed to deliver the cells composed of human pancreatic progenitor cells called PEC-01 TM cells. This system is currently being evaluated in phase I to II clinical trial called STEP ONE (Safety, Tolerability, and Efficacy of VC-01 Combination Product in Type One Diabetes).

Beta-O_2, also known as B air alginate macrocapsule protected by Teflon membrane, includes an oxygen-supplying technology to the islet-containing module. This design seeks to overcome the issue of overcrowded cells and their difficulty to receive enough oxygen when macroencapsulated. The animal studies have showed support of this system up to 10 months of the islets[34,35] and currently under clinical trial in United Kingdom.

In microencapsulation, alginate is the most commonly used material as hydrogel. The 2 common ways used to encapsulate islets are an air–syringe pump droplet generator or the electrostatic bead generator.[36,37] The first clinical experience reported with this technique dates back to 1992 by Calafiore.[38] Around 2011, promising results reported in 4 patients with type 1 diabetes who turned positive for C-peptide after receiving intraperitoneal microencapsulated islets, for 3 years. Their hemoglobin

A1c improved and total daily insulin use was lower.[39] Currently, multiple clinical trials are ongoing with microencapsulation with alginate.

The encapsulation technique enabled the usage of a new and exciting cell source for beta-cell therapy without compromising the immune system of the host, such as xenotransplantation and the use of embryonic stem cell lines. These new cell sources are extremely important to make the islet transplantation more widely available and accessible to a larger population in need.

One focus of investigation has been xenotransplantation, using animal pancreata such as the pig, as an islet source.[40] Using animal source cells have been very attractive because it can be limitless, but has its own challenges, like the immunogenicity of the products, and rejection by the host. Required immunosuppressive therapy so far has been very aggressive.[41] The possibility of transferring zoonotic diseases remains an additional concern. To overcome some of these road blocks, genetic engineering of the donor pig is used to decrease the instant blood-mediated inflammatory reaction. This is the detrimental reaction triggered by contact of the transplanted islet with blood of the recipient and causes destruction by complement and coagulation activation as well as other inflammatory pathways. Genetically engineered alpha Gal-deficient porcine donors, transgenic for human complement regulator CD55 and CD59, have been promising because they caused a minimum instant blood-mediated inflammatory reaction in baboon trials; however, aggressive immunosuppression was still required.[42] More research is needed to bring this field closer to clinical use.

In contrast, stem cell research once beyond our reach has entered a very exciting era. A variety of stem cells studies have been underway. Multiple different types currently exist, for example, human pluripotent stem cells, such as embryonic stem cells and human induced pluripotent stem cells, or mesenchymal stem cells isolated from adult tissues or directly programmed somatic cells.

Currently, stable cultures of pluripotent stem cells originating from ESC have been achieved, also maintaining their good genetic karyotype making them amenable for large production and cell banking.[19]

Another source for PSC is reprogramming of somatic cells by episomal vectors based on virus systems. Initial attempts to achieve insulin producing cells resulted in vitro polyhormonal glucose unresponsive type of structures.[43]

In the last few years, many groups reported achieving production of monohormonal and in vitro functional cells.[19] They have been also tested in reversing diabetes in mice model. The current trend is toward using these human pluripotent stem cell–derived pancreatic progenitors after maturing them into more functional islet like structures in vivo, so they transform into structures with subtypes of cells including alpha, beta, delta, and ghrelin and PP hormone-producing cells. This transformation produces tissue that could maintain glucose homeostasis in mice. The required length of time for this maturation is now down to 2 to 6 weeks. Cells currently being tested in human trial by ViaCYTE undergo this technique.

Another interesting result in this field is generating functional beta cells in vitro from partially reprogrammed somatic cells. This was possible by using murine fibroblast after multistep processing, which yielded 2% insulin positive and glucose responsive cells. Hyperglycemia in streptozotocin treated mice was improved with the transplantation of these cells.[44]

Also recently with a sophisticated multistep approach 2 different teams reported achieving in vitro production of beta cell–like structures from embryonic stem cells as well as human induced pluripotent stem cells.[45,46] This was followed by a study using these cells within a polymer encapsulation and showed normoglycemia in mice, which was maintained for 6 months.[47]

It has been very encouraging to witness these advances, although there remain multiple obstacles as safety and production difficulties remain to be solved.

SUMMARY

Both pancreas and islet cell transplantation are available as therapeutic options for patients with type 1 diabetes who are suffering severe hypoglycemia or worsening complications despite advanced medical therapy. Some countries like Canada have both therapies available as accepted medical treatment, whereas in the United States, islet transplantation remains experimental for type 1 diabetes. The advances and improvements achieved, especially since 2000, have brought this therapy much closer to clinical use. Many modifications in immunosuppressive regimens allowed islet transplantation to catch up with pancreas transplantation success rates. The encapsulation studies in humans with sources such as human pluripotent stem cells are underway, and results might open a path for many patients who would benefit replacement therapy without the unwanted side effects of immunosuppressive drugs. Current human trials will give us some answers in the very near future.

REFERENCES

1. Geiss LS, Wang J, Cheng YJ, et al. Prevalence and incidence trends for diagnosed diabetes among adults aged 20 to 79 years, United States, 1980-2012. JAMA 2014;312(12):1218–26.
2. Lipman TH, Levitt Katz LE, Ratcliffe SJ, et al. Increasing incidence of type 1 diabetes in youth: twenty years of the Philadelphia Pediatric Diabetes Registry. Diabetes Care 2013;36(6):1597–603.
3. Egro FM. Why is type 1 diabetes increasing? J Mol Endocrinol 2013;51(1):R1–13.
4. Kelly WD, Lillehei RC, Merkel FK, et al. Allotransplantation of the pancreas and duodenum along with the kidney in diabetic nephropathy. Surgery 1967;61(6): 827–37.
5. Farney AC, Rogers J, Stratta RJ. Pancreas graft thrombosis: causes, prevention, diagnosis, and intervention. Curr Opin Organ Transplant 2012;17(1):87–92.
6. Williams P. Notes in diabetes. BMJ 1894;2:1303–4.
7. Moskalewski S. Isolation and culture of the islets of Langerhans of the guinea pig. Gen Comp Endocrinol 1965;5:342–53.
8. Ballinger WF, Lacy PE. Transplantation of intact pancreatic islets in rats. Surgery 1972;72(2):175–86.
9. Sutherland DE, Matas AJ, Goetz FC, et al. Transplantation of dispersed pancreatic islet tissue in humans: autografts and allografts. Diabetes 1980;29(Suppl 1): 31–44.
10. Scharp DW, Lacy PE, Santiago JV, et al. Insulin independence after islet transplantation into type I diabetic patient. Diabetes 1990;39(4):515–8.
11. Bretzel RG, Brendel M, Eckhard M, et al. Islet transplantation: present clinical situation and future aspects. Exp Clin Endocrinol Diabetes 2001;109(Suppl 2): S384–99.
12. Shapiro AM, Lakey JR, Ryan EA, et al. Islet transplantation in seven patients with type 1 diabetes mellitus using a glucocorticoid-free immunosuppressive regimen. N Engl J Med 2000;343(4):230–8.
13. Ryan EA, Lakey JR, Rajotte RV, et al. Clinical outcomes and insulin secretion after islet transplantation with the Edmonton protocol. Diabetes 2001;50(4):710–9.
14. Available at: www.citisletstudy.org. Accessed March 2016.

15. Shapiro AM, Ricordi C, Hering BJ, et al. International trial of the Edmonton proto-col for islet transplantation. N Engl J Med 2006;355(13):1318–30.

16. Collaborative Islet Transplantation Registry (CITR). CITR 8th annual report. 2014. Available at: https://web.emmes.com/study/isl/reports/201502013citr. Accessed March 14, 2016.

17. Barton FB, Rickels MR, Alejandro R, et al. Improvement in outcomes of clinical islet transplantation: 1999-2010. Diabetes Care 2012;35(7):1436–45.

18. Gruessner RW, Gruessner AC. What defines success in pancreas and islet transplantation-insulin independence or prevention of hypoglycemia? A review. Transplant Proc 2014;46(6):1898–9.

19. Bartlett ST, Markmann JF, Johnson P, et al. Report from IPITA-TTS opinion leaders meeting on the future of beta-cell replacement. Transplantation 2016;100(Suppl 2):S1–44.

20. Hering BJ, Clarke WR, Bridges N, et al. Phase 3 trial transplantation of human is-lets in type 1 diabetes complicated by severe hypoglycemia. Diabetes Care 2016;39(7):1230–40.

21. Hering BJ, Kandaswamy R, Ansite JD, et al. Single-donor, marginal-dose islet transplantation in patients with type 1 diabetes. JAMA 2005;293(7):830–5.

22. Danielson KK, Hatipoglu B, Kinzer K, et al. Reduction in carotid intima-media thickness after pancreatic islet transplantation in patients with type 1 diabetes. Diabetes Care 2013;36(2):450–6.

23. Thompson DM, Meloche M, Ao Z, et al. Reduced progression of diabetic micro-vascular complications with islet cell transplantation compared with intensive medical therapy. Transplantation 2011;91(3):373–8.

24. Gruessner RW, Gruessner AC. The current state of pancreas transplantation. Nat Rev Endocrinol 2013;9(9):555–62.

25. Gerber PA, Pavlicek V, Demartines N, et al. Simultaneous islet-kidney vs pancreas-kidney transplantation in type 1 diabetes mellitus: a 5 year single centre follow-up. Diabetologia 2008;51(1):110–9.

26. Grulich AE, van Leeuwen MT, Falster MO, et al. Incidence of cancers in people with HIV/AIDS compared with immunosuppressed transplant recipients: a meta-analysis. Lancet 2007;370(9581):59–67.

27. Hering BJ, Kandaswamy R, Harmon JV, et al. Transplantation of cultured islets from two-layer preserved pancreases in type 1 diabetes with anti-CD3 antibody. Am J Transplant 2004;4(3):390–401.

28. Bellin MD, Kandaswamy R, Parkey J, et al. Prolonged insulin independence after islet allotransplants in recipients with type 1 diabetes. Am J Transplant 2008; 8(11):2463–70.

29. Bellin MD, Barton FB, Heitman A, et al. Potent induction immunotherapy promotes long-term insulin independence after islet transplantation in type 1 diabetes. Am J Transplant 2012;12(6):1576–83.

30. Vincenti F, Mendez R, Pescovitz M, et al. A phase I/II randomized open-label multicenter trial of efalizumab, a humanized anti-CD11a, anti-LFA-1 in renal trans-plantation. Am J Transplant 2007;7(7):1770–7.

31. Posselt AM, Bellin MD, Tavakol M, et al. Islet transplantation in type 1 diabetics using an immunosuppressive protocol based on the anti-LFA-1 antibody efalizu-mab. Am J Transplant 2010;10(8):1870–80.

32. Scharp DW, Marchetti P. Encapsulated islets for diabetes therapy: History, current progress, and critical issues requiring solution. Adv Drug Deliv Rev 2014;67-68: 35–73.

33. O'Sullivan ES, Vegas A, Anderson DG, et al. Islets transplanted in immunoisolation devices: a review of the progress and the challenges that remain. Endocr Rev 2011;32(6):827–44.
34. Ludwig B, Reichel A, Steffen A, et al. Transplantation of human islets without immunosuppression. Proc Natl Acad Sci U S A 2013;110(47):19054–8.
35. Barkai U, Weir GC, Colton CK, et al. Enhanced oxygen supply improves islet viability in a new bioartificial pancreas. Cell Transplant 2013;22(8):1463–76.
36. De Vos P, De Haan BJ, Van Schilfgaarde R. Upscaling the production of microencapsulated pancreatic islets. Biomaterials 1997;18(16):1085–90.
37. Farney AC, Sutherland DE, Opara EC. Evolution of islet transplantation for the last 30 years. Pancreas 2016;45(1):8–20.
38. Calafiore R. Transplantation of microencapsulated pancreatic human islets for therapy of diabetes mellitus. a preliminary report. ASAIO J 1992;38(1):34–7.
39. Basta G, Montanucci P, Luca G, et al. Long-term metabolic and immunological follow-up of nonimmunosuppressed patients with type 1 diabetes treated with microencapsulated islet allografts: four cases. Diabetes Care 2011;34(11):2406–9.
40. Ekser B, Ezzelarab M, Hara H, et al. Clinical xenotransplantation: the next medical revolution? Lancet 2012;379(9816):672–83.
41. Hering BJ, Wijkstrom M, Graham ML, et al. Prolonged diabetes reversal after intraportal xenotransplantation of wild-type porcine islets in immunosuppressed nonhuman primates. Nat Med 2006;12(3):301–3.
42. Phelps CJ, Koike C, Vaught TD, et al. Production of alpha 1,3-galactosyltransferase-deficient pigs. Science 2003;299(5605):411–4.
43. Hrvatin S, O'Donnell CW, Deng F, et al. Differentiated human stem cells resemble fetal, not adult, beta cells. Proc Natl Acad Sci U S A 2014;111(8):3038–43.
44. Zhu H, Yu L, He Y, et al. Nonhuman primate models of type 1 diabetes mellitus for islet transplantation. J Diabetes Res 2014;2014:785948.
45. Pagliuca FW, Millman JR, Gurtler M, et al. Generation of functional human pancreatic beta cells in vitro. Cell 2014;159(2):428–39.
46. Rezania A, Bruin JE, Arora P, et al. Reversal of diabetes with insulin-producing cells derived in vitro from human pluripotent stem cells. Nat Biotechnol 2014;32(11):1121–33.
47. Vegas AJ, Veiseh O, Gurtler M, et al. Long-term glycemic control using polymer-encapsulated human stem cell-derived beta cells in immune-competent mice. Nat Med 2016;22(3):306–11.

Understanding Population Health Through Diabetes Population Management

Joanna Mitri, MD, MS*, Robert Gabbay, MD, PhD

KEYWORDS

- Population health ● Population management ● Chronic disease ● Diabetes

KEY POINTS

- Chronic diseases, in particular diabetes, are major drivers of cost in health care.
- Most of the costs related to diabetes are a result of preventable complications.
- Population health management's goals in diabetes are to reduce cost and improve quality of care.
- Population health can address diabetes management challenges in many ways.

INTRODUCTION

There is a continued increase in the US population. Life expectancy and the proportion of individuals older than 65 year old are increasing.[1] Chronic diseases including diabetes are the leading cause of death and constitute 46% of the global disease burden.[2] Health care services are costly and complex for individuals with chronic diseases.[3] In parallel, there is a shortage of physicians in most medical specialties.[4] Specifically, the demand for endocrinologists is expected to increase secondary to the aging population with diabetes and obesity. It has been suggested that this demand will exceed the capacity of the endocrinology workforce. A more coordinated team based approach between endocrinologists, primary care providers, and other key team members will be needed to manage the population of patients with diabetes.

The United States health care system is facing quality and cost challenges, a major driver of cost being chronic disease. According to the Centers for Disease Control and Prevention, more than 75% of our nation's health care spending is on individuals with chronic conditions. Health systems are not oriented toward managing chronic diseases. Chronic disease management is complex and it entails multiple factors over

Disclosures: The authors have nothing to disclose.
Joslin Diabetes Center, Lipid Clinic, Adult Diabetes, 1 Joslin Place, Boston, MA 02215, USA
* Corresponding author. Joslin Diabetes Center, Lipid Clinic, Adult Diabetes, 1 Joslin Place, #239, Boston, MA 02215.
E-mail address: Joanna.mitri@joslin.harvard.edu

Endocrinol Metab Clin N Am 45 (2016) 933–942
http://dx.doi.org/10.1016/j.ecl.2016.06.006
0889-8529/16/© 2016 Elsevier Inc. All rights reserved.

a lifetime, as well as a more horizontal and integrated approach, with patient, family, and the community being active participants. The increasing global burden of chronic diseases necessitates stronger leadership by policymakers, advocates, and health care professionals. Developing effective strategies to prevent and manage these conditions is a global health priority.[5] In an effort to reduce cost and improve quality of care in patients with chronic diseases, population health management has to do with organization of the health care system delivery system in a way that meets these 2 goals.

Diabetes has often been an initial target disease for the key principles of chronic disease and population management given its high cost, prevalence, and available evidence-based quality metrics. This type of thinking requires a mental shift from simply focusing on individual patients one at a time to a broader perspective where the quality of care of a population of patients is tracked, and system based efforts are used to shift the health of that overall population of patients toward better quality and lower long-term costs by reducing complications. Herein, we describe several efforts to improve population management for diabetes, outline some of the challenges of measuring quality, and highlight system changes that can facilitate better care of those with chronic diseases such as diabetes.

DIABETES, A CHRONIC DISEASE

The worldwide prevalence of diabetes has been increasing over the past few decades.[6] The estimated prevalence of diabetes is 12% to 14% among US adults based on the National Health and Nutrition Examination Survey data. Diabetes represents a major threat to public health in many countries of the world. The costs associated with diabetes are sizable and noted to be 245 billion annually in the United States alone.[7]

Diabetes affects 29 million people—9.3% of the US population.[8] Out of these, only 21 million have been officially diagnosed; 8 million remain undiagnosed. More important, an estimated 79 million American adults aged 20 years or older have prediabetes. The leading cause of kidney failure, nontraumatic lower limb amputations, and new cases of blindness remains diabetes, and it remains the major cause of cardiovascular disease. Based on these numbers, there is an urgent need for national plans to improve diabetes prevention and quality of care. International health organizations are also monitoring quality of care indicators at the population level; however, this monitoring remains a challenge for many countries.[9] There are large gaps between what guidelines recommend and actual achievement of care goals.[10] Individualized glycemic control and multifactorial risk reduction are the cornerstones of high-quality diabetes care.

Despite national decline in hemoglobin A1c, 33% to 49% of patients still do not meet targets for glycemic, blood pressure or cholesterol control. Only 14% of patients meet targets for all 3 measures and nonsmoking status.[10] It is likely that patient factors play a role in this; however, the persistent variation in quality of diabetes care across providers and practice settings indicate a problem at the system level. The health care system is fragmented and poorly designed to coordinate care management for chronic diseases. There are unmet needs for an increasing number of people who have a chronic disease such as diabetes. Health care reform calls for new approaches to diabetes care delivery and greater emphasis on improving the efficiency and ability of health systems to respond to chronic disease to prevent diabetes and its complications in an equitable manner.

Reversing the diabetes epidemic requires remaking of our health care delivery system by focusing on proactive prevention, improved delivery of care, and continuous access to coordinated, evidence-based management of chronic diseases.

Diabetes management extends beyond blood glucose control. Regulation of metabolic risk factors such as body weight, blood pressure, and lipid profile is needed. In addition, preventative strategies such as annual eye and foot examinations, and lifestyle modifications such as physical activity, dietary modification, and smoking cessation require extensive counseling and coordination. Although there are guidelines for goals in diabetes management, there is a need to individualize care for patients, particularly when it comes to glycemic goals.

POPULATION MANAGEMENT

Despite increasing awareness of population health management, the concept remains unclearly defined and even less well-understood. Population health has been defined as the health outcomes of a group of individuals, including the distribution of such outcomes within the group. Whereas medical care is a key factor that affects health outcomes, other factors include public health interventions, social and physical environment, genetics, and individual behavior.[11] Based on this concept, there have been some efforts to combine health care with social services to improve population health.[12]

Population health management is an approach to medicine that improves patient access to care and helps patients to navigate the complex health care system. It facilitates care delivery across the general population and helps patients to make the best possible health care decisions. The goal is to improve care and reduce health care cost by keeping the patient population as healthy as possible and reducing the need for expensive interventions such as emergency department visits, hospitalizations, and procedures.

The advent of shared accountability financial arrangements between delivery systems and purchasers has created significant financial incentives to focus on population health management and measuring and reporting its outcomes. Accountable care organizations, at-risk contracting, and value-based payment all involve the continuum of US health care payment models that aim to reward health care systems beyond the traditional fee-for-service model. Fundamentally, these payment models incentivize better population management by rewarding health systems for better quality outcomes, and diabetes fits nicely in this framework because most of the costs associated with diabetes are related to long-term complications, which can be reduced significantly with better management of intermediate outcomes such as hemoglobin A1c, blood pressure, and lipids. Health care systems are shifting from fee-for-service to different types of value-based and shared risk alternative payments models like accountable care organizations. This shift provides an enormous opportunity for the health systems to invest in services that have traditionally been poorly reimbursed (eg, diabetes self-management education and support) to lower overall health care costs.

Population health management requires major changes at the system and provider levels. Providers have learned to care for an individual patient seeking care rather than managing an entire population of individuals. In a new era of value-based and shared risk payment, providers will need to learn how to work together by coordinating care and exchanging health information. Health care organizations, on the other hand, need to adapt to a new reimbursement models, change structure and leadership approaches. The Centers for Medicare and Medicaid Services reimbursement is shifting dramatically. The goal is to have 85% of all Medicare fee-for-service payments tied to quality by 2016% and 90% by 2018. Also, 30% of Medicare payments will be tied to quality or value through alternative payment models such as accountable care organizations and bundled payment arrangements by the end of 2016, and 50% of payments by the end of 2018. Health care providers will be accountable for the quality and cost of the care they deliver to patient populations under accountable care organizations and bundled payment arrangements (**Box 1**).[13]

THE CHALLENGES WITH MEASURING POPULATION HEALTH

Measuring is where successful population health management starts. One of the challenges lies in how to measure success and failure. The most common measures are:

1. Process measures: these measures are the specific steps in a process, ensuring appropriate processes have occurred, like yearly eye examinations.
2. Intermediate measures: these are physiologic or biochemical values, like control of hemoglobin A1c, blood pressure, or low-density lipoprotein cholesterol value. These precede and may lead to longer-range end result outcomes.
3. Finally, true disease outcomes are measures of a reduction of complications, for example, fewer amputations or cases of blindness.

The most widely used quality measures in the United States are The Healthcare Effectiveness Data and Information Set measures. These measures are used by more than 90% of America's health plans to measure performance on important dimensions of care and service. They also form the basis for the Provider Recognition Program by the National Center for Quality Assurance and used for provider recognition. The 81 Healthcare Effectiveness Data and Information Set measures are divided into 5 domains of care: effectiveness of care, access and availability of care, experience of care, utilization and relative resource use, and health plan descriptive information.[14]

These measures evolve over time but currently for diabetes include the percentage of patients:

- Testing blood glucose level (hemoglobin A1c test);
- Controlling hemoglobin A1c level;
- Screening for serum cholesterol level (low-density lipoprotein cholesterol screening);
- Controlling serum cholesterol level;
- Examining eyes for retinal disease;
- Monitoring for kidney disease;
- Controlling high blood pressure; and
- Medical assistance with smoking cessation.

Although Healthcare Effectiveness Data and Information Set measures have been reported for many years, there is a need for more refined measures for population

---

Box 1
Goals of population health management

1. Reduce the frequency of acute and chronic complications of chronic diseases.

2. Lower the cost per service through an integrated delivery of care team approach.

3. Improve the overall patient experience.

4. Promote patient engagement and empower patients to better self-manage their health, and participate in the decision making process.

health management. A consensus development conference was convened by the American Diabetes Association to discuss the future of performance measurement in diabetes. One of the raised questions was the future of quality measurement in diabetes. Several new opportunities for quality measurement in diabetes were identified, and included clinical action measures, weighted quality measures, personalized risk-based quality measures, measures of overtreatment, and quality measures for primary prevention of diabetes. Additional opportunities involve incorporating measures of adherence into performances measures, incorporating costs into quality measures, and using performance measurement to reduce, not worsen, health disparities.[15]

Data analysis is an integral part of population health management. Data should report on mortality rates, health status, disease prevalence, and even patient experience. These reports are the basis for quality reporting to payers or outside entities and they serve as a measure of provider's quality of care and patient outcomes. This only emphasizes the need of programs that can incorporate different types of data, include patient self-reports and be able to reports on different subpopulation. In this way, trends and gaps can be identified. Most of the measures neglect the distribution of outcomes within these subpopulations, which can only inevitably widen health gaps by improving the health of some, while leaving marginalized communities behind.

Most health care providers and organizations see the critical importance of population health management; however, they do not have the information technology infrastructure that is required to implement it successfully. To advance population health management, providers also must develop electronic registries with population-wide databases that are not limited to patients with specific diseases.

ROLE OF INFORMATION TECHNOLOGY

The current tools used by organizations do not have the ability to store, manage, and distribute comprehensive, timely, and relevant information to the degree needed for population management. There is a need for electronic registries with population-wide databases. Registries capture clinical data, claims data, administrative data, and self-reported patient data to power clinical decisions and identify gaps in care. There is a wealth of information at the disposal of health systems, but typically they are not integrated into a single system that can provide real time data for providers. Using this information will facilitate delivery of information-powered care to patients in real time to advance clinical outcomes, improve quality, and lower costs.

Organizations need to identify and invest in physician leaders, who can manage and drive the results. Sharing data on quality of care across provides can spur opportunities for "healthy competition," as different providers work to improve their outcomes compared with their peers. Appropriate leadership can promote better quality by highlighting those that have achieved better outcomes and spread their approaches to other providers who have been less successful. Ongoing outcome reporting can then ensure that the providers are continuously focused on improved population outcomes. Clinical information professionals are in the midst of the greatest transformation in the history of the US health care system.

POPULATION HEALTH AND DIABETES
Challenges in Diabetes

Timely diagnosis
One of the ongoing challenges in diabetes is timely diagnosis. The median delay from the onset of diabetes to physician diagnosis is 2.4 years, with more than 7% of cases remaining undiagnosed for at least 7.5 years.[16] By the time type 2 diabetes is

diagnosed, many patients have already developed microvascular complications. Population health management tools can be used to identify those at high risk for diabetes and ensure timely screening for diabetes occurs.

Transition of care

Diabetes is a complex disease requiring care by multiple specialists and care providers. It has been shown that errors could result from lack of communication and coordination among providers as well as lack of effective data sharing.[17] One particularly problematic area where disconnects can play a role is when transitioning from an acute care setting. Hospital readmissions can be reduced by better coordination of care from the inpatient to outpatient settings.[18] Patients with diabetes have a significantly higher hospital readmission rate and better coordination of care is key to reducing this trend.

Self-management

Behavioral management is a critical element in disease management. Providers face the major challenge of getting patients with chronic diseases to take more responsibility for their own health. Empowering patients is time consuming and cannot be achieved easily in a typically short visit. Engagement plays an important role in adherence to the care plan. Every individual must take responsibility for promoting his or her own health. However, individual's health behaviors are influenced by many factors, including the patient's family, culture, environment, socioeconomic status, insurance, care access, and health literacy. Many patients will require support and assistance to improve illness self-management. Diabetes self-management education improves psychosocial and clinical outcomes in patients with diabetes,[19] but is typically underused.

How Population Health Can Address Diabetes

Being a chronic and progressive illness, diabetes requires early diagnosis, effective coordination of care and self-management to stem its progression. Population health management strategies hold promise to improve outcomes.

Identification of high-risk patients

To achieve better diabetes outcomes at lower cost, the first step involves identifying relevant patients and stratifying them according to clinical risk. The greatest opportunity to lower health care costs is to focus on those at high risk, for example, those with a hemoglobin A1c of greater than 9%. Those who are furthest from evidence-based goals are most likely in the short term to contribute to health care costs through avoidable hospitalizations and emergency visits. Proactively identifying these patients can enable outreach efforts to address their needs. Care management where an individual within a practice focuses on these high-risk patients through outreach, engagement, self-management support, and problem solving has been shown to be one of the most effective quality improvement interventions for glycemic control.[8]

At-risk population identified from aggregated risk factor data should be screened to avoid delays in diagnosis. Early glycemic control can be achieved only after a timely diagnosis. Automated patient identification systems and surveillance applications that ingest data in near-real time can help health care organizations close this gap and begin intervention at the earliest possible time. In addition to speeding the diagnosis of diabetes, analytics can help to identify prediabetic individuals. Such early identification can prompt assignment to a lifestyle management program to prevent progression to type 2 diabetes. It has been shown in the Diabetes Prevention Program that intensive lifestyle intervention, including dietary modification, weight loss, and increases in physical activity, can prevent progression of type 2 diabetes.[20]

Once the diabetes population is stratified, one can design referral strategies and identify gaps in care that can ensure the right patient is seen in the right setting. One may think of this as a "pyramid of risk," with the highest risk patients at the top and being most appropriate for endocrinologist care and those at lower risk being cared for primarily in primary care with some guidance and education by endocrinologists (**Fig. 1**).

Coordination of care

Diabetes management involves a range of specialty physicians, dietitians, exercise physiologists, diabetes educators, primary care providers, and behavioral health specialists. Effective diabetes care requires collaboration across the care community to avoid miscommunication among providers and ineffective care transitions. It has been shown that proactive previsit preparation may be a key strategy for primary care practices to improve areas critical for chronic disease management, such as patient engagement, kept appointments, and adherence with recommended screenings, tests, and services.[11] Supporting primary care practices in practice redesign, and transforming practices into teams where doctors and other caregivers work to coordinate care for patients, improve both clinical outcomes and patient satisfaction.[21] The ultimate goal would be to keep high-risk individuals healthier and lower the overall costs for their care by preventing avoidable hospital visits.

Patient engagement

Through a team-based practice and with family support, patients are motivated to change their lifestyle, be adherent with medications, and build a support network. Identifying what team members can most effectively engage patents is a key step. Diabetes educators are well-suited to this role, but ongoing self-management support is critical to achieve optimal outcomes.

CHRONIC CARE DELIVERY

To target fragmentation of our health care delivery system, duplicate services, and lack of clinical information, the chronic care model[22] and the patient-centered medical home (PCMH) model[21] were developed to provide frameworks for effective care of diabetes and other chronic diseases. By incorporating team care as a vital component

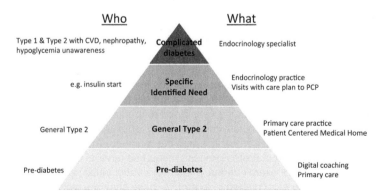

Fig. 1. Pyramid of risk. CVD, cardiovascular disease; PCP, primary care physician.

of delivery system design, these models will serve as guidance for health care reform initiatives aiming for an integrated health care delivery system.

The chronic care model provides patients with self-management skills and tracking systems. It represents a well-rounded approach to restructuring medical care through partnerships between health systems and communities. The model ensures that a prepared proactive practice team has productive interactions with an informed activated patient, and focuses on the domains needed to achieve this goal. It has been shown that the chronic care model is generally effective for managing diabetes in US primary care settings.[23]

The PCMH is a great example of a new health delivery system that developed out from the principles of the chronic care model framework. Leading primary care organizations introduced the PCMH to address high costs and poor health outcomes, particularly those related to chronic medical conditions, such as hypertension and diabetes. The objective of the PCMH model of care is to have a centralized setting that facilitates partnerships between patients and their personal physicians and, when appropriate, the patient's family.[24] Medically complex patients can be managed through an integrated care management program, which assigns nurse care managers to oversee complicated and chronically ill patients with multiple medical conditions, such as diabetes or heart disease. The PCMH has been shown to be a viable mechanism to improve the quality and costs of diabetes care.[25] The basic elements of a PCMH are care coordination, quality and safety, whole person orientation, personal physician, enhanced access, and payment reform. A critical component of a medical home practice is care with coordination and communication among its members and where information technology is essential to improve patient-centered care.[26,27] Efforts to transform diabetes care align with the aims of PCMH. In a typical workflow, the patient experience is improved when previous results and past medical records have been collected and merged across health care providers. One of the main goals of the visit is to empower patients enable to manage their own care. In summary, the PCMH has shown promise for improving outcomes through coordinated primary care and better coordination with others outside primary care—sometimes referred to as the medical neighborhood.[28]

IMPROVING QUALITY THROUGH POPULATION HEALTH

The framework of the PCMH has been the focus of the most recent efforts to drive better diabetes care in the primary care. Some attributes of the PMCH is for practices to assess care quality at the population level uses evidence-based measures, identify high-risk patients for outreach and care management, and enhance patient engagement—all key aspects of population management. Many of the early PCMH pilots focused on diabetes as a target disease and have showed improvements in both process and outcome measures.[21]

For example, a large multipayer supported PMCH initiative in Pennsylvania had its initial focus on diabetes. More than 100 primary practices across the state were transformed to National Center for Quality Assurance reconfigured PCMHs through practice facilitation, monthly population level reporting of clinical quality measures and implementation of care management for high risk patients. After 1 year, there was a significant improvement in diabetes process measures (annual eye examination, nephropathy screening, foot examinations, pneumonia vaccination, and smoking cessation) and clinical measures of diabetes control.[25] These changes were also associated with improvements on health care use.[14]

SUMMARY

In an era of accountable care organizations, health care systems need to be redesigned to care for the chronically ill. Diabetes is a great example of a chronic disease that could be partly prevented, but more important most of its complications that are costly and burdensome could be prevented. Population health management, which seeks to decrease health care cost and improve quality of care, can address most of the challenges in diabetes management. However, it cannot be achieved successfully without information technology system in place and a mental shift of provider who has been trained on treating the acutely ill and typically incentivized by reimbursement for every provided service. Stratifying populations based on risk is an important step to ensuring the right patient receives the right care from the right provider. Better measurement tools for assessing diabetes quality continue to evolve, and systems to better coordinate care within a medical neighborhood will be important elements to refine. As has happened so often in the history of health care delivery changes, the field of diabetes care has the opportunity to lead the way in developing this more comprehensive approach to care. Health care organizations, payers, and stakeholders have a big challenge to find the best delivery and payment model to meet populations' needs.

REFERENCES

1. National Center for Health Statistics. Health, United States, 2012: with special feature on emergency care. Hyattsville (MD): 2013.
2. Coleman K, Austin BT, Brach C, et al. Evidence on the chronic care model in the new millennium. Health Aff (Millwood) 2009;28(1):75–85.
3. McColl MA, Shortt S, Gignac M, et al. Disentangling the effects of disability and age on health service utilisation. Disabil Rehabil 2011;33(13–14):1253–61.
4. Dill MJ, Salsberg ES. Association of American Medical Colleges. The complexities of physician supply and demand: Projections through 2025. Available at: https://members.aamc.org/eweb/upload/The%20Complexities%20of%20Physician%20Supply.pdf. Accessed March 29, 2016.
5. Yach D, Hawkes C, Gould CL, et al. The global burden of chronic diseases: overcoming impediments to prevention and control. JAMA 2004;291(21): 2616–22.
6. Danaei G, Finucane MM, Lu Y, et al. National, regional, and global trends in fasting plasma glucose and diabetes prevalence since 1980: systematic analysis of health examination surveys and epidemiological studies with 370 country-years and 2.7 million participants. Lancet 2011;378(9785):31–40.
7. American Diabetes Association. Economic costs of diabetes in the U.S. in 2012. Diabetes Care 2013;36:1033–46.
8. Shojania KG, Ranji SR, McDonald KM, et al. Effects of quality improvement strategies for type 2 diabetes on glycemic control: a meta-regression analysis. JAMA 2006;296(4):427–40.
9. OECD. Cardiovascular disease and diabetes: policies for better health and quality of care. Paris: OECD Publishing; 2015.
10. Ali MK, Bullard KM, Saaddine JB, et al. Achievement of goals in U.S. diabetes care, 1999-2010. N Engl J Med 2013;368(17):1613–24.
11. Kindig D, Stoddart G. What is population health? Am J Public Health 2003;93(3): 380–3.

12. Shortell SM, Zukoski AP, Alexander JA, et al. Evaluating partnerships for community health improvement: tracking the footprints. J Health Polit Policy Law 2002; 27(1):49–91.

13. Burwell SM. Setting value-based payment goals–HHS efforts to improve U.S. health care. N Engl J Med 2015;372(10):897–9.

14. Friedberg MW, Rosenthal MB, Werner RM, et al. Effects of a medical home and shared savings intervention on quality and utilization of care. JAMA Intern Med 2015;175(8):1362–8.

15. O'Connor PJ, Bodkin NL, Fradkin J, et al. Diabetes performance measures: current status and future directions. Diabetes Care 2011;34(7):1651–9.

16. Samuels TA, Cohen D, Brancati FL, et al. Delayed diagnosis of incident type 2 diabetes mellitus in the ARIC study. Am J Manag Care 2006;12(12):717–24.

17. Elhauge E. The Fragmentation of U.S. Health Care: causes and solutions. New York, NY: Oxford University press; 2010.

18. Naylor MD, Kurtzman ET, Grabowski DC, et al. Unintended consequences of steps to cut readmissions and reform payment may threaten care of vulnerable older adults 2012;31(7):1623–32.

19. Norris SL, Lau J, Smith SJ, et al. Self-management education for adults with type 2 diabetes: a meta-analysis of the effect on glycemic control. Diabetes Care 2002;25(7):1159–71.

20. Diabetes Prevention Program Research Group, Knowler WC, Fowler SE, et al. 10-year follow-up of diabetes incidence and weight loss in the Diabetes Prevention Program Outcomes Study. Lancet 2009;374(9702):1677–86.

21. Bojadzievski T, Gabbay RA. Patient-centered medical home and diabetes. Diabetes Care 2011;34(4):1047–53.

22. Wagner EH, Austin BT, Von Korff M. Improving outcomes in chronic illness. Manag Care Q 1996;4(2):12–25.

23. Stellefson M, Dipnarine K, Stopka C. The chronic care model and diabetes management in US primary care settings: a systematic review. Prev Chronic Dis 2013; 10:E26.

24. Martsolf GR, Kandrack R, Gabbay RA, et al. Cost of transformation among primary care practices participating in a Medical Home Pilot. J Gen Intern Med 2016;31(7):723–31.

25. Gabbay RA, Bailit MH, Mauger DT, et al. Multipayer patient-centered medical home implementation guided by the chronic care model. Jt Comm J Qual Patient Saf 2011;37(6):265–73.

26. Cohn KH, Berman J, Chaiken B, et al. Engaging physicians to adopt healthcare information technology. J Healthc Manag 2009;54(5):291–300.

27. Weber V, Bloom F, Pierdon S, et al. Employing the electronic health record to improve diabetes care: a multifaceted intervention in an integrated delivery system. J Gen Intern Med 2008;23(4):379–82.

28. Spatz C, Gabbay R. The patient-centered medical neighborhood and diabetes care. Diabetes Spectr 2014;27(2):131–3.

Evidence-based Mobile Medical Applications in Diabetes

Andjela Drincic, MD[a],*, Priya Prahalad, MD, PhD[b],
Deborah Greenwood, PhD, RN, CDE[c],
David C. Klonoff, MD, FRCP (Edin)[d]

KEYWORDS

- Mobile • Medical • Applications • Diabetes • mHealth • Glucose • Telemedicine

KEY POINTS

- Many mobile medical applications (apps) are available to consumers with diabetes, but only 14 currently have clinical outcomes data published in the peer-reviewed literature or have been cleared by the US Food and Drug Administration or have received a Conformité Européenne (CE) mark in Europe.
- Apps provide guidance for insulin management and feedback based on blood glucose pattern analysis, and can permit data sharing with family members and health care professionals.
- Apps can positively affect such outcomes, such as hemoglobin A1C, hypoglycemia incidence, and diabetes self-care measures.

BACKGROUND

Management of chronic diseases such as diabetes mellitus (DM) is difficult. People living with chronic diseases face challenges related to knowledge deficiencies, inability to sustain lifestyle modifications, and scarce access to specialists for timely advice. In addition, people with DM need to master reading and mathematics skills to effectively incorporate the principles of basal, bolus, and correction insulin doses

Disclosures: Dr A. Drincic is a consultant for Bayer. Dr D. Greenwood is a scientific advisor for Welkin Health. Dr D.C. Klonoff is a consultant for Bayer, Insuline, Lifecare, and Voluntis. Dr P. Prahalad has nothing to disclose.
[a] Nebraska Medicine, Diabetes Center, 4400 Emile Street, Omaha, NE 68198, USA; [b] Division of Endocrinology and Diabetes, Pediatrics, Stanford University, 300 Pasteur Drive, Room G313, MC 5208, Stanford, CA 94305, USA; [c] Sutter Health Integrated Diabetes Education Network, Quality and Clinical Effectiveness Team, Office of Patient Experience, Sutter Health, 2200 River Plaza Drive, Sacramento, CA 95833, USA; [d] Diabetes Research Institute, Mills-Peninsula Health Services, 100 South San Mateo Drive, Room 5147, San Mateo, CA 94401, USA
* Corresponding author.
E-mail address: andjela.drincic@unmc.edu

Endocrinol Metab Clin N Am 45 (2016) 943–965
http://dx.doi.org/10.1016/j.ecl.2016.06.001
0889-8529/16/© 2016 Elsevier Inc. All rights reserved.

endo.theclinics.com

to effectively manage their disease. Health care professionals who care for patients with diabetes face challenges related to having inadequate time and ability to view and effectively analyze patient glucose and insulin dosing data, which is usually provided in a format too cumbersome for a quick analysis. An Institute of Medicine report from 2001 identified 3 major factors contributing to the gap in care of patients with chronic illnesses: (1) increased demands on medical care from the rapid increases in chronic disease prevalence and the complexity of underlying science and technology; (2) the inability of the system to meet these demands because of poorly organized delivery systems; and (3) constraints in using modern information technology.[1] Fifteen years later, these 3 factors are no less important.

Mobile health (mHealth), a subset of telemedicine and health information technology, encompasses the use of mobile communication devices (such as mobile phones and other wireless devices) for health services and information.[2] mHealth facilitates remote monitoring and delivery of timely recommendations for health care. The promise of this approach is to improve care through enhanced access to health information.[2] Specifically, for individuals with DM, mHealth could increase the capacity for self-management; facilitate decision-making processes needed for optimal insulin dosing; help sustain necessary lifestyle modifications; and improve communication between patients, family members, and health care professionals. Therefore, this approach has the potential to improve outcomes such as hemoglobin A1C (A1C), hypoglycemia incidence, and quality of life (QOL). In addition, self-management aims to involve patients in their own long-term care, which empowers individuals, increases self-efficacy, and reduces health care costs.

Smartphone technology provides an obvious platform for the development of mobile medical applications (apps) intended to help people with DM improve self-management and facilitate communication with their health care teams. Reviews have been published elsewhere that have evaluated commercially available mobile medical apps with a focus on functionality, usability, and outcomes[3–6] (including those focusing on specific populations, such as the very young and those >50 years old).[4,6] However, most of the more than 1100 currently available apps[7] are similar, offer only 1 or 2 functions, and lack published outcome studies in peer-reviewed medical journals. Therefore, aside from US Food and Drug Administration (FDA) clearance, there is little evidence to guide health care professionals in helping their patients choose the best DM app. Furthermore, additional platforms, such as computer tablets and glucose monitoring devices, including continuous glucose sensors and meters, can be used to provide digital health solutions. All of these devices can be produced containing decision support software that organizes data, analyzes data, and has the capability to further transmit the data to end users, including patients, families, and the health care team.

This article reviews mobile medical apps for DM that are commercially available in the United States or European Union (EU) and either have had clinical outcomes data published in peer-reviewed literature in the past 5 years or have been cleared by the FDA in the United States or have received a CE (Conformité Européenne) Mark in the EU. Identification of mobile medical apps was based on a search of 2 commercially available platforms: Apple and Android app stores. The PubMed database was searched for studies based on randomized controlled trials (RCTs), observational studies, post hoc analyses, and survey studies. Our search encompassed articles published between January 2010 and December 2015. Our search was completed on 3/10/16. The authors included apps intended to support blood glucose (BG) monitoring and DM self-management in patients with type 1 DM (T1DM) and type 2 DM (T2DM). Mobile medical apps and products were analyzed according to the criteria outlined in **Box 1**.

Box 1
Criteria used to evaluate mobile apps
Platform
Smartphone
Meter
Insulin pump
Computer: Web-based software
Other
Function/description
Insulin dose calculator
Basal bolus: pattern adjustment
Activity diary
Education
End user
T1DM
T2DM
Data collection: data source and mode of collection
Glucose
Carbohydrate/nutrition
Activity
Manual versus automatic
Connectivity:
Cloud
Web
Electronic medical record
Other: SMS (short message service)
Availability/regulatory
US Government or EU
FDA cleared or CE marked
Clinical evidence
Study design
Outcomes: safety, efficacy, and QOL

A total of 14 mobile medical apps (summarized in **Table 1**) were identified. They can be divided into 2 major categories: smartphone-based apps and glucose meter (smart meter)–based apps.

A. Smartphone-based apps (and their developers)
1. Blue Star (WellDoc)
2. Share (Dexcom)
3. Diabeo (Voluntis)
4. Diabetes Diary (Norwegian Centre for Integrated Care and Telemedicine)

Table 1
Summary of commercially available mobile medical apps for DM management (N = 14)

Name	Platform	Function/Description	End User	Data Collection	Connectivity: Cloud Web EMR Communication	Availability/ Regulatory	Clinical Evidence/ Reference
Blue Star by WellDoc	App (Android and iOS) or Web based	• Real-time feedback • Touch point messages • Video education • Education library • Longitudinal reporting • The Easy Carb Education library • The Easy Carb Estimator and Restaurant Helper to support healthy eating	T2DM	Manual data entry into app Automatic BG entry with Bluetooth adapter	Cloud: yes Web: yes EMR: no Can send reports to provider	FDA cleared in United States Needs MD Rx	A1C reduction[9] Improvement in self-efficacy[8]
Dexcom Share	App (iOS) for Share (upload to cloud)	Share real-time CGM data with followers	T1DM; T2DM	Dexcom G4 Platinum CGM uploads data to cloud via Bluetooth-enabled receiver	Cloud: yes Web: yes EMR: no	FDA cleared in United States	None
Diabeo	App (Android and iOS)	• Bolus calculator • Adjusts for exercise • Basal bolus pattern recognition • Real-time feedback	T1DM; T2DM on insulin	Manual data entry into app	Cloud: no Web: yes for MD EMR: no Patient can communicate with provider for real-time assistance	Developed in France CE marked in EU	A1C reduction[10-12]

Name	Platform	Features	Type	Data entry	Connectivity	Regulatory	Outcomes
Diabetes Diary	App (Android and iOS)	• Bolus calculator • Tracks BG level, insulin, food, and activity • Provides historical data to facilitate decision making	T1DM	Manual data entry Automatic BG entry with Bluetooth adapter	Cloud: no Web: no EMR: no	Developed in Norway CE marked in EU	A1C reduction[13]
Diabetes Interactive Diary (DID) (Il Diario Interattivo per il Diabete)	App (iOS)	• Logbook for blood sugar, insulin dosing, and events • Nutritional database for counting carbohydrates • Food exchange data • Insulin dose calculator • Physical activity diary • Annual screening reminder • SMS to diabetes provider	T1DM	Manual data entry • BG • CHO selection • Physical activity	Cloud: no Web: no EMR: no Other: SMS sent to diabetes provider	Developed in Italy CE marked in EU	No A1C reduction[14,15] Improved QOL[14] Reduction in hypoglycemia[15]
Glooko	App (Android and iOS)	• Downloads diabetes data from 40+ meters, insulin pumps and CGMs • Integrates health and fitness apps • Nutrition database for CHO counting • Data sharing with providers • Analytics data on clinic population for providers • Hypoglycemia prediction algorithms • Reminders	T1DM/T2DM	BG upload data via cellular network and MeterSync Blue cable Dexcom CGM data obtained via Apple HealthKit Obtains data from fitness tracking devices	Cloud: yes Web: yes EMR: yes Can email, print, or fax standardized reports to provider	FDA cleared in United States	None

(continued on next page)

Table 1
(continued)

Name	Platform	Function/Description	End User	Data Collection	Connectivity: Cloud Web EMR Communication	Availability/ Regulatory	Clinical Evidence/ Reference
Accu-Chek Aviva Expert	Glucose meter	• Bolus calculator embedded in the meter • Accounts for CHO and insulin on board • Minimizes insulin stacking	T1DM; T2DM on insulin	Glucose data automatic Hand enter CHO and insulin dose	Cloud: no Web: yes Accu-Chek 360 diabetes management software for MD and patient EMR: no	FDA cleared in United States Needs MD Rx	ABACUS 1 RCT clinical trial with A1C reduction[17] Survey results[16]
Accu-Chek Connect (Roche)	Glucose meter and app (Android and iOS or Web based)	• Integrated meter, app, and online portal • Meter automatically transmits data to app • App incorporates bolus calculator • Data shared with health care provider	T1DM; T2DM	Glucose data automatic Hand enter CHO and insulin dose Meal photographs can be attached to BG	Cloud: no Web: yes Uses Accu-Chek 360 View tool for 3-d profile EMR: no	FDA cleared in United States Needs MD Rx	Bolus calculator studied in ABACUS 1 trial[17]
Dario	Glucose meter app (Android and iOS)	• Downloads BG when connected to a smartphone • App contains insulin calculator • Can chart CHO intake, insulin doses, notes • Share results with family, provider	T1DM; T2DM	Glucose data automatic Nutrition, activity, insulin doses manual	Cloud: yes Web: yes	FDA cleared in United States CE marked in EU	None

Diabetes Insulin Guidance System	Glucose meter	• Bolus calculator • Adjusts insulin dosing plan based on historical data • Uses time of day to suggest CHO bolus	T1DM; T2DM on insulin	Glucose data automatic Initial insulin dosing entered manually	Cloud: no Web: no EMR: no Other: connect device to computer to download data	CE marked in EU	A1C reduction, decreased hypoglycemia[18]
FreeStyle InsuLinx	Glucose meter	• Bolus calculator embedded in the meter • Easy mode for fixed CHO meals • Advanced mode for CHO counting • Real-time feedback • Trending reports	T1DM; T2DM on insulin	Glucose data automatic Hand enter CHO	Cloud: no Web: yes FreeStyle Auto-Assist diabetes management software for MD and patient EMR: no	CE marked in EU Needs MD Rx	More accurate meal bolus[19] Confidence in bolus calculation[20]
Gmate	Glucose meter App (Android and iOS)	Downloads BG when connected to a smartphone BG	T1DM; T2DM	Glucose automatic nutrition, activity manual	Cloud: yes Web: yes EMR: yes Data sharing with family, provider via texts, email	FDA cleared in United States	None
Livongo	Glucose meter (In Touch) App (Android and iOS)	• Cellular-enabled glucose meter with touch screen • Tags meals, exercise, medications • Real-time scripted feedback about BG • Displays logbook and patterns • Share results with family, provider, and coach via touch screen	T1DM; T2DM	Glucose and activity data automatically uploaded via cellular network	Cloud: yes Web: yes EMR: yes Patient can communicate with CDE for real-time assistance	FDA cleared in United States	None

(continued on next page)

Table 1
(continued)

Name	Platform	Function/Description	End User	Data Collection	Connectivity: Cloud Web EMR Communication	Availability/ Regulatory	Clinical Evidence/ Reference
Telcare	Glucose meter App (Android and iOS) Web portal	• Cellular-enabled glucose meter • Uploads BG automatically to cloud and from there to Web or smartphone • Real-time contextual feedback via text messages • Share data with diabetes care provider • Two-way text messaging between patient and health care professional	T1DM; T2DM; GDM	Glucose data automatic	Cloud: yes Web: yes EMR: yes	FDA cleared in United States	Potential for cost savings when used with disease management program[21] A1c reduction when used with FDA-cleared glucose management software Glucommander[24]

Abbreviations: ABACUS, Automated Bolus Advisor Control and Usability Study; CDE, certified diabetes educators; CGM, continuous glucose monitoring; CHO, carbohydrate; EMR, electronic medical record; GDM, gestational DM; iOS, iPhone operating system; MD, Doctor of Medicine; Rx, therapy; SMS, short message service.

5. Diabetes Interactive Diary (DID) (METEDA)
6. Glooko Mobile App (Glooko)

B. Glucose meter–based mobile apps (and their developers)
7. Accu-Chek Aviva Expert (Roche)
8. Accu-Chek Connect (Roche)
9. Dario (LabStyle Innovations)
10. Diabetes Interactive Guidance System (Hygeia)
11. FreeStyle InsuLinx (Abbott)
12. Gmate (Philosys)
13. Livongo (Livongo Health)
14. Telcare (Telcare)

Fourteen studies are included in this article. These studies were published between January 2010 and August 2015, and they evaluated a total of 8 mobile medical app products: Blue Star[8,9] Diabeo,[10–12] Diabetes Diary,[13] DID,[14,15] Accu-Chek Aviva Expert,[16,17] Diabetes Insulin Guidance Systems,[18] FreeStyle InsulLinx,[19,20] and Telcare.[21] Six apps (Dexcom Share, Glooko, Accu-Chek Connect, Dario, Livongo, and Telcare) have received FDA clearance for use but do not have studies on efficacy and safety in peer-reviewed literature. A summary of studies is presented in **Table 2**. Only 6 out of the 14 studies were RCTs.[9,10,13–15,17] Sample size in RCT or observational studies ranged from to 7 to 203 subjects; a single survey study had 1412 subjects.[16] The interventions lasted from 4 weeks to 1 year, but the duration of most studies was 3 to 6 months. Most studies involved subjects with mean age 40 to 50 years, with an age range of 13 to 83 years. One small study targeted older adults more than 65 years of age.[8] Eight out of 14 studies enrolled only subjects with T1DM. A summary of the 14 studies, including design, methodology, and results, is provided in **Table 2**.

BRIEF OVERVIEW OF PRODUCTS
Smartphone-based Mobile Medical Applications

Blue Star (WellDoc)
This automated patient coaching system is an algorithm-driven app, based on patient-reported data. The mobile device is connected to the Web portal, and patients can use a mobile phone and/or a computer to access the app. Patients enter their medical history, medications, and clinical data. The Blue Star clinical/behavioral analytical engine automatically delivers real-time messages and contextually relevant content to the patient through proprietary algorithms when clinical data, such as BG values, are entered. Options exist to use a Bluetooth-enabled OneTouch Ultra BG meter, which transmits the patient's glucose values directly to the patient's cell phone. If the BG value is more or less than a target value, then the patient is provided with real-time feedback, including suggestions on how to bring values into the target range. Blue Star also performs blood sugar pattern analysis and uses this information to provide general suggestions for lifestyle or medication interventions. This product is indicated only for T2DM. Patients can send a SMART Visit report by fax to their health care professionals by clicking on an icon within the product. It is FDA cleared and available by prescription as mobile prescription therapy (MPT). The definition of MPT is a treatment prescribed by a health care professional and generated by a mobile device that is (1) automated and personalized, (2) associated with published outcomes, (3) adherent to governing regulations or standards, and (4) reimbursed by a health plan.[22] Studies have shown A1C level reduction with Blue Star.[9]

Table 2
Summary of 14 published studies evaluating mobile medical apps in the period January 2010 to December 2015

Author, (Reference), Year	Design Country Time Frame	Sample Type of Diabetes Mean Age	Platform/Name I and C Groups	Outcome Measures	Main Results
Barnard,[16] 2012	Survey United Kingdom 4–12 wk	n = 1412 T1DM <18–70 y	• *Glucose meter app: Accu-Chek Aviva Expert* • Survey 270 hospitals • Patients using Accu-Chek Aviva Expert BG meter for at least 4 wk • Bolus advisor with integrated BG meter • Electronic log book		• 588 (41.6%) responded • 80% (n = 456) ↑ ability to act on SMBG data • ↑ of 28% in frequency of checking BG 4–5 times/d (n = 257–331) • ↑ of 42% in frequency of checking BG >6 times/d (n = 133–189) • ↓ fear of hypoglycemia
Bergenstal et al,[18] 2012	Observational United States 3 mo	n = 46 T1DM and T2DM (T1DM 43%)	• *Glucose meter app: DIGS by Hygeia* • DIGS provides weekly insulin dose adjustment based on sugar patterns 3 groups: • I: T1DM on basal bolus • II: T2DM on basal bolus • III: T2DM on twice-daily premixed insulin	Primary: % dose adjustments approved by study team Secondary: ↓ in mean BG A1C	• 99.9% DIGS adjustments approved • ↓ A1C 0.5% (P<.05)
Charpentier,[10] 2011	RCT TeleDiab 1 France 6 mo	n = 180 T1DM 33 y	• *Smartphone app: Diabeo* • Diabeo software with basal and prandial insulin dose advisor • 3 groups (G1, G2, G3) C: G1 paper log book with in-person visit at 3 and 6 mo I: 2 groups • G2 Smartphone with electronic logbook with in-person visit at 3 and 6 mo • G3 Smartphone with electronic logbook + teleconsultation every 2 wk and visit at 6 mo	Primary: A1C	• A1C ↓ 0.91 G3–G1 (P≤.001) • A1C ↓ 0.67 G2–G1 (P≤.001) • No difference in hypoglycemia • G1 and G2 had 5-h ↑ hospital appointments

Study	Design	Sample	Intervention	Outcomes	Results
Franc,[12] 2012	Observational France 4 mo	n = 35 T1DM 39 y	*Smartphone app: Diabeo* • 1 group • Diabeo Software on smartphone with electronic logbook • Insulin bolus calculator using BG, CHO, and physical activity to suggest mealtime insulin dose • Algorithm calculated a 30% to 50% reduction in prandial insulin for the meal closest to the physical activity based on intensity of activity reported.	Primary: mean BG	• Significant ↑ in 2-h PPBG after physical activity ($P<.042$) • Returned to FBS/premeal levels by next meal ($P = .29$) • No difference in hypoglycemia with or without physical activity
Franc,[11] 2014	Post hoc analysis of TeleDiab 1 France 6 mo	n = 180 T1DM 33 y	*Smartphone app: Diabeo* • See description of TeleDiab 1 Charpentier, 2011 • G1 high system users (greater than the median) • G2 low system users (less than the median)	Primary: high users vs low users on A1C and impact of teleconsultation	• High users had lower A1C at baseline ($P = .008$) and more familiar with CHO counting ($P{\leq}.001$) • High users ↓ A1C 0.05% with no difference between G2 and G3 ($P = .89$) • Low users ↓ A1C 0.93% in G3 vs 0.46% in G2 ($P = .084$)
Javitt,[21] 2013	Retrospective	n = 141 T1DM and T2 DM GDM	*Glucose meter app: Telcare* • I: used Telcare for bolus calculations and call center monitoring for those with high or low BG • C: did not use product	Primary: change in allowed claims	↓ for $1600/y per person who used the product

(continued on next page)

Table 2
(continued)

Author, (Reference), Year	Design, Country, Time Frame	Sample, Type of Diabetes, Mean Age	Platform/Name, I and C Groups	Outcome Measures	Main Results
Quinn,[9] 2011	Cluster RCT, United States, 12 mo	n = 163, T2DM, 53 y	*Smartphone app: Blue Star WellDoc* C: UC I: 3 groups G1 • Mobile phone hand enter BG, CHO, medications • Automated real-time feedback with virtual coaching G2: • No analysis of log book data • No PCP Web access to log book G3: • PCP access to log book data via Web portal G4: • SMBG real-time analysis with feedback using computerized decision support • PCP receives summary via fax or email • Fax or email to review an analyzed report of all patients	Primary: A1C	A1C ↓ 1.2% G4–UC (P<.001)
Quinn,[8] 2015	Observational, United States, 1 mo	n = 7, T2DM, 70 y	*Smartphone app: Blue Star WellDoc* • 1 group • Entered glucose and self-care data and received automated feedback	Primary: self-efficacy SF-36 Depression	Trends in improvement in self-efficacy (P = .2), SF-36, and depression (P = .043)
Rossi,[14] 2010	RCT, Italy, United Kingdom, Spain, 6 mo	n = 130, T1DM, 36 y	*Smartphone app: DID* I: DID software installed in patient's smartphone that works as a CHO/insulin bolus calculator • Data sent to MD every 1–3 wk, reviewed, and new regimen texted to the patient C: received traditional education on CHO counting and bolusing (were not previously educated)	Primary: A1C Secondary: QOL Satisfaction with Rx Hypoglycemia	• No difference in A1C • No severe hypoglycemia in either group • Improved in some mental health components • Improved treatment satisfaction (P = .04)

Rossi,[15] 2013	RCT Italy 6 mo	n = 127 T1DM 37 y	*Smartphone app: DID* • DID software installed in patient's smartphone that works as a CHO/insulin bolus calculator • Data sent to MD every 1–3 wk, reviewed, and new regimen texted to the patient C: received traditional education on CHO counting and bolusing (were not previously educated)	Primary: A1C Secondary: glucose variability Mean daily insulin dose Hypoglycemia	• No difference in A1C (A1C ↓ 0.5% both groups, *P* = .73) • I: lower mean insulin dose (*P* = .04) • No reduction in glycemic variability • 86% decrease in severe hypoglycemia (requiring third-party assistance)
Skrovseth,[13] 2015	RCT Norway 6 mo	n = 30 T1DM 40 y	*Smartphone app: DD* • DD is a bolus calculator in its basic version. Diastat module can be added to allow a wireless transfer of BG values via Bluetooth and feedback module with BG graphs, trends I: DD + Diastat C: DD	Primary: number of hypoglycemia and hyperglycemia events Secondary: A1C	• No difference in A1C or out-of-range BG • All patients had ↓ A1C 0.6% (*P* = .001)
Sussman,[19] 2012	Observational United States 1 d	n = 205 T1DM and T2DM (T1DM: 48%) 51 y	*Glucose meter app: FreeStyle InsuLinx* • 1 group • 2 modes of operation: easy mode with fixed doses of rapid-acting insulin; advanced mode for patients who count CHO and calculate insulin doses • Subjects had to calculate 2 prandial insulin doses: manually and via FreeStyle InsuLinx • Compared accuracy of bolus calculation	Primary: frequency of insulin errors	• 63% (n = 256) manually calculated doses were incorrect • 10 times fewer errors using meter (*P*<.0001)

(continued on next page)

Table 2
(continued)

Author, (Reference), Year	Design Country Time Frame	Sample Type of Diabetes Mean Age	Platform/Name I and C Groups	Outcome Measures	Main Results
Ziegler,[17] 2013	RCT United Kingdom Germany 6.5 mo	n = 193 T1DM (93%) 42 y	*Glucose meter app: Accu-Chek Aviva Expert* C: Enhanced UC • Standard glucose meter, manual bolus calculation per individualized parameters • 7-point BG profiles over 3 d • Clinic visits focusing on diabetes care • BG data downloaded for therapy adjustments I: • Accu-Chek Aviva Expert meter with integrated bolus advisor to calculate insulin dosages • 7-point BG profiles over 3 d • BG data downloaded for therapy adjustments • Prandial and correction bolus recommendations based on BG, CHO intake, and individualized therapy	Primary: A1C Secondary: hypoglycemia	• ↓ A1C 0.2% (I – UC) (P<.05 1 sided) • 56% (C) vs 34.4% (I) had >0.5% A1C reduction (P<.01) • Improved treatment satisfaction (11.4% vs 9%; P<.01) • ↑ hypoglycemia in I compare to UC (P<.05)
Neil,[20] 2014	Observational United States 6 mo	n = 203 T1DM and T2DM (T1DM:64%) Age not reported	*Glucose meter app: FreeStyle InsuLinx* • One group • 2 modes of operation: easy mode with fixed doses of rapid-acting insulin; Advanced mode for patients who count CHO and calculate insulin doses	Primary: A1C Secondary: Confidence	• ↓ A1C 0.17% (P = .033) • ↑ confidence in insulin calculation(P<.01)

Abbreviations: C, control; DD, Diabetes Diary; DID, Diabetes Interactive Diary; DIGS, Diabetes Insulin Guidance System; FBS, fasting blood sugar; I, intervention; PCP, primary care physician; PPBG, postprandial blood glucose; SF-36, Short Form 36; SMBG, self-monitoring BG; UC, usual care.

Share (Dexcom)

Dexcom continuous glucose monitoring (CGM) system with Share is an FDA-approved CGM system with Bluetooth technology built into the receiver that allows uploading of real-time CGM data via an iOS device onto a Health Insurance Portability and Accountability Act (HIPAA)–compliant server that can be shared with family and the care team. Data can be shared with up to 5 designated recipients (followers) who can remotely monitor the patient's glucose information and receive alert notifications. CGM systems have been shown to achieve A1C level reduction; however, no studies of outcomes using the Share product as a standalone intervention have been published.

Diabeo (Voluntis)

Diabeo provides a bolus calculator with a validated algorithm for insulin dosage adjustments based on premeal BG, carbohydrate intake, and anticipated physical activity. It also has an algorithm for adjustment of insulin/carbohydrate ratio and basal insulin doses or insulin pump infusion rates based on postprandial or fasting glucose levels. If the patient desires, data can be uploaded to a Web site for a teleconsultation with a professional. It was initially reported for use by patients with T1DM (including pump users), but can also be used for T2DM. Diabeo does not offer electronic medical record connectivity. It is currently available only in Europe, but its developer has announced plans to introduce this product in the United States.[23] A1C reduction has been reported with this product.[10,11]

Diabetes Diary (Norwegian Centre for Integrated Care and Telemedicine)

Diabetes Diary is a mobile phone app designed for patients with T1DM. The app functions as a bolus calculator and allows wireless transfer of BG values, which is achieved by pairing the mobile phone with a Bluetooth adapter connected to a BG meter. The Diabetes Diary allows BG levels, insulin, food, and activity to be registered. It stores historical data so patients can analyze previous events by searching for similar situations in the database. The events are identified by several factors, including the amount of carbohydrate ingested, time of day, physical activity, and the most recently registered BG, which aids decisions regarding food and medicine. It is available in Europe only. A study has shown A1C level reduction.[13]

Diabetes Interactive Diary (DID) (Meteda)

DID is an iOS app that serves as a logbook for BG, insulin dosing, physical activity, and notes.[14,15] The app also provides a nutritional database for carbohydrate counting and food exchanges. The app contains a built-in insulin dose calculator. When DID is downloaded, it is immediately active as a food diary. In order to become a bolus calculator, it needs to be activated remotely by the health care team, using My Star Connect software. The health care professional sets the insulin/carbohydrate ratio, correction factor, and target BG level. The app allows patients to send text messages to their DM care professionals. All the data and graphs are received and managed through My Star Connect software. DID has obtained a CE mark in Europe and is available through the Apple App store in Italy only. Studies have not shown A1C level reduction[14,15] but have shown improvement in QOL and a reduction in hypoglycemia.[15]

Glooko (iOS and Android)

Glooko is a smartphone app and transmission device for BG meters, CGMs, and insulin pumps that syncs with an HIPAA-compliant server, whose data is shared with the patient's DM care team. Glooko also integrates with many commonly used lifestyle apps and automatically incorporates activity/exercise, blood pressure, and weight data. Patients can use the smartphone app to enter carbohydrate intake, insulin doses, and exercise. The app contains a nutrition database to aid carbohydrate counting. Data are displayed in an integrated fashion using graphs, charts, and trends to allow patients and health care professionals to gain insights needed for management decisions. Glooko is an FDA-cleared app, but no outcome studies have been published.

Glucose Meter–based Mobile Medical Applications

Accu-Chek Aviva Expert (Roche)

Accu-Chek Aviva Expert is a bolus calculator embedded in the Accu-Chek meter. It helps with accuracy of preprandial and correction insulin dosing, reduces stacking, and provides real-time feedback. The meter is indicated for use by individuals with T1DM, and those with T2DM using insulin. There is Web access for health care professionals and patients through Accu-Chek 360 View software to help patients evaluate a 3-day glucose profile to view trends and to learn how activity, food, and treatment affect BG levels. It is FDA cleared in the United States and available with a prescription from a health care professional. Studies have shown improvement in glycemic control and treatment satisfaction.[16,17]

Accu-Chek Connect (Roche)

Accu-Chek Connect is a glucose meter that wirelessly transfers test results to the Accu-Chek Connect app on a smartphone or an online portal. The Bolus Insulin Advisor, which needs to be activated by the patient's health care professional, is an FDA-cleared insulin calculator embedded in the Accu-Chek Connect app. Meal photographs can be attached to any BG result to help check the accuracy for patients learning to count carbohydrates. Results can be shared with a designated other person, such as a parent or caregiver, by using autogenerated texts. The app includes the Accu-Chek 360 View tool software described earlier. Data are automatically uploaded to a health care professional portal for access during and between visits. The Accu-Chek Aviva Connect meter is available at retail stores. Accu-Chek Connect app can be downloaded from Apple App store and Google Play. The use of this bolus calculator has been shown to improve A1C levels.[17]

Dario (LabStyle innovations)

Dario is a coin-sized glucose meter that plugs directly into an Android or iOS phone jack and transmits glucose readings directly to these smartphones using a downloaded app. The Dario app automatically syncs with the Dario meter each time it is connected to the mobile device, and stores the information in the cloud. Through the app, activity or medication data can be entered and there is easy access to tools for insulin bolus calculating and carbohydrate counting. Dario's cloud-based software allows patients to record, save, track, analyze, manage, and share diabetes-related information with caregivers and family members. Dario has obtained FDA clearance in the United States as well as the CE mark in EU. No outcome studies have been published in peer-reviewed literature.

Diabetes Insulin Guidance System (Hygieia)

The Diabetes Insulin Guidance System (DIGS) is a service provided by Hygieia for people with T1DM and T2DM on insulin therapy. Following a visit with a diabetes health care professional, the insulin plan is entered into the d-Nav device, which functions as both a glucose meter and an insulin dose calculator. Patients use the d-Nav device to monitor their BG level before a dose of insulin. Based on the patient's historical BG patterns and insulin dosing, the device automatically adjusts the insulin plan and displays a recommended dose incorporating a correction factor, prandial dose, and insulin on board. As a safety feature, a company service nurse is able to periodically view the data and provide follow-up with patients. This product has a CE mark in Europe. One observational study has shown improvement in A1C.[18]

FreeStyle Insulinx (Abbott)
FreeStyle Insulinx is a bolus calculator embedded in the Insulinx BG meter. The focus is on insulin dosing and real-time feedback. There are 2 modes: the easy mode for a fixed dose of rapid-acting insulin with standard meals, and the advanced mode for carbohydrate counting. The meter is indicated for use by people with T1DM and those with T2DM on insulin therapy. There is Web access for health care professionals and patients through FreeStyle Auto-Assist DM management software. It is not available in the United States. Insulinx has a CE mark in Europe, and is prescribed by health care professionals. Studies have shown improvement in confidence and in the accuracy of prandial insulin dosing.[19,20]

Gmate (Philosys)
The Gmate meter (which is approximately the size of a US quarter dollar) plugs into the headphone jack of an iOS or Android device. The Gmate SMART app, which is downloaded from the iTunes or the Google Play app store, interfaces directly with the phone's operating system. BG results are displayed on the screen of the iOS or Android device. In addition, the data are uploaded to the cloud and can be accessed by a caregiver for real-time patient management. Alternatively, BG results can be emailed or sent via text to the health care team or a single caregiver. This FDA-cleared app is available for iOS, and soon it will be available for Android. No efficacy outcomes have been published in the peer-reviewed literature.

Livongo (Livongo Health)
Livongo is a disease management program that offers coaching support as a covered benefit by health insurance plans. It uses a cellular-enabled, connected BG meter (In Touch) that uploads BG readings and important contextual information (eg, the time of day, the type of meal, and physical activity) in real time to the company cloud system. An instant feedback message tells the patient whether the BG level is in range, and provides tailored educational messages from the American Association of Diabetes Educators (AADE) curriculum. In addition (and if desired), cloud connectivity allows for real-time coaching by certified diabetes educators (CDEs) located in Livongo's call center. It is FDA cleared and also accredited by the AADE Diabetes Education Accreditation Program, indicating that the diabetes self-management education program meets the national standards. No efficacy outcomes have yet been published in the peer-reviewed literature.

Telcare (Telcare)
Telcare is an FDA-cleared BG monitor that uses cellular technology to transmit data directly to an HIPAA-compliant data repository for sharing with the patient's family and health care team. Following each BG check, the meter receives automatic contextual messages to provide feedback. Telcare has its own 3G cellular antenna and automatically uploads BG values to the central cloud system. Users can access their data through a Web browser or use the partner app Diabetes Pal for Android or iOS. Because data are uploaded to the cloud, users do not need to own an Android device or an iOS device. Telcare has been evaluated for use in patients with T1DM, T2DM, and gestational DM (GDM). Users can grant read-only access to family members and full access to health care professionals who are then able to monitor the service

and provide messaging. Telcare has shown a potential for cost savings when used with a diabetes management call center in an employer-sponsored disease management intervention.[21] According to a recent press release, when Telcare was used with a recently FDA-cleared software program for outpatient disease and pattern management, Glucommander (Glytec), in a small study a reduction in A1C was noted.[24]

DISCUSSION

The authors reviewed the current status of mobile medical apps with the goal of understanding the content, common design features, evidence for efficacy, and benefits as well as regulatory requirements governing mobile medical apps. This article addresses the following 7 questions.

What Are the Common Characteristics of High-quality Mobile Medical Applications?

The apps that were selected for review based on the outlined criteria (peer-reviewed literature data, FDA clearance, or CE marking) have the potential to benefit individuals with both T1DM and T2DM. Not only do many of the apps function as basal/bolus calculators, incorporating carbohydrate/insulin ratios, but some also provide feedback regarding the insulin regimen or behavior change.

What Are the Benefits of Using Digital Health Applications (What Are the Efficacy Outcomes)?

Despite design features instilling hope for achieving favorable disease management outcomes with digital health apps, limited supporting data are available in the peer-reviewed literature. Fourteen articles published in the past 5 years, summarized in **Table 1**, evaluated following outcomes.

Efficacy outcomes

- A1C (as a change in A1C level from baseline to end point or the proportion of patients reaching A1C target)[9–11,13–15,17,18,20]
- Self-efficacy (following a healthy eating plan, choosing healthy foods, exercise, confidence in ability to control DM as reported by patients), and self-management[8,12,19,20]
- Change in self-monitoring frequency[16]
- Change in QOL as assessed by diabetes QOL questionnaire[8,14,15]
- Cost of care[21]

Safety outcomes

- Major hypoglycemic episodes (requiring third-party assistance) and minor hypoglycemic episodes (defined as symptomatic hypoglycemia with BG level <70 mg/dL, self-reported by the participant)[10,14,15,17]
- Fear of hypoglycemia[16]

Historically, the impact on A1C of many digital health systems has been disappointing because of multiple factors. Earlier interventions involved electronic transmission of data that did not incorporate a complete feedback loop with recommendations for actionable treatment or specific behavior changes for the patient to follow. Telehealth remote monitoring interventions that incorporate multiple elements of structured self-monitoring of BG have been shown to be the most effective in achieving A1C level reduction.[25]

Overall, the impact on A1C varies widely from study to study, depending not only on the intervention but on the design, population studied, and baseline A1C level. Some studies reported no improvement in A1C,[14,15] 1 reported a modest A1C reduction,[17] and some reported larger A1C decreases of up to 1.9%.[9,10] However, even modest A1C reductions, of as little as 0.4 percentage points, are all that are required for a new medication to receive FDA approval.[26] In some of the studies it was difficult to distinguish the health care professional effect from the technology effect on the A1C level. Patients receiving Diabeo support via teleconsultation had a greater improvement in A1C than those who did not (-0.93% vs -0.46% respectively).[11] Similarly the Blue Star system showed a greater decrease in A1C level when health care professional support was added to the treatment.[9] The clinical significance of these differences is unclear and there is a need for further studies incorporating analyses of the clinical benefits and economic impact of providing professional support along with mobile diabetes apps. Technology enables productive interactions between patients and the health care teams, so it is useful to design studies that can evaluate digital health interventions as a whole. Furthermore, in studies in which there was a beneficial effect on A1C level, it is unclear whether this effect continued after the study period ended. Similar to A1C data, hypoglycemia outcomes varied widely from study to study, with some showing no improvement[21] and others reporting substantial decrease in hypoglycemia.[15]

Overall, RCTs of mobile apps for diabetes have tended to be underpowered to show a large clinical benefit and have tended to be too short to exclude a novelty effect. Large adequately powered studies of at least a 1-year duration are needed to establish the clinical and economic impacts of this type of intervention.

What Are the Barriers to Mobile Medical Application Adoption?

Limited data are available to answer this question, because none of the studies included in this article were specifically designed to evaluate barriers. However, some indirect observations can be made from the data presented. Ability to afford, use, understand, and adjust to technology are important barriers to consider. Smartphone apps are easily adopted because today 68% of US adults have a smartphone[27] and the price of most DM apps is modest. The capability to adopt apps associated with BG meters and insulin pumps is likely to depend on insurance coverage for those products. Education level may influence the adoption of apps, as suggested by 56% of Diabeo participants in one study having a university degree.[10] In addition, because smartphone ownership significantly declines after the age of 50 years,[28] age greater than 50 years may be another potential barrier to consider. In a survey of more than 1400 patients evaluating the use of an automated bolus calculator (Accu-Chek Aviva Expert), almost 90% of participants were younger than 50 years.[16] In addition, language is a barrier to consider because most smartphone apps are written in English, which limits access for non–English speakers.

What Are the Regulatory Requirements Governing Mobile Medical Application Use?

All of the 14 mobile apps reviewed have FDA clearance and/or a CE mark, highlighting the issue of regulatory requirements governing certification of apps. FDA guidance on mobile medical apps, released in February 2015, states: "When the intended use of a mobile app is for the diagnosis of disease or other conditions, or the cure, mitigation, treatment, or prevention of disease, or is intended to affect the structure or any function of the body of man, the mobile app is a device."[29] In a similar way, the European Commission Medical Devices Directive covers the regulatory requirements of the EU for medical devices. Therefore, although FDA/CE clearance is not mandatory for all mobile medical apps, it is the opinion of many prescribing health care professionals that cleared apps may be better than noncleared apps.

What Is the Spectrum of New Innovations Offered via mHealth?

Although technologically the apps appear to be similar, they all offer unique characteristics that may fit individual needs in specific ways. For instance, the bolus calculator feature, which is available in Diabeo, Diabetes Diary, DID, Accu-Chek Aviva Expert, Accu-Chek Connect (Roche), Dario, DIGS, and FreeStyle InsuLinx, may be a particularly desirable feature for patients with T1DM or insulin-treated patients with T2DM, but may not provide value to other patients. In addition, some patients may prefer bolus calculators embedded in meters (FreeStyle InsuLinx, Accu-Chek Aviva, DIGS) versus those available through an app (Diabeo, Diabetes Diary, DID Accu-Chek Connect [Roche]). The data sharing feature, especially one intended for sharing with family members (eg, Blue Star, Dexcom Share, Telcare, Gmate, Dario, Livongo), may offer additional advantages for treatment of children, young adults, patients with intellectual impairment, and those with hypoglycemia unawareness. The ability to share data with the health care team (Blue Star, Diabeo, Glooko, Dexcom Share, Livongo, as shown in **Table 2**) and the option for real-time feedback by a professional (Diabeo, DID, Livongo, Telcare) provide an additional layer of safety.

Apps that do not necessarily require ownership of smartphones (eg, apps embedded in the Accu-Chek Aviva, Telcare, DIGS d-Nav device, FreeStyle InsuLinx, Livongo) provide a particular advantage to patients who do not own an Android or iOS device. In contrast, the design of some new meters (Gmate, Dario) challenges the traditional concept of a meter as a device that displays a BG value. With their exceptionally small size and close integration with smartphones, they turn the smartphone into a meter.

Education features are innovative, from standardized feedback messages available on many apps to the ability to attach mealtime photographs to BG (Accu-Chek Connect [Roche]), which can further help estimate adequacy of carbohydrate counting.

Perhaps the most intriguing (and least intuitive) innovation that the new technology offers is the creation of new medical management paradigms and business models that emerge with the development of technology. The Telcare glucose meter has been combined with a disease management call center and offered as an employer-sponsored benefit. Livongo has created a new disease management and business model by offering a comprehensive program that encompasses access company–employed CDEs for a BG review and feedback as needed, through services that are covered by the participating insurance company. Glytec offers integrated outpatient technology with computerized glucose management decision support software (Glucommander) based on glucose data from the Telcare cellular-enabled meter. This system can effectively adjust insulin therapy.

What Is Desired for the Future of Mobile Medical Apps?

Technology is continuing to develop and adoption of medical mobile apps is becoming widespread, which provides an opportunity to consider the requirements for future app designs and research. A useful app cannot be merely a static repository of information; it must provide real-time feedback to the patient independent of the health care professional and foster a complete feedback loop.[30] In addition, the ability to integrate and analyze multiple sets of data is needed (in addition to that obtained from glucose meters), such as from sensors measuring exercise, sweat, and cardiovascular physiology. Interoperability is needed to allow all devices to communicate and be compatible with each other and with electronic medical records. For health care professionals, work flows and time constraints as well as reimbursement for time spent reviewing the data need to be considered. The capability of apps to provide real-time feedback without health care professionals' input in real time provides a potential solution to this dilemma, but raises the issue of safety and accuracy as well as liability in the event of a risky recommendation by the software program.

What Are the Directions for Future Research?

Most studies evaluated short-term outcomes, thus a longer-term impact on glycemic control and A1C levels needs to be evaluated. Clinicians need to know whether the A1C outcomes seen in initial studies are sustainable over time, after the excitement over novel technology subsides. In addition, it is important to find whether (and to what degree) some interaction with a health care professional is needed for the A1C benefit to be achieved.

Other outcomes, including incidence of hypoglycemia, time in range, QOL, and self-management behaviors, are equally important to evaluate. Additional studies need to be conducted to determine the features that improve adoption and the needs of special populations, including children and older adults.

In conclusion, several mobile medical apps are available to patients with DM on various platforms. In general, the 3 main features of these apps are (1) guidance for insulin management via a dose calculator, (2) feedback based on BG pattern analysis independent of the health care team, and (3) data sharing with family and health care professionals. Mobile medical apps have been shown to positively affect outcomes, including A1C level. More long-term studies are needed to identify best practices and evaluate the sustainability of the effects of technology on A1C level and hypoglycemia. Consumers need practical evidence-based guidance when selecting the best mobile medical app for their specific needs. Until more data are available, consumers and health care professionals can consider guidance based on FDA/CE status. Digital technology and mobile medical apps, when incorporated within an expanded mHealth enhanced chronic care model, can revolutionize diabetes management.[31] Patients with diabetes need to self-manage. Mobile medical apps that can increase the frequency and value of feedback to initiate behavior change or treatment adjustment may affect the clinical outcomes, and more importantly QOL, of patients living with diabetes. Diabetes is a dynamic condition needing more than glycemic management alone to improve health quality. In future, the glucose-oriented apps that are reviewed here will need to be integrated with other health-related apps to be even more effective.

REFERENCES

1. Institute of Medicine. Crossing the quality chiasm: a new health system for the 21st century. Washington, DC: National Academy Press; 2001.
2. Klonoff DC. The current status of mHealth for diabetes: will it be the next big thing? J Diabetes Sci Technol 2013;7(3):749–58.
3. El-Gayar O, Timsina P, Nawar N, et al. Mobile applications for diabetes self-management: status and potential. J Diabetes Sci Technol 2013;7(1):247–62.
4. Arnhold M, Quade M, Kirch W, et al. Mobile applications for diabetics: a systematic review and expert-based usability evaluation considering the special requirements of diabetes patients age 50 years or older. J Med Internet Res 2014;16(4): e104.
5. Silva B, Rodriguez J, de la Torre Díez I, et al. Mobile-health: a review of current state in 2015. J Biomed Inform 2015;56:265–72.
6. Sheehy S, Cohen G, Owen KR. Self-management of diabetes in children and young adults using technology and smartphone applications. Curr Diabetes Rev 2014;10(5):298–301.

7. mHealth. University of Florida Diabetes Institute; 2016. Available at: http://diabetes.ufl.edu/my-diabetes/diabetes-resources/diabetes-apps/. Accessed March 31, 2016.

8. Quinn C, Khokhar B, Weed K, et al. Older adult self-efficacy study of mobile phone diabetes management. Diabetes Technol Ther 2015;17(7):455–61.

9. Quinn C, Shardell M, Terrin M, et al. Cluster-randomized trial of a mobile phone personalized behavioral intervention for blood glucose control. Diabetes Care 2011;34(9):1934–42.

10. Charpentier G, Benhamou P, Dardari D, et al. The Diabeo software enabling individualized insulin dose adjustments combined with telemedicine support improves HbA1c in poorly controlled type 1 diabetic patients: a 6-month, randomized, open-label, parallel-group, multicenter trial (TeleDiab 1 Study). Diabetes Care 2011;34(3):533–9.

11. Franc S, Borot S, Ronsin O, et al. Telemedicine and type 1 diabetes: Is technology per se sufficient to improve glycaemic control? Diabetes Metab 2014; 40(1):61–6.

12. Franc S, Dardari D, Biedzinski M, et al. Type 1 diabetes: dealing with physical activity. Diabetes Metab 2012;38(5):466–9.

13. Skrovseth S, Arsand E, Godtliebsen F, et al. Data-driven personalized feedback to patients with type 1 diabetes: a randomized trial. Diabetes Technol Ther 2015; 17(7):482–9.

14. Rossi M, Nicolucci A, Bartolo P, et al. Diabetes interactive diary: a new telemedicine system enabling flexible diet and insulin therapy while improving quality of life an open-label, international, multicenter, randomized study. Diabetes Care 2010;33(1):109–15.

15. Rossi M, Nicolucci A, Pellegrini F, et al. Impact of the "diabetes interactive diary" telemedicine system on metabolic control, risk of hypoglycemia, and quality of life: a randomized clinical trial in type 1 diabetes. Diabetes Technol Ther 2013; 15(8):670–9.

16. Barnard K, Parkin C, Young A, et al. Use of an automated bolus calculator reduces fear of hypoglycemia and improves confidence in dosage accuracy in patients with type 1 diabetes mellitus treated with multiple daily insulin injections. J Diabetes Sci Technol 2012;6(1):144–9.

17. Ziegler R, Cavan D, Cranston I, et al. Use of an insulin bolus advisor improves glycemic control in multiple daily insulin injection (MDI) therapy patients with suboptimal glycemic control: first results from the ABACUS trial. Diabetes Care 2013; 36(11):3613–9.

18. Bergenstal R, Bashan E, McShane M, et al. Can a tool that automates insulin titration be a key to diabetes management? Diabetes Technol Ther 2012;14(8): 675–82.

19. Sussman A, Taylor E, Patel M, et al. Performance of a glucose meter with a built-in automated bolus calculator versus manual bolus calculation in insulin-using subjects. J Diabetes Sci Technol 2012;6(2):339–44.

20. Niel JV, Geelhoed-Duijvestijn PH, on behalf of the Dutch Insulinx Study Group. Use of a smart glucose monitoring system to guide insulin dosing in patients with diabetes in regular clinical practice. J Diabetes Sci Technol 2014;8(1):188–9.

21. Javitt JC, Reese CS, Derrick MK. Deployment of an mHealth patient monitoring solution for diabetes—improved glucose monitoring leads to reduction in medical expenditure. US Endocrinol 2013;9(2):119–23.

22. Iyer A. Mobile prescription therapy evolving mHealth from mobile to mainstream. 2014. Available at: http://www.himss.org/ResourceLibrary/GenResourceDetail. aspx?ItemNumber=30696. Accessed March 31, 2016.

23. Comstock J. Voluntis raises $29M to bring diabetes app to US. 2014. Available at: http://mobihealthnews.com/32499/voluntis-raises-29m-to-bring-diabetes-app-to-us. Accessed March 31, 2016.

24. BusinessWire. Study of Glytec's Glucommander™ in an outpatient setting indicates dramatic A1C reductions. 2015. Available at: http://www.businesswire.com/news/home/20151103006391/en/Study-Glytec%E2%80%99s-Glucommander%E2%84%A2-Outpatient-Setting-Dramatic-A1C. Accessed March 31, 2016.

25. Greenwood DA, Young HM, Quinn CC. Telehealth remote monitoring systematic review: structured self-monitoring of blood glucose and impact on A1C. J Diabetes Sci Technol 2014;8(2):378–89.

26. US Department of Health and Human Services. Food and Drug Administration Center for Drug Evaluation and Research (CDER). Guidance for industry diabetes mellitus: developing drugs and therapeutic biologics for treatment and prevention. Clinical/Medical. 2008. Available at: http://www.fda.gov/downloads/Drugs/.../Guidances/ucm071624.pdf Accessed March 22, 2016.

27. Anderson M. Technology device ownership. 2015. Available at: http://www.pewinternet.org/2015/10/29/technology-device-ownership-2015/. Accessed March 31, 2016.

28. Anderson M. The demographics of device ownership. Available at: http://www.pewinternet.org/2015/10/29/the-demographics-of-device-ownership/. Accessed March 31, 2016.

29. U.S. Department of Health and Human Services Food and Drug Administration. Mobile Medical Applications: guidance for industry and Food and Drug Administration staff. Available at: http://www.fda.gov/downloads/UCM263366.pdf. Accessed March 31, 2016.

30. Greenwood DA, Blozis SA, Young HM, et al. Overcoming clinical inertia: a randomized clinical trial of a telehealth remote monitoring intervention using paired glucose testing in adults with type 2 diabetes. J Med Internet Res 2015; 17(7):e178.

31. Gee PM, Greenwood DA, Paterniti DA, et al. The eHealth enhanced chronic care model: a theory derivation approach. J Med Internet Res 2015;17(4):e86.

Transcultural Endocrinology

Adapting Type-2 Diabetes Guidelines on a Global Scale

Ramfis Nieto-Martínez, MD, MSc[a,b,*], Juan P. González-Rivas, MD[c], Hermes Florez, MD, PhD[d], Jeffrey I. Mechanick, MD[e]

KEYWORDS

- Diabetes • Global • Guidelines • Implementation • Type-2 diabetes • Prevention
- Transcultural

KEY POINTS

- Health care professionals must consider both biological and ethno-cultural factors to provide specific recommendations for optimal adherence and outcomes.
- White papers, such as guidelines, algorithms, and checklists, synthesize the best evidence available to guide decision-making by clinicians and policy makers regarding organization and provision of health care, but unfortunately, most remain underused and poorly validated in many international target settings.
- It is necessary to develop objective protocols for transcultural adaptations and their respective implementation strategies that address specific barriers to improve white paper utilization.
- The development of clinical practice algorithm templates with node-specific adaptations should be emphasized as the best way to facilitate the entire transculturalization process.

The authors have nothing to disclose.
[a] Department of Physiology, School of Medicine, Universidad Centro-Occidental "Lisandro Alvarado" and Cardio-metabolic Unit 7, Av. Andrés Bello con Av. Libertador, Apartado 516, Barquisimeto, Venezuela; [b] Department of Physiology, School of Medicine, University of Panamá, Vía Transísmica, Apartado 0824, Estafeta Universitaria, Panamá, República de Panamá; [c] The Andes Clinic of Cardio-Metabolic Studies, Av. Miranda entre calles Bermúdez y Arismendi, Apartado 3112, Timotes, Venezuela; [d] Miami Veterans Affairs Medical Center, University of Miami Miller School of Medicine, 1201 Northwest 16th Street, CLC 207, Miami, FL 33125, USA; [e] Division of Endocrinology, Diabetes, and Bone Disease, Icahn School of Medicine at Mount Sinai, 1192 Park Avenue, New York, NY 10128, USA
* Corresponding author. Universidad de Panamá, Facultad de Medicina, Departamento de Fisiología, Vía Transísmica, Apartado 0824, Estafeta Universitaria, Panamá, República de Panamá.
E-mail address: nietoramfis@gmail.com

Endocrinol Metab Clin N Am 45 (2016) 967–1009
http://dx.doi.org/10.1016/j.ecl.2016.06.002
0889-8529/16/© 2016 Elsevier Inc. All rights reserved.

INTRODUCTION

Type-2 diabetes (T2D) and its complications impose a heavy burden to public health systems worldwide.[1,2] Combating T2D on any scale requires effective implementation and prevention strategies.[2] However, on a global scale, these strategies need to be robust and applicable to a host of varying socioeconomics, political settings, cultures, and lifestyles. White papers are systematically developed authoritative documents by professional organizations to address a specific topic, usually complex, and assist with decision-making. Examples of white paper formats include position papers, consensus reports, conference proceedings, clinical practice guidelines (CPGs), clinical practice algorithms (CPAs), and clinical checklists (CCs). Evidence-based CPGs written by experts improve quality of care by translating research findings and clinical observations into specific recommendations to optimize clinical practice.[3] Specific methodologies to develop effective CPGs have been adopted[4] and updated,[5,6] with visually and graphically simpler instruments, such as clinical CPAs and CCs, increasingly used.[6] Despite calls for culturally sensitive applications,[7] CPGs are generally resistant to policy mandates or clinical practice variances.[8] Thus, global implementation of CPGs, adapted to individual patients with different cultures, represents an onerous challenge and requires a new paradigm of white paper development.

In 2000, approximately 10 years after CPGs were defined, the quality of CPGs developed by scientific specialty societies was cataloged as unsatisfactory, and only a small proportion met any high-quality criteria.[9] In fact, the gap between CPG recommendations, and their expected impact, and current clinical practice and their outcomes is substantial. This is reflected by studies reporting that only a relatively small proportion of patients with T2D reach combined goals for glycemia, blood pressure, and lipid control.[10,11]

Translating a complex field of research into effective interventions for a target population consists of 2 distinct processes: transcultural adaptation and implementation (**Table 1**).[12] National CPGs of non-Western countries are largely based on existing international guidelines.[13] In general, the direct application of western CPGs to other cultures is ineffective without a transculturalization process.[14,15] This review addresses the portability issue of CPGs and other white papers and outlines the general principles of transculturalization for T2D.

WHY TRANSCULTURALIZE: THE GLOBAL DIMENSION OF TYPE 2 DIABETES CARE
Global Epidemiology of Type 2 Diabetes

The worldwide prevalence of diabetes was 415 million adults in 2015 and predicted to rise to 642 million by 2040.[16] The International Diabetes Federation (IDF) estimates that almost half (46.5%) of all people with diabetes are unaware of their condition; and 318 million adults have impaired glucose tolerance.[16] In 2012, an estimated 29.1 million (9.3%) US adults had diabetes, of whom 8.1 million (27.8%) were unaware of their diagnosis.[17] In 2013, diabetes represented the 12th leading cause of disability-adjusted life years (DALYs)[18] and the 17th leading cause of death globally.[19]

T2D imposes an economic burden on individuals and health care systems, with conspicuous differences among various countries and regions. Eighty percent of people with diabetes live in low-to-middle-income countries (LMICs),[20] but these countries spend only 19% of global health expenditure on diabetes.[16] Direct costs related to diabetes are positively associated with a country's gross domestic product.[21] In LMICs, out-of-pocket costs represent a larger share of health care expenditures.[21]

Table 1
Terminology and definitions

Term	Definition	Reference
Translation research	Development and application of scientific methods on dissemination of efficacious interventions to a target individual or population, including transcultural adaptation and implementation of the intervention.	12
Translation strategies	Systematic processes, activities, and resources that are used to integrate interventions into usual settings. Includes preservice and in-service training, ongoing consultation and coaching, staff and program evaluation, administrative support, and systems interventions.	117
Culture	Belief systems and values that influence customs, standards, practices, and social institutions, including psychological aspects (language, care, practices, media, educational systems) and organizations.	118
Race	Clustering of only physical or genetic attributes common to a category of people.	43
Ethnicity	Clustering that incorporates not only culture and race, but also emphasizes on genealogy, ancestry, geography (region), linguistics, and political ideology.	
Transculturalization	Process of adapting concepts from one culture to another, without changing either culture.	
Acculturation	Changes in culture that occur when 2 or more cultures interact.	
Deculturation	Process of adapting one culture to another losing the previous culture.	
Neoculturation	Process of adapting one culture to another creating a new culture.	
Transculturation	Creation of a new culture when 2 or more cultures merge.	
Transcultural adaptation	Systematic modification of an evidence-based intervention to consider language, culture, and context to be compatible with the participant's cultural patterns, meanings, and values. Transcultural adaptation offers guidance on how to adapt an intervention to increase its fit for the target population.	42,119
Implementation research	Development and application of scientific methods to promote incorporation of evidence-based interventions into routine health care in clinical, organizational, public health, or policy contexts. Answer the question of how implementation of an effective program works in specific contexts.	42,44

The greatest impact of T2D has been observed in the Middle East, sub-Saharan Africa, the Indian subcontinent, and China.[22] In fact, one of the epicenters of T2D is Asia, accounting for 60% of the world's diabetic population, which is mostly a consequence of urbanization, nutritional transition, and economic development, all over a short period of time.[23] Global epidemiology, drivers, and challenges in diabetes care are summarized in **Table 2**.

Table 2
Global dimensions of diabetes

Epidemiology		Reference
Global prevalence to 2015 (20–79 y)	8.8% (7.2%–11.4%)	16
Number of people with diabetes in 2015 (20–79 y)	415 million (340–536)	16
Global DALYs to 2013	55 million (46.3–66.8)	18
Global mortality to 2013	1.3 million (1.2–1.4)	19
Global health expenditure	USD $673 billion	16
Direct cost range	USD $242 to $11,917	21
Indirect cost range	USD $45 to $16,914	21

Risk Factor	Impact on Diabetes	Reference
Obesity	Obesity is a chronic disease characterized by increased adipose tissue mass that can increase morbidity and mortality by T2D. Obesity affects most adult populations in developed countries and it is increasing rapidly in developing countries. In Asia, excess body fat impacts the risk of diabetes at a lower BMI than people in other regions.	120,121
Diet	Excessive caloric intake and diet with low-quality foods lead to overweight/obesity and diabetes. In particular, higher dietary glycemic load, transfats, sugar-sweetened beverages, and foods from animal sources can lead to increased insulin demand, dyslipidemia, and chronic inflammation. Globalization and economic development promote the nutritional transition in many developing nations.	24
Physical activity	Regular physical activity consistently prevents or delays T2D. At least 150 min of exercise at week is recommended, associated with a healthy diet to reach and maintain 7% of weight loss.	45,122
Smoking	Cigarette smoking increased the risk of diabetes in 37.0%, and can cause 11.7% of cases of T2D in men and 2.4% in women. The link between smoking cigarettes and diabetes could be explained by the β-cell dysfunction due to nicotine exposure mediated by neuronal nicotinic acetylcholine receptors.	123,124
Alcohol use	A meta-analysis of prospective observational studies showed that moderate alcohol consumption lowers the risk of T2D, with a U-shaped relationship. Heavy users and nonusers have higher risk of diabetes.	125
Genetic	Multiple genetic loci and environmental/behavioral risk factors interact in a complex way in the diabetes. For example, the transcription factor 7-like 2 (TCF7L2) gene is the T2D risk locus with the largest effect size per risk allele and the most replicated across studies.	126

Abbreviations: BMI, body mass index; DALYs, disability-adjusted life years; T2D, type 2 diabetes; USD, US dollar.

Global Drivers of Type 2 Diabetes and Challenges with Clinical Practice Guideline Implementation

Biological factors govern the final pathways through which a toxic diabetogenic environment is expressed. Beta-cell defects and insulin resistance, conferred by genetic and epigenetic factors, contribute to the pathophysiology of T2D, but the dominant drivers for disease expression are excess body fat and lifestyle.[24] Although dietary indiscretion and physical inactivity are the main adverse lifestyle factors, other unhealthy behaviors include heavy alcohol use and cigarette smoking, especially in Asia.[24] In the Middle East region, an unhealthy dietary pattern was the leading cardiometabolic risk factor for mortality due to cardiovascular disease (CVD) and/or T2D in 11 countries, including 48% of CMD (cardiometabolic disease) deaths in Morocco and 72% in the United Arab Emirates.[25]

Evidence suggests that much of the T2D burden can be prevented or delayed by population-wide dietary modifications and an increase in physical activity levels,[26] and therefore, it is advisable to investigate how to best simplify and adapt recommendations for these interventions. A few population-wide polices have been effective, including promoting subsidies on production, transportation, and accessibility of low-cost healthy foods[27]; discouraging unhealthy food products through taxes and regulatory measures[28,29]; offering nutrition labeling to improve health messaging to consumers[30]; and promoting large-scale educational campaigns advocating healthy lifestyles.[26]

In addition to biological factors, health care systems can impact diabetes care, especially in LMICs where there are relatively low levels of income as well as insufficient health care expenditures.[31] The most important barriers to diabetes management in these settings include poor infrastructure and organization of the health care system, ever-increasing population needs, insufficient human resources, inadequate information for proper decision-making, limited availability/accessibility of pharmaceutics and medical equipment, intrusive or even ineffective government policies, and an overall insurmountable burden of care.[31] Race and ethnic factors may complicate this picture. For example, in New York City, the diabetes prevalence rate in foreign-born South Asians (13.6%) was almost twice that of other foreign-born Asians (7.4%); moreover, normal-weight foreign-born South Asians had 5 times the diabetes prevalence rate of US-born non-Hispanic whites (14.1% vs 2.9%, respectively).[32] These data are meaningful when considering that racial and ethnic minorities are at much higher risk for T2D, hospitalization due to diabetes-related complications, morbidity, and mortality than the predominant white non-Hispanic population.[33]

Specific cultural barriers represent additional challenges. A recent systematic review described the following barriers to T2D management in South Asia: language and a discordant communication with the health care provider, inconsistent willingness to participate in self-management, misconceptions on the components and resistance to adopting a new "anti-diabetic" diet, lack of gender-specific exercise facilities and fear of injury, lack of understanding about diabetes medication management, preference for folk and phytotherapy, concerns about the long-term safety of diabetes medications, and lack of any cultural adaptation of evidence-based recommendations.[34] Thus, CPG implementation confronts great challenges because cultural differences impose many layers of uncertainty that need to be addressed and reconciled independent of a particular geographic region.

HOW TO TRANSCULTURALIZE: GENERAL PROCESS AND RECOMMENDATIONS

The process of transculturalization begins with an evidence-based template. Among the most diligent, CPGs are evidence-based documents written by experts and systematically developed to provide information to guide decisions about health care in specific clinical topics.[35] Despite the widespread recognition of this utility, CPGs are not always translated to public health policies or clinical practice.[8]

In 2004, The American Association of Clinical Endocrinologists (AACE) published a "guidelines for guidelines" (G4G) that standardized production of CPGs[4] with a formal evidence-based methodology, recommendation cascades, incorporation of subjective factors, and other explicit attributes outlined in **Table 3**. The 2010[5] and 2013[6]

Table 3
White paper formats on diabetes

Tool	Goal	Content	Reference
Production			
AACE Guidelines for Guidelines (G4G; also see AMA G4G)	To establish a protocol for standardized production of CPGs	Criteria for the evaluation of CPGs: 1. Involvement of HCP organization(s): provide participant names and professional affiliations 2. Evidence-based methodology: uses middle-range literature searching and rigorous a priori set of rules for assigning evidence levels to recommendation grades 3. Credentials of experts: document expertise by providing curricula vitae and academic positions 4. COI: each author/reviewer submits multiplicity of interests and potential conflicts; reviewed by COI committee; relevant COI are not permitted 5. Generalizability: include disclaimers, limitations, and discussion of the degree of generalizability, especially when interpreting evidence from RCTs 6. Relevance: recommendations must be current and applicable to real-life clinical patient-oriented issues 7. Subjective factors: incorporation of information beyond evidence; including cost-effectiveness, risk-benefit analysis, patient/HCP preferences, and resource availability, evidence gaps, relevance 8. Review process: multilevel for critiques by experts and nonexperts; increased diligence 9. Distribution: ensure that CPGs are readily available to all HCPs influenced by the recommendations 10. Updating: time-stamping; describe the update mechanism 11. Cascades: provide alternative recommendations based on resource availability, cost constraints, and cultural differences; must be consistent with the evidence 12. Electronic: CPGs must be able to be converted to an electronic format for enhanced implementation	4–6,127

Transcultural adaptation			
Ecological Validity Model (EVM)	Modification of the intervention content using an ecological validation model.	Describes 8 dimensions of an intervention that can be adapted.	128

1. Language: adaptation of the materials in a culturally sensitive way, ensuring the message is received as intended.
2. Persons: patient and provider variables and the relationship between them
3. Metaphors: symbols and concepts shared with the target population
4. Content: cultural knowledge (ie, social, economic, historical, and political values, customs, and traditions)
5. Concepts: constructs of a theoretic model how the problem/intervention is conceptualized and communicated with the participant
6. Goals: objectives of the intervention that should be aligned between the provider and the participant, with support from the cultural values of the target population
7. Methods: procedures for achieving the intervention goals
8. Context: consideration of the clients' environment (eg, economic, political, developmental) during the intervention

Implementation			
Framework to guideline implementability	To guide implementation of guidelines	Seven domains and its elements (in parenthesis) include the following:	129

1. Usability: content is presented, organized, or formatted to facilitate the use of the guide (navigation, evidence format, recommendation format)
2. Adaptability: the guideline is available in a variety of versions for different users or purposes (alternate versions)
3. Validity: evidence is summarized and presented to be easily reviewed, understood, and interpreted (number of references, evidence graded, number of recommendations)
4. Applicability: contextual or supplementary clinical information is provided to interpret and apply the recommendations for individual subjects (individualization)
5. Communicability: information is included to support discussions with patients, or patient involvement in decision making (patient education or involvement)
6. Accommodation: to identify costs, resources, competencies and training, technical specifications, and anticipated impact required to accommodate use (objective, users, user need/values, technical, regulatory, human resources, professional, impact, and costs)
7. Implementation: strategies for identifying barriers of use, and selecting, planning, and applying strategies to overcome barriers (barriers/facilitators, tools, strategies)
8. Evaluation: consists of including performance measures for audit or monitoring (monitoring)

(continued on next page)

Table 3
(continued)

Tool	Goal	Content	Reference
Conceptual framework for implementation outcomes	Taxonomy of implementation outcomes	Implementation outcomes help improve our understanding regarding the implementation strategies that work best with specific interventions, settings, and conditions. These outcomes include the following: 1. Acceptability: perception that a given treatment, service, practice, or innovation is agreeable or satisfactory 2. Adoption: intention, initial decision, or action to use an innovation or evidence-based practice 3. Appropriateness: perceived fit of the innovation to address a particular issue or problem 4. Cost: cost impact of an implementation effort 5. Feasibility: extent to which a new treatment, or an innovation, can be successfully used or carried out within a given agency or setting 6. Fidelity: degree to which an intervention was implemented as it was prescribed in the original protocol or as it was intended by the program developers 7. Penetration: integration of a practice within a service setting and its subsystems 8. Sustainability: extent to which a newly implemented treatment is maintained or institutionalized within a service setting's ongoing stable operations	42,130
The Reach, Effectiveness, Adoption, Implementation, Maintenance (RE-AIM) Model	Evaluation of effectiveness of health care interventions	RE-AIM elements follow a sequence beginning with adoption and reach, followed by implementation and efficacy and finally maintenance 1. Reach: is the absolute number, proportion, and representativeness of individuals who are willing to participate in an intervention 2. Effectiveness: is the impact of an intervention on outcomes; this includes negative effects, quality of life, and economic outcomes 3. Adoption: is the absolute number, proportion, and representativeness of settings and HCPs who are willing to initiate an intervention 4. Implementation: refers to the capacity of intervention agents to deliver the program as intended (consistency), that is, being faithful to the protocol; this includes the time and cost of the intervention 5. Maintenance: is the extent to which a program or policy passes the test of time and becomes institutionalized or part of the routine organizational practices and policies	131

Abbreviations: AACE, American Association of Clinical Endocrinologists; AMA, American Medical Association; COI, conflicts of interest; CPG, clinical practice guidelines; G4G, guidelines for guidelines; HCP, health care professional; RCTs, randomized controlled trials.

updates advanced and optimized the protocol while also including provisions for CPAs and CCs. Implementation strategies has been described but found to be difficult to validate.[36,37] Barriers, or "determinants of practice,"[38] include financial and human resources, time constraints, and resistance to change by the medical community.[39] Barriers are seldom used to tailor interventions to achieve necessary changes.[40] However, one barrier to implementing a theoretic sound, evidence-based template deserving special mention is the complex effect of culture.

Transculturalization describes the process of adapting concepts from one culture to another, without changing either culture (see **Table 1**).[41] In other words, transculturalization in diabetes care involves the incorporation of cultural factors to optimize implementation of a scientific template for diabetes care. In a CPG or CPA, cultural adaptation should explicitly include culture, ethnicity, and race of the individuals, as well as the biological and social determinants of their health. Adaptations should not only be broad-strokes, but nuanced-based to account for subtle, although impactful population-based and individualized factors. For comparison, efforts that merely translate template content into a different language, with nominal inclusion of obvious cultural differences, are not considered to be a substantive cultural adaptation expected to have transformative effects.[42] Overall, a bona fide transculturalization process in diabetes care and prevention includes the following:

1. Development of evidence-based (scientifically substantiated) white papers by credentialed experts and professional societies.
2. Validated protocols for cultural adaptation to optimize white paper implementation to specific target regions.
3. Discussion and incorporation of demonstrable and relevant biological variables at the physiologic and molecular levels.
4. Focus on socioeconomic status and ethno-cultural characteristics of the target region.
5. Focus on epidemiology and disease burdens.
6. Focus on lifestyle, particularly healthy eating habits according to typical food available; food safety, preparation, and the culinary arts; physical activity; tobacco cessation; stress reduction and management; and sleep care.
7. Focus on toxicology in the environment, particularly the effects of pollutants and other endocrine disrupting compounds (EDCs).
8. Focus on resource availability and affordability, particularly hemoglobin A1c (A1C), glucose measurements, pharmaceuticals, and other technologies.
9. Focus on diabetes education programs for patients and health care professionals.[43]

Implementation science is an emerging field involving complex and multilevel processes that apply evidence-based actions into routine health care.[44] Implementation strategies are based on available evidence, taxonomies, and frameworks that capture the essential components of a discipline. Although not all frameworks and taxonomies are validated with effectiveness, they provide a systematic way to adapt interventions and facilitate replications in different settings (see **Table 3**; **Fig. 1**).[42]

ADAPTING EVIDENCE-BASED INTERVENTIONS TO PREVENT AND TREAT DIABETES
Diabetes Prevention

Emblematic controlled studies in the United States (Diabetes Prevention Program [DPP]),[45] Finland (Diabetes Prevention Study [DPS]),[46] China (DaQing),[47] and India (Indian DPP)[48] using structured interventions in subjects at high risk for T2D demonstrated that lifestyle changes can prevent or delay the development of T2D. The

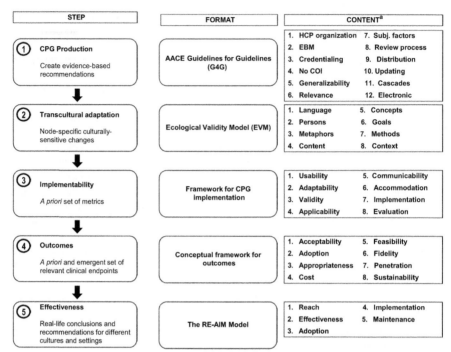

Fig. 1. Stepwise approach to transculturalization process. [a] See **Table 3** for content definitions. See references (AACE; AMA),[4,128] (EVM),[129] (Framework for CPG implementation),[130] (Conceptual framework for outcomes),[131] and (RE-AIM).[132] AMA, American Medical Association; COI, conflicts of interest; EBM, evidence-based medicine; HCP, health care professional.

initial reports in the United States and Finland showed reductions of 58% in the risk of T2D.[45,46] The long-term follow-up in these studies have shown durable effects in the Chinese study at 20 years (43%),[49] in the US study at 10 years (34%),[50] and the Finnish study at 7 years (36%).[51] Despite this efficacy evidence, the obvious challenge is to translate these study interventions into routine clinical practice for different settings.

A systematic review and meta-analysis that included 40 eligible studies evaluated the feasibility and effectiveness of lifestyle interventions using different endpoints: anthropometrics, metabolic, behavioral (physical activity and/or nutrition), and diabetes incidence among subjects with impaired glucose regulation or at high-risk of T2D, as determined by validated risk scores.[52] Seven of the studies were replications of the US DPP and the Finnish DPS. Although 8 studies concluded that translation to real life was feasible, effectiveness was lower than the reference studies.[52] The meta-analysis showed that the pooled weight loss at 1 year (−1.82 kg; 95% confidence interval −2.7 to −0.99 kg) was lower than that reported in the original DPP (5.6 kg) and DPS (4.2 kg) trials; also, the percentage of subjects who reached the weight goal was half compared with the reference studies.[52] The reductions of diabetes incidence, in the only 2 studies reporting them, at 1 year follow-up (37% and 23%), were lower than those reported in the DPP and DPS (58%) over 4 and 6 years, respectively.[52] Once again, the conclusion of these analyses was recommending improved translation research.

The initial efforts for the implementation of the Finnish DPS in local primary care settings demonstrates that T2D can be prevented in real-life conditions.[53,54] Exporting this experience to Australia[55] and sharing implementation experiences with Finland, the *Life!* program successfully translated this preventive intervention to a larger scale in subjects at high-risk of T2D using community facilitators.[55,56] The Diabetes in Europe—Prevention using Lifestyle, Physical Activity and Nutritional intervention (DEPLAN)[57] intervention is developing a prevention management model to be implemented in routine clinical practice settings. This project was shown to be practical, feasible, and effective in Poland[58] and Greece,[59] where recruitment from workplaces was the most successful strategy.

The US DPP[60,61] was based on behavioral strategies, and several systematic reviews[42,62–65] have translated the results of the protocol to various settings (**Table 4**). Of the 44 studies in the review by Tabak and colleagues,[42] 34 (86.4%) explored implementation, 15 (34.1%) described transcultural adaptation, and, of these, only 5 included a framework. In general, effectiveness varied substantially among programs and it was lower than the original US DPP. Another study demonstrated that the implementation of DPP-based lifestyle intervention leads to moderate improvements in overall cardiovascular health among Latinos with prediabetes in Venezuela.[66] In addition to the studies testing DPP implementation, this protocol is being implemented nationally through initiatives supported by the Young Men's Christian Association (YMCA)[67] and the Centers for Disease Control and Prevention (CDC)'s National DPP authorized by the US Congress in 2010.[68] The CDC (http://www.cdc.gov/diabetes/prevention/index.html), American Diabetes Association (ADA), and American Medical Association recently launched a national campaign to promote screening for prediabetes (https://doihaveprediabetes.org/) and the implementation of culturally sensitive revised curricula for the diabetes prevention in the US population.

Diabetes Care

Diabetes clinical practice guidelines worldwide
Various scientific societies and health institutions have dedicated enormous efforts to produce CPGs, CPAs, and position statements for the diagnosis, control, and management of diabetes,[13] covering a range of different components of diabetes care, with comparisons provided in **Table 5**. The CPGs are purposed to optimize clinical decision making[69] and realize aspirational targets for diabetes outcomes.[70] All of the CPGs cover similar aspects of care and agree on the classification and specified diagnostic cutpoints with minor differences for gestational diabetes mellitus. The CPGs promote structured lifestyle interventions (eg, weight reduction, healthy eating, and physical activity), as well as a stepwise approach for the pharmacologic management of T2D. All CPGs support a multidisciplinary/comprehensive approach to diabetes, which represents a major paradigm change from a more linear approach of simply targeting glycemic control and introduces many more decision points amenable to transculturalization.

Home and colleagues[13] reviewed the established national CPGs in non-Western countries (outside North America, western Europe, and Australasia), finding that 44% (33 of 75 countries studied) had national CPGs in diabetes. Most of these CPGs (58%) were supported by national diabetes societies/associations, whereas 36% were endorsed by the ministries of health.[13] Most of the CPGs were largely based on preexisting domestic or international CPGs: the most cited were from the ADA (55%), IDF (36%), European Association for the Study of Diabetes (EASD) (12%), AACE (9%), and Latin American Diabetes Association (ALAD) (3%).[13]

Table 4
Translations of the diabetes prevention program to different settings

Author (Reference)	Goals/Outcomes	Trial Design	Endpoints	Results/Recommendations
Diabetes Prevention Program Research Group[a,45,60]	Primary goal: To compare 3 interventions (intensive lifestyle or standard lifestyle recommendations combined with metformin or placebo) in prevention or delay of T2D • 7% weight loss and moderate physical activity for at least 150 min per wk	Randomized clinical trial/3234 participants from 27 clinical centers in the United States	Behavioral strategies • Collaborative, educational, supportive and motivational approach in a 16-week core curriculum provided individually by trained health coaches followed by monthly meetings and a long-term maintenance program, including additional strategies and incentives[60]	Results: • Lifestyle intervention reduced the T2D incidence by 58% • Weight loss: − 6.9% • Attendance: 95% • Attrition: 7% • Diversity: 46% non-White
Whittemore,[62] 2011	To review translational research of the DPP protocol in adults at-risk for T2D	SR/16 studies/2005 participants in 4 settings: • Hospital outpatient • Primary care • Community • Work and church	The Reach, Efficacy, Adoption, Implementation, Maintenance (RE-AIM) Model[131]	Results: • Weight loss: −2.7% to −6% • Attendance: 54%–96% • Attrition: 0%–43% • Diversity: 0%–100% non-White Recommendations: • Ongoing development of innovative programs for subjects with low health literacy and low socioeconomic status • More rigorous evaluation of program using RE-AIM model

| Tabak et al,[42] 2015 | To evaluate the cultural adaptations used by studies on diabetes prevention • Inventory implementation search within translation studies | SR/44 studies/Most in 3 settings: • Churches (n = 8) • Medical settings (n = 18) • Community centers (n = 10) | • Ecological Validity Model (EVM)[128] to evaluate if adaptations were made to meet the need of study subjects • Bernal et al[132] to establish how the adaptation was made • Proctor et al[130] to evaluate implementation outcomes | Results: • Translation strategies: large variability; modifications in words of the program, mostly group-based interventions, changes in administration (reducing timeline and frequency of meetings) • Cultural adaptation: reported in only 5 studies all in community centers, more frequent in specific population studies; adaptations of content and 67% of studies matched ethnicity of staff • Implementation outcomes most reported: adoption (individual level) and feasibility (organization level) |
| Aziz et al,[65] 2015 | Identifying success factors for implementing diabetes prevention programs in real-world settings | SR/38 studies/12,136 participants over the past 15 y; Mainly based on either the US-DPP or Finnish-DPS • Implemented in the United States (n = 17), United Kingdom (n = 4), Netherlands (n = 4), other countries in Europe (n = 8), Australia (n = 3), and Japan (n = 2) | Penetration, implementation, participation, and effectiveness (PIPE) impact metric to evaluate outcomes[133] | Results: • Participation: 92% • Coverage of their target population (penetration): 18% • Program intensity or implementation: 100% • Implementation fidelity: 84% • Employment of quality assurance measures: 18% • Effectiveness: 16% "highly" and 26% "moderately" positive changes based on weight loss • Program intensity plays a major role in weight loss outcomes • Programs with high uptake maintain considerable impact even with a low intensity intervention Recommendations: • Important finding to apply in resource constrained settings • More use of the PIPE framework components |

(continued on next page)

Table 4
(continued)

Author (Reference)	Goals/Outcomes	Trial Design	Endpoints	Results/Recommendations
Ali et al,[63] 2012	• To estimate the magnitude of weight loss achieved • To determine program features (number of core sessions, type of intervention staff, and inclusion of the maintenance component) influencing weight loss	SR-M/28 US studies/3797 participants	Quality assessment framework.[134] Criteria: 1. High diabetes risk target population was clearly defined 2. Actions to minimize attrition were reported (ITT analysis, completers vs noncompleters comparisons) 3. Data limitations were reported 4. Practical translatability of interventions was informed	Results: • Weight loss at 12 mo: −4% from baseline • Similar results regardless facilitator (clinically trained professionals or lay educators) Recommendations: • Costs can be lowered maintaining effectiveness, using nonmedical personnel and motivating subjects to attend at program sessions
Dunkley et al,[64] 2014	• To determine the effectiveness of pragmatic interventions on weight loss • To examine the relationship between adherence to guideline recommendations and effectiveness (meta-regression analysis)	SR-M/25 studies. In the United States (n = 11), Australia (n = 11), Europe (n = 2), and Japan (n = 1)/9211 participants (5500 subjects in meta-analysis)	Quality assessment: • NICE guidance score: UK National Institute for Health and Clinical Excellence (NICE) quality appraisal checklist for quantitative intervention studies[135] • IMAGE guidance score[136]	Results: • Weight loss at 12 mo: −2.6% • Adherence to guideline recommendations was associated with a greater weight loss (for each 1-point increase on the 12-point scale for adherence to NICE an additional 0.4 kg of weight loss was achieved (P = .008) Recommendation: • Maximizing guideline adherence improve its effectiveness

Abbreviations: DPP, Diabetes Prevention Program; ITT, intention to treat; M, meta-analysis; SR, systematic review; T2D, type 2 diabetes.
^a DPP is the reference to compare implementation studies.

Table 5
Diabetes CPG comparisons

CPG (Region-Country)	AACE/ACE (United States)[137]	ADA (United States)[122]	ESC/EASD (Europe)[138]	CDA (Canada)[139]	IDF (World)[140–143]
Classification and diagnosis	T2D: comprise >90% of cases, typically related to risk factors. T1D: absolute insulin deficiency. Levels of insulin and C-peptide and immune markers help distinguish between them. There are another atypical presentations.	T2D: progressive loss insulin secretion/ insulin resistance. T1D: β-cell destruction/ absolute insulin deficiency GDM: diabetes on the 2nd or 3rd trimester of pregnancy. Other specific causes (eg, MODY syndrome)	T2D: combination of insulin resistance and β-cell failure, associated with major risk factors. T1D: deficiency of insulin due to destruction of pancreatic β-cells. GDM: develops during pregnancy, increased risk for T2D. Other specific types of diabetes.	T2D: insulin resistance and insulin deficiency. T1D: β-cell destruction/ absolute insulin deficiency, prone to ketoacidosis. GDM: glucose intolerance onset or first during pregnancy. Other specific and uncommon types.	T2D: insulin resistance and insulin deficiency. T1D: Individuals have an absolute deficiency of insulin secretion and are prone to ketoacidosis. GDM: any degree of glucose intolerance with onset or first recognition during pregnancy.
Testing for diabetes in asymptomatic patients	FPG ≥126 mg/dL or 2-h PG ≥200 mg/dL during an OGTT or A1C ≥6.5%.	FPG ≥126 mg/dL (7.0 mmol/L) or 2-h PG ≥200 mg/dL (11.1 mmol/L) during an OGTT or A1C ≥6.5% (48 mmol/mol).	FPG ≥126 mg/dL (7.0 mmol/L) or 2-h PG ≥200 mg/dL (11.1 mmol/L) during an OGTT or A1C ≥6.5% (48 mmol/mol).	FPG ≥7.0 mmol/L; 2-h PG- 75 g OGTT ≥11.1 mmol/L or A1C ≥6.5%.	Step 1: identify high-risk individuals using a risk assessment questionnaire; Step 2: glycemic measure in high-risk individuals - FPG ≥7.0 mmol/L (126 mg/dL) or, 75 g OGTT ≥11.1 mmol/L (200 mg/dL) or, A1C ≥6.5%.

(continued on next page)

Table 5
(continued)

CPG (Region-Country)	AACE/ACE (United States)[137]	ADA (United States)[122]	ESC/EASD (Europe)[138]	CDA (Canada)[139]	IDF (World)[140–143]
Detection and diagnosis of gestational diabetes mellitus (GDM)	In patients with risk factors at 24–28 wk of gestation should be screened. Criteria diagnosis for GDM: FPG ≥92 mg/dL or 1 h: ≥180 mg/dL or 2 h: ≥153 mg/dL	In patients with risk factors perform a 75-g OGTT. Criteria diagnosis for GDM: FPG ≥92 mg/dL (5.1 mmol/L) or 1 h: ≥180 mg/dL (10.0 mmol/L) or 2 h: ≥153 mg/dL (8.5 mmol/L)	NA	All pregnant women should be screened for GDM at 24–28 wk of gestation. Screening at 2-stage diagnostic 50 g GCT (nonfasting state): PG ≥7.8 mmol/L at 1 h will be considered screening positive and most indicate 75 g OGTT confirmatory, if the PG is ≥11 mmol/L do not require 75g OGTT to confirm DMG diagnosis.	Diagnosis could be established by 1-stage (preferred) or 2 steps. 75 g 2 h. World Health Organization (WHO) test.

Prevention or delay of T2D	Persons with prediabetes should modify their lifestyle. In overweight/obesity lose 5%–10% weight and moderate physical activity (150 min/wk). Included in lifestyle change programs to follow-up. Medications including metformin, acarbose, or TZDs, should be considered.	Patients with prediabetes counseling DPP targets: 7% weight loss, 150 min/wk moderate-intensity physical activity, with long-time follow-up. Metformin should be considered in prediabetes.	Encourage modest weight loss and increased physical activity, to prevent or delay progression in high-risk individuals with IGT.	Establish intensive and structured lifestyle modification resulting in weight loss (5%). Dietary modification and moderate-intensity physical activity. Pharmacologic therapy could be considered with metformin, acarbose, and TZD.	Population approach to develop and implement a National Diabetes Prevention Plan. Encourage all population at least 30 min of moderately intense physical activity and to maintain a healthy weight. High-risk approach: Step 1: identification of subjects at elevated risk and apply the Finnish Diabetes Risk Score (FINDRISC). Step 2: measurement of risk, including anthropometric and biochemical variables. Step 3: intervention, lifestyle, exercise, weight reduction, and metformin in some cases.

(continued on next page)

Table 5
(continued)

CPG (Region-Country)	AACE/ACE (United States)[137]	ADA (United States)[122]	ESC/EASD (Europe)[138]	CDA (Canada)[139]	IDF (World)[140–143]
Diabetes care					
Initial evaluation		To include patients in diabetes self-management education (DSME) and support (DSMS).	Patient-centered care is recommended to facilitate shared control and decision making within the context of patient priorities and goals.	Diabetes care should be organized around the patient using the chronic care model, by a multidisciplinary team.	Offer care with sensitivity to cultural wishes and desires, with a collaborative relationship, using a multidisciplinary team.
Management					
Glycemic control	Glucose target must be individualized. Goal in general <6.5%; FPG <110 mg/dL; 2-h PPG <140 mg/dL.	Could be assessed by patient SMBG and A1C.CGM or interstitial glucose in selected patients. Goals A1C <7% most of patients; <6.5% selected patients; <8.5% selected patients with comorbid conditions.	Glycemic targets: Generally <7.0% (<53 mmol/mol). FPG: <7.2 mmol/L (<120 mg/dL). PPG <9–10 mmol/L (<160–180 mg/dL). More stringent targets could be considered in the young for a long life expectancy and nonsignificant CVD.	Glycemic targets should be individualized. Most patients with T1D or T2D should be targeted A1C ≤7.0%. Some patients with T2D with an A1C ≤6.5%. Less stringent A1C targets (7.1%–8.5%) in some conditions.	Targets: A1C <7.0%/ 53 mmol/mol. Fasting/ premeal capillary plasma glucose: 6.5 mmol/L (115 mg/dL). Postmeal capillary Plasma glucose: 9.0 mmol/L (160 mg/dL). Lower or higher A1C levels could be adapted according to the patients.

MNT	Individualized MNT in all patients with diabetes/prediabetes. Teaching by a trained nutritionist or registered dietitian or a physician knowledgeable in nutrition. Goals: to improve health by teaching to eat a diet, adapted to cultural and personal differences.	Individualized MNT, preferably provided by a registered dietitian. Goals: To promote and support healthful eating patterns, adapted to cultural and personal preferences, maintaining the pleasure of eating and providing practical tools.	Is recommended any diet with low energy intake to reduce weight in excess body weight. Fat intake should be <35%, saturated fat <10%, and monounsaturated fatty acids >10% of total energy. Dietary fiber intake should be >40 g/d.	Nutrition therapy should be administered by registered dietitian. Implement nutrition education a small group or one-on-one settings. Encourage to follow "Eating Well with Canada's Food Guide." Macronutrient distribution: 45%–60% carbohydrate, 15%–20% protein and 20%–35% fat.	Provide access to a dietitian or other health care professional trained in the principles of nutrition. Individualize advice on food/meals to match needs, preferences, and culture.
DSME	DSME should be administrated at the time of diagnosis, and subsequently as appropriate. This includes MNT, prescribed exercise, avoid tobacco, and proper sleep.	DSME includes clinical content and skills, behavioral strategies, and engagement with psychosocial concerns, culturally sensitive, these elements are critical to prevent complications.	Multidisciplinary teams and nurse-led programs should be considered to support lifestyle change and self-management.	Offer timely diabetes education to enhance self-care management and education, incorporating cognitive-behavioral educational interventions, in small and/or one-on-one settings.	Provide ongoing self-management support, taking account of culture, ethnicity, psychosocial, and disability issues.

(continued on next page)

Table 5
(continued)

CPG (Region-Country)	AACE/ACE (United States)[137]	ADA (United States)[122]	ESC/EASD (Europe)[138]	CDA (Canada)[139]	IDF (World)[140–143]
Physical activity	Adapting at least 150 min/wk of moderate-intensity exercise, such as brisk walking. Also incorporate flexibility and strength training exercises.	• Children with diabetes or prediabetes at least 60 min of physical activity each day. • Adults with diabetes at least 150 min/wk of moderate-intensity aerobic physical activity. Reduce sedentary time. Two times per week resistance training if there is no contraindication.	Moderate-vigorous physical activity of ≥150 min/wk is recommended for the prevention and control of T2D, and prevention of CVD in diabetes. Aerobic and resistance exercise are best combined.	At least 150 min/wk of moderate-vigorous aerobic exercise 3 d/wk and resistance exercise at least twice a week. Structural exercise programs should be implemented.	Introduce physical activity gradually and individualized. Encourage increased duration and frequency of physical activity, up to 30–45 min on 3–5 d/wk, or 150 min/wk of moderate-intensity aerobic activity. If not contraindicated, resistance training 3 times/week.
Psychosocial Assessment and Care	Screening for depression should be performed routinely due to highly frequent association.	Routinely screen for psychological and social situation. Older adults must be considered for evaluation of cognitive function and depression.	Cognitive behavioral strategies, including problem-solving, goal-setting, self-monitoring, ongoing support and feedback/positive reinforcement.	Regular screening for subclinical psychological distress and psychiatric disorders. Incorporate psychological interventions to diabetes care plans.	Explore the social situation, attitudes, beliefs, and worries related to diabetes and self-care issues. Refer to a mental health care professional if is necessary.

Hypoglycemia	Oral administration of rapidly absorbed glucose should be used to treat hypoglycemia. In severe hypoglycemia to administer carbohydrates or glucagon.	Every visit evaluate symptomatic and asymptomatic hypoglycemia. Glucose treatment for mild hypoglycemia. Glucagon in risk of severe hypoglycemia.	Most be avoided, it has been related to increased risk of CVD events.	Patients with mild to moderate: oral ingestion of 15 g carbohydrate. Severe (conscious): oral ingestion of 20 g carbohydrate. Severe (unconscious) 1 mg glucagon or 10–25 g of IV glucose.	Assessment of hypoglycemia unawareness. Avoid secondary hypoglycemia.
Bariatric surgery	Considered if BMI $\geq$35 kg/m^2 associated with severe obesity-related complications including T2D.	May be considered for adults with BMI $\geq$35 kg/m^2 and T2D, especially in difficult control with lifestyle or drugs therapy.	NA	Considerer bariatric surgery when weight goals are not met in patients with T2D and BMI $\geq$35 kg/m^2.	Eligible patients: T2D and BMI $\geq$35 kg/m^2; or with a BMI 30–35 kg/m^2 and uncontrolled diabetes, especially in high-risk patients.
Immunization	All patients with diabetes should be vaccinated for influenza and pneumococcal infection.	Provide routine vaccinations for children and adults according to age-related recommendations.	NA	Recommend annual influenza immunization and pneumococcal immunization.	NA

(continued on next page)

**Table 5
(continued)**

CPG (Region-Country)	AACE/ACE (United States)[137]	ADA (United States)[122]	ESC/EASD (Europe)[138]	CDA (Canada)[139]	IDF (World)[140-143]
Prevention and management of diabetes complications					
Prevention and management of diabetes complications (CVD, renal, eye, neuropathy, foot).	Recommendations included.	Recommendations included.	Recommendations included.	Recommendations included.	Recommendations included.
Assessment of common comorbid conditions	Recommendations included.	Recommendations included.	Recommendations included.	Recommendations included.	Recommendations included.
Diabetes care in specific populations and settings	Recommendations included.	Recommendations included.	Recommendations included.	Recommendations included.	Recommendations included.
Strategies for improving diabetes	Recommendations included.	Recommendations included.	Recommendations included.	Recommendations included.	Recommendations included.

Abbreviations: A1C, glycated hemoglobin A1c; BMI, body mass index; CGM, continuous glucose monitoring; CPG, clinical practice guideline; CVD, cardiovascular disease; DPP, Diabetes Prevention Program; DSME, diabetes self-management education; DSMS, diabetes self-management support; FPG, fasting plasma glucose; GCT, glucose challenge test; GDM, gestational diabetes mellitus; IGT, impaired glucose tolerance; MNT, medical nutrition therapy; MODY, maturity onset diabetes of the young; NA, not available; OGTT, oral glucose tolerance test; PG, plasma glucose; PPG, post prandial glucose; SMBG, self-monitoring of blood glucose; T1D, type-1 diabetes; T2D, type-2 diabetes; TZDs, thiazolinediones; WHO, World Health Organization.

The implementation of diabetes care on a global scale is more difficult than local T2D prevention strategies due to the sheer increase in variables requiring transculturalization. As a starting point, CPG implementation to improve diabetes care increases the number of patients to have A1C and low-density lipoprotein (LDL)-cholesterol levels in the target range,[71] while also being cost-effective in primary[72] and secondary care[73] settings. CPGs also facilitate adherence with national standards of diabetes care.[74] A recent review of the trends in guideline implementation, including 21 studies on diabetes, reported that most studies (87%) achieved positive impact and education for health care professionals or patients; print materials were the most commonly used strategies for translating guidelines to practice.[8]

Case studies
According to the IDF, the world is divided into 7 regions: Africa, Europe, Middle East and North Africa, North America and Caribbean, South-East Asia, South and Central America, and the Western Pacific.[16] Although the rule is diversity within any given region, many populations living in a given region share biological and ethno-cultural characteristics.[16] Information for diabetes transculturalization from Vietnam,[75] India,[76] Peru,[77] Panama,[78] Egypt,[79] Brazil,[80] Italy,[81] Nigeria,[82] Venezuela,[83] Colombia,[84] the Philippines,[85] and Iran,[86] as well as a core set of recommendations for optimizing diabetes care on a global scale,[87] has been recently reviewed.

Many factors need to be accounted for in the transculturalization process because cultural differences (genetics, phenotypic expression and natural history of disease, nutrition and food preferences, physical activity, health care management, religion, socioeconomic status, politics, availability of preventive and care resources, and patient adherence, among others) exist globally both among countries and within a country. It has been demonstrated that acculturation, the change of individual or group behavior due to contact with another culture, can affect some cardiometabolic risk factors.[41] Analysis of longitudinal[88,89] and case control[90] studies in immigrant populations have confirmed that acculturation increases the incidence of overweight/obesity probably due to racial/ethnic disparities in feeding behavior, and physical activity[91] and/or the time living in the country,[92] among other factors. Cultural disparities in dietary preferences due to availability, customs, or religion, and the adoption of dietary patterns (eg, Mediterranean and Korean, Western high saturated fat, Asian-Indian high *trans*fat dietary patterns, among others) also should also be considered to establish nutrition recommendations.

Examples of CPG transculturalizations in different regions of the world are presented in **Table 6**. Most of these transculturalizations acknowledge the difficulties associated with implementation and the potential benefits of overcoming barriers.[93–95] Common barriers in these examples include fragmentation of the health care system,[96] need to adapt to chronic disease management,[97,98] and education.[99] Strategies to overcome barriers include the development of local recommendations[100–102] and translation to selected centers, physicians, and patients. For instance, educational intervention programs were launched through seminars, audits, structured records, and pocket guides.[99,103,104] Most of the strategies improved diabetes care[103,105] and optimized metabolic parameters by increasing knowledge[95,96] and by promoting participation, integration,[102,106] and self-management.[95,98] In other cases, failure to recognize local needs and effectively address barriers compromised implementation.[15,93,100,101]

In a recent example, AACE/ACE standardized a methodology to guide local development of CPAs in endocrinology in Latin America, specifically for glycemic control in diabetes, weight loss in obesity, thyroid nodule evaluation, and postmenopausal

Table 6
Transculturalization case studies by IDF regions

Region/Country (Reference)	Background	Strategy	Adaptation	Outcomes/Results	Success
Africa (AFR)					
South Africa[93]	Demonstrated local deficiency in diabetes care.	Introducing a structured clinical record that includes the national CPG strategies and recommendations.	Design a structured record and training of health care providers in its use.	No impact on diabetes or hypertension control, due to the record was not used as expected.	- -
Europe (EUR)					
Germany[96]	Educational meetings slightly improved professional practice and patients outcomes.	Implementation of interactive, team-based continuing professional development concept.	Launched it in a series of seminars on endocrinology and diabetes care, on case-based related to medical practice.	Increased short-term knowledge and referral diabetes specialist. Other professional behavior did not change.	+ -
Germany[106]	Need for integration care across primary and secondary care sectors.	CPG developed and sent to GPs and SPs, to integrate diabetes management.	Incentive-based system to participating GPs in collecting information. Continuous quality management of GPs by SPs. Education programs to patients	Decrease of median A1C. More patients achieved targets.	+ +
Italy[95]	Management of a chronic disease requires more active participation from patients about control of their illness.	Implement a work patient–provider "partnership" that involves effective treatment within an integrated system of collaborative care that includes self-management education and follow-up.	To integrate, physicians from primary and secondary care, and patients through care managers. Patients received: (1) initial and follow-up assessments, (2) an individualized care plan, (3) educational materials, (4) assistance with service coordination, (5) regular health coaching sessions.	Feasible application. Increasing of the patient's knowledge, self-management skills, and readiness to make health changes.	+ +

Italy[144]	Patients managed by SP and primary care are more adherent to CPGs than only attended by GP.	Implement a surveillance population-based program monitoring diabetes.	Collected data to compare quality of care levels based on CPG adherence.	Patients with lower quality of care had increased risk of diabetes-related complications. + +
Netherlands[74]	Evaluated the role of a facilitator to implement local CPGs.	Nurses were trained as facilitators. They analyzed structured care, trained staff, introduced barriers, gave performance feedback, and encouraged to treat patients according to local CPGs.	Implementation of local CPGs based on national guidelines for the treatment T2D of the Dutch College of General Practitioners.	Improvement on diabetes care. No improved on A1C, blood pressure or cholesterol levels. + -
Spain[94]	Lack attachment for CGPs for inpatients,	Medical evidence-based educational intervention program for inpatient management.	On weekdays, 20-min seminar about ADA statements, addressed to physicians and nurses. Pocket guides and posters were distributed.	Increased attachment to CPG recommendations. Reduction in median glycemia at discharge. + +
United Kingdom[145]	Cost of diabetes care is increasing, management in primary care level is cost-effective.	Integrated primary and secondary care levels. Diabetes specialist nurse support to primary care professionals.	Implement referral guidelines to secondary care.	Decrease in referrals from GPs to SPs. + +
Middle East and North Africa (MENA)				
Kuwait[105]	In Kuwait, diabetes has rapidly emerged as a public health problem.	Implementation of the Kuwait Diabetes Care Program (KDCP) in the primary health care setting.	Develop, publish, and disseminate local CPGs, conduct training courses, standards for diabetes care, and introduce a monitoring and evaluation system.	Improvement the process of diabetes care + +
United Arab Emirates[103]	Clinical audit has not been completely evaluated.	Clinical audit evaluated quality of care and identified gaps between practice and goals.	Implementation of local CPGs based on data collection, establishment of adapted goals, and evaluated patient satisfaction.	Improvement of diabetes care and metabolic control. + +

(continued on next page)

Table 6
(continued)

Region/Country (Reference)	Background	Strategy	Adaptation	Outcomes/Results	Success
North America and Caribbean (NAC)					
Canada[100]	In the long-care setting there is no standardized diabetes care.	Implementation of a flow sheet after educational intervention.	1-h diabetes education seminar. Design and implementation of flow sheet.	Flow sheet was not found useful for attending physicians.	- -
Canada[146]	Limited evidence nursing guideline implementation.	Nursing best practice guidelines implementation.	Structured educational sessions. Toolkit describing strategies for implementation.	Improved practice and patient outcomes.	+ -
Mexico[147]	Rapid increase of prevalence and diabetes-related mortality, and poor control.	Structured patient diabetes education program, training in foot care and in-service training for primary care personnel.	3 learning sessions using the breakthrough series methodology. Selected patients for learning sessions.	Increased glycemic control and higher proportion of patients achieving goals.	+ +
United States[148]	High clinical inertia leading to failure in intensifying treatment.	Electronic medical record (EMR) implementation.	EMR provides basic information for clinic support to trained primary care physicians.	Increased number of A1C and LDL tests, but not to better metabolic control.	+ -
United States[99]	African Americans in the United States are more likely to develop diabetes-related complications than whites.	Diabetes self- management education (DSME) program.	12-week church-based DSME intervention. Incentives for participants.	Improvement in medication adherence, healthy eating, and foot care.	+ +
United States[149]	There is lack evidence about the incorporation of clinical pharmacist management to diabetes care.	Clinical pharmacists are credentialed providers with rights to prescribe medication, order laboratory tests, place consults to other services, and order immunizations.	Patients are referred to the pharmacist-run clinic by their primary care provider for diabetes education and medication management.	Positive improvement in diabetes control in patients treated by pharmacists.	+ +

South and Central America (SACA)

Brazil[15]	Test the ADA/EASD algorithm in real-life setting.	Delivery orientation and a folder of diet plan and exercise recommendations. Achieve capillary glucose goal according to algorithm sequence.	Medications were administrated free of charge by the public health care system: 1st metformin: 2nd glibenclamide; 3rd NPH insulin.	Increased number of drugs administrated. No improvement on A1C levels.	− −
Ten Latin American Countries[104]	Lack of participation of the patients in the management of the disease.	Implement an educational program in 10 Latin American countries.	Training local educators in an intensive 10-person 2-day session. Application of structured education model to selected patients and family. Main goal to improve health behavior.	Improvement of metabolic control and risk factors related to diabetes.	+ +

South-East Asia (SEA)

India[101]	Need to improve health care system focused on chronic diseases.	Health services intervention with facilitators.	Interventions were applied on delivery of cultural diabetes education to patients, prescription of generic medication, and use of CPGs.	No improvement on diabetes care or patient outcomes.	− −
Philippines[98]	Many developing countries have not adapted the chronic care model system of health.	Integration of chronic care model in primary care activities.	Taking account of the capabilities of the local health system and making use of preexisting health care personnel.	Personal improved knowledge and self-assessed skills. Metabolic controls of patients were optimized.	+ +
Philippines[97]	Need for diabetes self-management education and training for chronic disease.	Incorporate a chronic disease care model-based.	Training the preexisting local government health care personnel.	Patients included improved metabolic control and risk factors related to diabetes.	+ +

(continued on next page)

Table 6
(continued)

Region/Country (Reference)	Background	Strategy	Adaptation	Outcomes/Results	Success
Western Pacific (WP)					
Australia[102]	Indigenous Australians have high diabetes-related complications, and a complex care system.	Intervention of assessment, feedback workshops, action planning, and implementation of system changes in 12 indigenous community health centers.	Adapted version of the Assessment of Chronic Illness Care (ACIC) scale and applied to selected health care centers. Adherence to guideline-scheduled services and medication adjustment.	Significant improvement in health care system, processes of care and intermediate outcomes.	+ +

IDF region abbreviations are provided in parentheses.

Abbreviations: − −, objective not reached; + −, objective partly reached; + +, objective reached; ADA, American Diabetes Association; CPG, clinical practice guideline; DSME, diabetes self-management education; EASD, European Association for the Study of Diabetes; EMR, electronic medical record; GP, general physicians; LDL, low-density lipoprotein; SP, specialist physicians; T2D, type-2 diabetes.

osteoporosis.[43] This transculturalization process incorporated the processes outlined in **Fig. 1**, and consisted of (1) published AACE CPGs and CPAs on the topics, (2) a modified Delphi method to identify areas with and without consensus,[107] (3) a face-to-face half-day workshop in Costa Rica to focus on areas of disagreement, and (4) production of a final written document.[43] Other examples in Latin America are in progress, such as an adaptation of the Mediterranean pyramid for Venezuela using local foods and preparations.[108]

The transcultural diabetes nutrition algorithm initiative

In 2010, an international core committee of diabetes specialists and endocrinologists developed an evidence-based algorithmic template of diabetes care, primarily based on US CPGs from the AACE/ACE and ADA, with a focus on nutritional management and with the intent to transculturalize for any setting on a global scale.[109] This activity was triggered by (1) a recognition that CPGs/CPAs at that time were not portable to other cultures owing to poor implementation strategies, and (2) a provision for cascades of recommendations in AACE/ACE G4G. The logical flow for this CPA template consisted of screening, risk stratification, intervention, and follow-up, and included a comprehensive array of nutritional and other lifestyle factors. The process of developing a transcultural Diabetes Nutrition Algorithm (tDNA) proceeded through 4 stages and is currently in the last stage:

1. Development of the evidence-based algorithm template with a focus on having each node strategically amenable to cultural adaptation.
2. Organization of local conferences with local and international thought leaders, participation of core committee members, and followed by smaller working sessions of local thought leaders to transculturalize, node-by-node, the algorithm template; this was conducted in North, Central, and South America, Europe, the Persian Gulf, India, and southeast Asia.
3. Production of an in-office toolkit, in a variety of formats, for implementation; content validation of the toolkit.
4. Clinical validation of the toolkit with relevant implementation and outcome metrics in diverse countries.[100]

A comparison of the transcultural adaptations of the tDNA in 7 countries (South-East Asia,[110] Asian-India,[111] Malaysia,[112] Canada,[113] Venezuela,[108] Mexico,[114] and Brazil[115]) is presented in **Table 7**. The tDNA toolkit content was validated using a questionnaire provided to 837 health care providers from the United States, Mexico, and Taiwan.[116] Overall, 61% of respondents thought that the toolkit could help medical nutrition therapy implementation, 91% indicated positive impressions, 83% believed they would use the toolkit, and 80% thought the toolkit would be fairly easy to implement.[116]

The tDNA project has revealed many emergent and interesting findings. For instance, the unique phenotype of T2D in India is characterized by increased insulin resistance and postprandial hyperglycemia, sarcopenic obesity with decreased muscle mass, and increased WC (Waist circumference) even at normal body mass index (BMI) (transculturalized normal range: 18.5–22.9 kg/m^2), and inflammation, contextualized with a high-carbohydrate, low glycemic index, low protein eating pattern, sedentary lifestyle, high stress, poverty, spirituality, and frequent festivals.[111] This Asian-Indian exemplar requires specific lifestyle management pathways that are patently different from those for the general American population with T2D (eg, inability to overly restrict rice, less costly interventions, examples of healthy menus, an emphasis on strength training, and a priority of stress reduction). Other examples comprise the effects of economic,

Table 7
Main transcultural nutrition algorithm (tDNA) adaptations in several countries

Region/ Country (Reference)	Epidemiology	Nutrition	Physical Activity	Anthropometric Cut Points	Risk Identification	Bariatric Surgery
Brazil[115]	Rapid increasing rate prevalence reaching 11.7%, with only 1 of every 5 diabetic patients controlled (A1C <7%).	Healthy and high-quality diet: complex CHOs and rich in fiber, with a very low amount of sugar, low in unsaturated and transfats, rich in monounsaturated and polyunsaturated fats, and with an adequate amount of protein from good sources.	Moderate and intense aerobic exercise, resistance, and stretching, are recommended several days a week, individualized.	Cutoff for obesity: BMI: overweight 25–29.9 kg/m² and obesity ≥30 kg/ m²; WC: men ≥102 cm and women ≥88 cm.	To evaluated diabetes risk FPG and A1C testing for prediabetes or T2D should always be performed.	NA
Canada[113]	Diabetes affecting more than 3 million people and another 6 million had elevated risk. Non-Caucasian populations comprise more than 25% of Canadian population.	To replace high glycemic index carbohydrate foods by low glycemic index carbohydrate foods in mixed meals, based on their effect on postprandial blood glucose.	People with diabetes should be encouraged to perform 150 min/ wk of moderate-to-vigorous aerobic exercise and resistance exercise 3 times a week.	Same than reported for US Cutoff for obesity: BMI: overweight 25–29.9 kg/m² and obesity ≥30 kg/ m²; WC: men ≥102 cm and women ≥88 cm.	Ethno-cultural and geographic classification must be obtained.	May be considered for adults with clinically severe obesity (BMI ≥40 kg/ m² or ≥35 kg/m² with severe comorbid disease).

Country	Epidemiology	Diet	Physical Activity	Obesity Cutoffs	Notes
India[111]	Rapidly increasing diabetes prevalence. Currently has the second largest number of people with T2D (69.2 million).	Rapid nutritional transition. Excess consumption of calories, saturated fats, trans fatty acids, simple sugars, and salt, with low intake of fiber, monounsaturated fatty acids, and n-3 polyunsaturated fatty acids.	Asian Indians tend to be more sedentary than whites. Sixty minutes of physical activity per day has been recommended for healthy Asian Indians.	High proportion of low birth weight. Smaller muscle mass and centrally obese. Cutoff for obesity: BMI: overweight >23–24.9 kg/m^2 and obesity ≥25 kg/m^2; WC: men ≥90 cm and women ≥80 cm.	WC or WHR tend to be a better indicator of the risk of developing diabetes than BMI.	NA
Malaysia[112]	Prevalence of T2D of Malaysian adults (≥30 y) increased from 14.9% in 2006 to 20.8% in 2011. Diverse ethnic groups represent different T2D prevalence.	Calories: overweight/obese a reduced calorie diet of 20–25 kcal/kg body weight. Recommendation daily energy intake: CHO 45%–60%; protein 15%–20%; fat 25%–35%; saturated fat <7% of total calories; cholesterol <200 mg/d; fiber 20–30 g/d; sodium <2400 mg/d.	Exercise 5 d a week with no more than 2 consecutive days without physical exercise of moderate-intensity activities, 150 min/wk and/or at least 90 min/wk of vigorous aerobic physical activity.	Cutoff for obesity: BMI: overweight >23–27.4 kg/m^2 and obesity ≥27.5 kg/m^2; WC: men ≥90 cm and women ≥80 cm.	T2D appears at a lower BMI, at younger age, and with lower WC than whites.	NA
Mexico[114]	More than 10 million adults had diabetes and 16 million had prediabetes.	Hypocaloric (weight loss) diet: 250–1000 kcal/d deficit. Daily intake: CHO (preferably low-glycemic index): 45% to 65%; protein: 15% to 20%, dietary fat: <30%, saturated fat: <7%, cholesterol: <200 mg/d, fiber: 25–50 g/d, transfats: minimize or eliminate.	Moderate aerobic activity for ≥150 min/wk or vigorous aerobic activity for ≥75 min/wk.	Cutoff for obesity: BMI: overweight 25–29.9 kg/m^2 and obesity ≥30 kg/m^2; WC: men ≥90 cm and women ≥80 cm.	Ethno-cultural and geographic classification must be obtained. Individual risk stratification.	Suggested if BMI >35 kg/m^2 and any other comorbid conditions, including T2D.

(continued on next page)

Table 7
(continued)

Region/Country (Reference)	Epidemiology	Nutrition	Physical Activity	Anthropometric Cut Points	Risk Identification	Bariatric Surgery
Southeast Asia[110]	60% of the global population of people with T2D resides in Asia.	Provide information about foods with higher glycemic indices or glycemic loads. Medical nutrition therapy should be started, led by registered dietitians.	Asian professionals recommend 150 min/wk of moderate-intensity exercise for patients with diabetes.	Cutoff for obesity: BMI: overweight >23–24.9 kg/m² and obesity ≥25 kg/m²; WC: men ≥90 cm and women ≥80 cm.	Asians populations tend to develop T2D at a younger age, and with lower BMI and WC than western populations.	In patients with T2D with BMI ≥27.5 kg/m² could be appropriate.
United States[109]	Avoid the problem of generalizability and implemented recommendation adapted to geographic and ethno-cultural factors. Optimization of nutritional care for patients with T2D and prediabetes on a global scale.	Cultural factors should guide the selection of local foods and meals. Hypocaloric diet: 250–1000 kcal/d deficit; decrease weight by 5%–10% for overweight/obese, 15% for class 3 obesity. Daily energy intake: CHO (preferably low-glycemic index): 45%–65% and not <130 g/d in patients on a low-calorie diet. Protein: 15%–20%. Fat: <30%. Saturated fat: <7%. Cholesterol: <200 mg/d. Fiber: 25–50 g/d. Transfats: minimize or eliminate.	Encourage to achieve an active lifestyle of ≥150 min/wk of moderate-intensity activity, or ≥75 min/wk of vigorous-intensity aerobic activity, or some combination of equivalent moderate/vigorous activity.	Include weight, BMI, WC, and/or WHR, according to local preference/custom. For US: Cutoff for obesity: BMI: overweight 25–29.9 kg/m² and obesity ≥30 kg/m²; WC: men ≥102 cm and women ≥88 cm.	Location, ethnicity, and culture individualized recommendations.	BMI ≥40 kg/m² or BMI 35–39.9 kg/m² and an obesity-related comorbidity, such as T2D. BMI 30–34.9 kg/m² under special circumstances.

Venezuela[108]	Diabetes affecting ~1.7 million people. Prevalence diabetes 7,7% and prediabetes 11,2% and 76% is uncontrolled (A1C ≥7%)	• Nutrient composition with minor variations regarding other CPGs. • Promote components of the Mediterranean food pyramid by using local foods: Avocado and olive oil; legumes (beans as "caraotas"), whole grain (oats, corn as "cachapa"), abundant fruits served as "Tizana" (mixed), and vegetables, soups of vegetables and chicken ("sancocho") instead barbecues at weekends, fish (tuna, saltines) and poultry (chicken), avoid sugars and sweets, reduce complex CHOs, such as starch ("arepas," rice, potatoes, pasta, and so forth), prefer low glycemic index CHOs.	It is prescribed: • Type: aerobic, resistance, stretching, balance and general physical activity, are recommended several days a week. • Intensity: Low, medium, high individualized. • Prefer more common local activities (dancing, local sports).	Cutoff for obesity: BMI: overweight 25–27.4 kg/m² and obesity ≥27.5 kg/m²; WC: men ≥94 cm and women ≥90 cm.	Applied routinely screening of diabetes with the Latin America Modified FINDRISC score.	BMI 35–39.9 kg/m² and an obesity-related comorbidity, such as T2D. BMI 30–34.9 kg/m² under special circumstances.

Abbreviations: BMI, body mass index; CHO, carbohydrates; CPG, clinical practice guideline; FPG, fasting plasma glucose; NA, not available; T2D, type 2 diabetes; WC, waist circumference; WHR, waist-hip ratio.

demographic, and nutritional transitions, prevalent in Latin America, the Persian Gulf, and Asia, that require tailored approaches.

The ultimate goal of the tDNA project is that in every country of the world primary care providers and specialists have a validated portable tool, in electronic or printed format, that is culturally adapted and inclusive of the best scientific evidence available in each country or region.

FUTURE DIRECTIONS

T2D is a multifactorial disease with a heavy global burden and cultural descriptors. Optimizing a T2D care plan to improve outcomes requires the application of evidence-based tools, but implementation of these tools on a global scale is hampered by these cultural factors. The transculturalization process can help overcome implementation barriers.

Future advancements in transculturalization will be based on new information from clinical trials performed in local settings with application of culturally adapted decision-making tools. The time is ripe now for the recognition that diabetes care is overtly affected by nonbiological drivers that require new skill sets and understandings to grasp and manage different patient scenarios. A comprehensive approach is recommended, consisting of research focused on sound validation studies, education about nontraditional fields, such as social and behavioral sciences, and translation into clinical practice incorporating emergent information and tools. This approach can impel transcultural activities to a more integral role in global medicine. This is the future of diabetes, where neither innovative technologies nor original care models are sufficient; rather, each is a necessary component for success.

REFERENCES

1. Guariguata L, Whiting DR, Hambleton I, et al. Global estimates of diabetes prevalence for 2013 and projections for 2035. Diabetes Res Clin Pract 2014;103(2): 137–49.
2. Zimmet PZ, Magliano DJ, Herman WH, et al. Diabetes: a 21st century challenge. Lancet Diabetes Endocrinol 2014;2(1):56–64.
3. Shekelle P, Woolf S, Grimshaw JM, et al. Developing clinical practice guidelines: reviewing, reporting, and publishing guidelines; updating guidelines; and the emerging issues of enhancing guideline implementability and accounting for comorbid conditions in guideline development. Implement Sci 2012;7:62.
4. Mechanick JI, Bergman DA, Braithwaite SS, et al. American Association of Clinical Endocrinologists protocol for standardized production of clinical practice guidelines. Endocr Pract 2004;10(4):353–61.
5. Mechanick JI, Camacho PM, Cobin RH, et al. American Association of Clinical Endocrinologists Protocol for standardized production of clinical practice guidelines–2010 update. Endocr Pract 2010;16(2):270–83.
6. Mechanick JI, Camacho PM, Garber AJ, et al. American Association of Clinical Endocrinologists and American College of Endocrinology Protocol for standardized production of clinical practice guidelines, algorithms, and checklists—2014 update and the AACe G4G Program. Endocr Pract 2014;20(7):692–702.
7. U.S. Department of Health & Human Services. HHS action plan to reduce racial and ethnic health disparities. Washington, DC. Available at: http://www.hhs.gov/ocr/civilrights/resources/specialtopics/health_disparities/.
8. Gagliardi AR, Alhabib S. Trends in guideline implementation: a scoping systematic review. Implement Sci 2015;10:54.

9. Grilli R, Magrini N, Penna A, et al. Practice guidelines developed by specialty societies: the need for a critical appraisal. Lancet 2000;355(9198):103–6.

10. Jenssen TG, Tonstad S, Claudi T, et al. The gap between guidelines and practice in the treatment of type 2 diabetes. A nationwide survey in Norway. Diabetes Res Clin Pract 2008;80(2):314–20.

11. Chan JCN, Gagliardino JJ, Baik SH, et al. Multi-faceted determinants for achieving glycemic control: The International Diabetes Management Practice Study (IDMPS). Diabetes Care 2009;32(2):227–33.

12. Rabin B, Brownson R. Developing the terminology for dissemination and implementation research. In: Brownson R, Colditz G, Proctor E, editors. Dissemination and implementation research in health: translating science to practice. New York: Oxford University Press; 2012. p. 23–51.

13. Home P, Haddad J, Latif ZA, et al. Comparison of National/Regional Diabetes Guidelines for the management of blood glucose control in non-western countries. Diabetes Ther 2013;4(1):91–102.

14. Vaccaro O, Boemi M, Cavalot F, et al. The clinical reality of guidelines for primary prevention of cardiovascular disease in type 2 diabetes in Italy. Atherosclerosis 2008;198(2):396–402.

15. Viana LV, Leitao CB, Grillo Mde F, et al. Are diabetes management guidelines applicable in 'real life'? Diabetol Metab Syndr 2012;4(1):47.

16. International Diabetes Federation. IDF diabetes atlas. 7th edition. Brussels (Belgium): International Diabetes Federation; 2015.

17. National Diabetes Statistics Report. Centers for Disease Control and Prevention (CDC). Diagnosed and undiagnosed diabetes in the United States 2014. Available at: http://www.cdc.gov/diabetes/data/statistics/2014StatisticsReport.html. Accessed July 29, 2016.

18. Murray CJ, Barber RM, Foreman KJ, et al. Global, regional, and national disability-adjusted life years (DALYs) for 306 diseases and injuries and healthy life expectancy (HALE) for 188 countries, 1990-2013: quantifying the epidemiological transition. Lancet 2015;386(10009):2145–91.

19. GBD. Global, regional, and national age-sex specific all-cause and cause-specific mortality for 240 causes of death, 1990-2013: a systematic analysis for the Global Burden of Disease Study 2013. Lancet 2015;385(9963):117–71.

20. Shaw JE, Sicree RA, Zimmet PZ. Global estimates of the prevalence of diabetes for 2010 and 2030. Diabetes Res Clin Pract 2010;87(1):4–14.

21. Seuring T, Archangelidi O, Suhrcke M. The economic costs of type 2 diabetes: a global systematic review. Pharmacoeconomics 2015;33(8):811–31.

22. Chen L, Magliano DJ, Zimmet PZ. The worldwide epidemiology of type 2 diabetes mellitus–present and future perspectives. Nat Rev Endocrinol 2012;8(4): 228–36.

23. Chan JC, Malik V, Jia W, et al. Diabetes in Asia: epidemiology, risk factors, and pathophysiology. JAMA 2009;301(20):2129–40.

24. Hu FB. Globalization of diabetes: the role of diet, lifestyle, and genes. Diabetes Care 2011;34(6):1249–57.

25. Afshin A, Micha R, Khatibzadeh S, et al. The impact of dietary habits and metabolic risk factors on cardiovascular and diabetes mortality in countries of the Middle East and North Africa in 2010: a comparative risk assessment analysis. BMJ Open 2015;5(5):e006385.

26. WHO. Global status report on noncommunicable diseases 2014. World Health Organization. Geneva (Switzerland): WHO Library Cataloguing-in-Publication Data; 2014. www.who.int/about/licensing/copyright_form/en/index.html.

27. Phipps EJ, Braitman LE, Stites SD, et al. The use of financial incentives to increase fresh fruit and vegetable purchases in lower-income households: results of a pilot study. J Health Care Poor Underserved 2013;24(2):864–74.

28. Sharma A, Hauck K, Hollingsworth B, et al. The effects of taxing sugar-sweetened beverages across different income groups. Health Econ 2014; 23(9):1159–84.

29. Snowdon W, Thow AM. Trade policy and obesity prevention: challenges and innovation in the Pacific Islands. Obes Rev 2013;14(Suppl 2):150–8.

30. Capacci S, Mazzocchi M, Shankar B, et al. Policies to promote healthy eating in Europe: a structured review of policies and their effectiveness. Nutr Rev 2012; 70(3):188–200.

31. Beran D. The impact of health systems on diabetes care in low and lower middle income countries. Curr Diab Rep 2015;15(4):20.

32. Gupta LS, Wu CC, Young S, et al. Prevalence of diabetes in New York City, 2002-2008: comparing foreign-born South Asians and other Asians with U.S.-born whites, blacks, and Hispanics. Diabetes Care 2011;34(8):1791–3.

33. Chow EA, Foster H, Gonzalez V, et al. The disparate impact of diabetes on racial/ethnic minority populations. Clin Diabetes 2012;30(3):130–3.

34. Sohal T, Sohal P, King-Shier KM, et al. Barriers and facilitators for type-2 diabetes management in South Asians: a systematic review. PLoS One 2015; 10(9):e0136202.

35. Field MJ, Lohr KN. Committee to Advise the Public Health Service on Clinical Practice Guidelines IoM: Clinical practice guidelines: directions for a new program. Washington, DC: National Academy Press; 1990.

36. Gagliardi AR, Brouwers MC. Integrating guideline development and implementation: analysis of guideline development manual instructions for generating implementation advice. Implement Sci 2012;7:67.

37. Gagliardi AR, Brouwers MC, Bhattacharyya OK. A framework of the desirable features of guideline implementation tools (GItools): Delphi survey and assessment of GItools. Implement Sci 2014;9:98.

38. Krause J, Van Lieshout J, Klomp R, et al. Identifying determinants of care for tailoring implementation in chronic diseases: an evaluation of different methods. Implement Sci 2014;9:102.

39. Ellen ME, Leon G, Bouchard G, et al. Barriers, facilitators and views about next steps to implementing supports for evidence-informed decision-making in health systems: a qualitative study. Implement Sci 2014;9:179.

40. Kajermo KN, Bostrom AM, Thompson DS, et al. The BARRIERS scale—the barriers to research utilization scale: a systematic review. Implement Sci 2010; 5(32):1748–5908.

41. Hegazi RA, Devitt AA, Mechanick JI. The transcultural diabetes nutrition algorithm: from concept to implementation. In: Watson RR, Dokken BB, editors. Glucose intake and utilization in pre-diabetes and diabetes implications for cardiovascular disease. Amsterdam: Elsevier Inc.; 2015. p. 269–80.

42. Tabak RG, Sinclair KA, Baumann AA, et al. A review of diabetes prevention program translations: use of cultural adaptation and implementation research. Transl Behav Med 2015;5(4):401–14.

43. Mechanick JI, Harrel RM, Aschner P, et al. Transculturalization recommendations for developing Latin American Clinical Practice Algorithms in Endocrinology—proceedings of the 2015 Pan-American Workshop by the American Association of Clinical Endocrinologists and American College of Endocrinology. Endocr Pract 2016;22(4):476–501.

44. Eccles MP, Foy R, Sales A, et al. Implementation science six years on—our evolving scope and common reasons for rejection without review. Implement Sci 2012;7:71.

45. Knowler WC, Barrett-Connor E, Fowler SE, et al. Reduction in the incidence of type 2 diabetes with lifestyle intervention or metformin. N Engl J Med 2002; 346(6):393–403.

46. Tuomilehto J, Lindstrom J, Eriksson JG, et al. Prevention of type 2 diabetes mellitus by changes in lifestyle among subjects with impaired glucose tolerance. N Engl J Med 2001;344(18):1343–50.

47. Pan XR, Li GW, Hu YH, et al. Effects of diet and exercise in preventing NIDDM in people with impaired glucose tolerance. The Da Qing IGT and Diabetes Study. Diabetes Care 1997;20:537–44.

48. Ramachandran A, Snehalatha C, Mary S, et al. The Indian Diabetes Prevention Programme shows that lifestyle modification and metformin prevent type 2 diabetes in Asian Indian subjects with impaired glucose tolerance (IDPP-1). Diabetologia 2006;49:289–97.

49. Li G, Zhang P, Wang J, et al. The long-term effect of lifestyle interventions to prevent diabetes in the China Da Quing Diabetes Prevention Study: a 20-year follow-up study. Lancet 2008;371:1783–9.

50. Knowler WC, Fowler SE, Hamman RF, et al. 10-year follow-up of diabetes incidence and weight loss in the Diabetes Prevention Program Outcomes Study. Lancet 2009;374(9702):1677–86.

51. Lindstrom J, Ilanne-Parikka P, Peltonen M, et al. Sustained reduction in the incidence of type 2 diabetes by lifestyle intervention: follow-up of the Finnish Diabetes Prevention Study. Lancet 2006;368(9548):1673–9.

52. Cardona-Morrell M, Rychetnik L, Morrell SL, et al. Reduction of diabetes risk in routine clinical practice: are physical activity and nutrition interventions feasible and are the outcomes from reference trials replicable? A systematic review and meta-analysis. BMC Public Health 2010;10:653.

53. Uusitupa M, Tuomilehto J, Puska P. Are we really active in the prevention of obesity and type 2 diabetes at the community level? Nutr Metab Cardiovasc Dis 2011;21(5):380–9.

54. Saaristo T, Moilanen L, Korpi-Hyovalti E, et al. Lifestyle intervention for prevention of type 2 diabetes in primary health care: one-year follow-up of the Finnish National Diabetes Prevention Program (FIN-D2D). Diabetes Care 2010;33(10): 2146–51.

55. Oldenburg B, Absetz P, Dunbar JA, et al. The spread and uptake of diabetes prevention programs around the world: a case study from Finland and Australia. Transl Behav Med 2011;1(2):270–82.

56. Reddy P, Rankins D, Timoshanko A, et al. Life! in Australia: translating prevention research into a large-scale intervention. Br J Diabetes Vasc Dis 2011;11(1): 193–7.

57. Schwarz PE, Lindstrom J, Kissimova-Scarbeck K, et al. The European perspective of type 2 diabetes prevention: diabetes in Europe—prevention using lifestyle, physical activity and nutritional intervention (DE-PLAN) project. Exp Clin Endocrinol Diabetes 2008;116(3):167–72.

58. Gilis-Januszewska A, Szybinski Z, Kissimova-Skarbek K, et al. Prevention of type 2 diabetes by lifestyle intervention in primary health care setting in Poland: Diabetes in Europe Prevention Using Lifestyle, Physical Activity and Nutritional Intervention (DE-PLAN) project. Br J Diabetes Vasc Dis 2011;11:198–203.

59. Makrilakis K, Liatis S, Grammatikou S, et al. Implementation and effectiveness of the first community lifestyle intervention programme to prevent type 2 diabetes in Greece. The DE-PLAN study. Diabet Med 2010;27(4):459–65.

60. The Diabetes Prevention Program. Design and methods for a clinical trial in the prevention of type 2 diabetes. Diabetes Care 1999;22(4):623–34.

61. Herman WH, Hoerger TJ, Brandle M, et al. The cost-effectiveness of lifestyle modification or metformin in preventing type 2 diabetes in adults with impaired glucose tolerance. Ann Intern Med 2005;142(5):323–32.

62. Whittemore R. A systematic review of the translational research on the Diabetes Prevention Program. Transl Behav Med 2011;1(3):480–91.

63. Ali MK, Echouffo-Tcheugui J, Williamson DF. How effective were lifestyle interventions in real-world settings that were modeled on the Diabetes Prevention Program? Health Aff (Millwood) 2012;31(1):67–75.

64. Dunkley AJ, Bodicoat DH, Greaves CJ, et al. Diabetes prevention in the real world: effectiveness of pragmatic lifestyle interventions for the prevention of type 2 diabetes and of the impact of adherence to guideline recommendations: a systematic review and meta-analysis. Diabetes Care 2014;37(4):922–33.

65. Aziz Z, Absetz P, Oldroyd J, et al. A systematic review of real-world diabetes prevention programs: learnings from the last 15 years. Implement Sci 2015;10(1):172.

66. Florez H, Stepenka V, Castillo-Florez S, et al. Lifestyle intervention improves global cardiovascular health in Latinos with prediabetes in Maracaibo, Venezuela. Circulation 2012;125:AP162.

67. Ackermann RT, Marrero DG. Adapting the Diabetes Prevention Program lifestyle intervention for delivery in the community: the YMCA model. Diabetes Educ 2007;33(1):69, 74–5, 77-8.

68. CDC. Diabetes: successes and opportunities for population-based prevention and control: at a glance 2011. Atlanta (GA): US Department of Health and Human Services; 2011.

69. Wollersheim H, Burgers J, Grol R. Clinical guidelines to improve patient care. Neth J Med 2005;63(6):188–92.

70. Sloan FA, Bethel MA, Lee PP, et al. Adherence to guidelines and its effects on hospitalizations with complications of type 2 diabetes. Rev Diabet Stud 2004;1(1):29–38.

71. McCraw WM, Kelley PW, Righero AM, et al. Improving compliance with diabetes clinical practice guidelines in military medical treatment facilities. Nurs Res 2010;59(1 Suppl):S66–74.

72. Szmurlo D, Schubert A, Kostrzewska K, et al. Economic analysis of the implementation of guidelines for type 2 diabetes control developed by Diabetes Poland: what increase in costs is justified by clinical results? Pol Arch Med Wewn 2011;121(10):345–50.

73. Dijkstra RF, Niessen LW, Braspenning JC, et al. Patient-centred and professional-directed implementation strategies for diabetes guidelines: a cluster-randomized trial-based cost-effectiveness analysis. Diabet Med 2006;23(2):164–70.

74. van Bruggen R, Gorter KJ, Stolk RP, et al. Implementation of locally adapted guidelines on type 2 diabetes. Fam Pract 2008;25(6):430–7.

75. Khue NT. Diabetes in Vietnam. Ann Glob Health 2015;81(6):870–3. Available at: www.annalsofglobalhealth.org.

76. Joshi SR. Diabetes care in India. Ann Glob Health 2015;81(6):830–8. Available at: www.annalsofglobalhealth.org.
77. Villena JE. Diabetes mellitus in Peru. Ann Glob Health 2015;81(6):765–75. Available at: www.annalsofglobalhealth.org.
78. Mc Donald Posso AJ, Bradshaw Meza RA, Mendoza Morales EA, et al. Diabetes in Panama: epidemiology, risk factors and clinical management. Ann Glob Health 2015;81(6):754–64. Available at: www.annalsofglobalhealth.org.
79. Hegazi R, El-Gamal M, Abdel-Hady N, et al. Epidemiology and risk factors of type 2 diabetes in Egypt. Ann Glob Health 2015;81(6):814–20. Available at: www.annalsofglobalhealth.org.
80. Coutinho WF, Silva Júnior WS. Diabetes care in Brazil. Ann Glob Health 2015; 81(6):735–41. Available at: www.annalsofglobalhealth.org.
81. Disoteo O, Grimaldi F, Papini E, et al. State-of-the-art review on diabetes care in Italy. Ann Glob Health 2015;81(6):803–13. Available at: www.annalsofglobalhealth.org.
82. Fasanmade OA, Dagogo-Jack S. Diabetes care in Nigeria. Ann Glob Health 2015;81(6):821–9. Available at: www.annalsofglobalhealth.org.
83. Nieto-Martínez R, González JP, Lima-Martínez M, et al. Diabetes care in Venezuela. Ann Glob Health 2015;81(6):776–91. Available at: www.annalsofglobalhealth.org.
84. Vargas-Uricoechea H, Casas-Figueroa LÁ. An epidemiologic analysis of diabetes in Colombia. Ann Glob Health 2015;81(6):742–53. Available at: www.annalsofglobalhealth.org.
85. Tan GH. Diabetes care in the Philippines. Ann Glob Health 2015;81(6):863–9. Available at: www.annalsofglobalhealth.org.
86. Noshad S, Afarideh M, Heidari B, et al. Diabetes care in Iran: where we stand and where we are headed. Ann Glob Health 2015;81(6):839–50. Available at: www.annalsofglobalhealth.org.
87. Mechanick JI, Leroith D. Synthesis: deriving a core set of recommendations to optimize diabetes care on a global scale. Ann Glob Health 2015;81(6):874–83.
88. Popkin BM, Udry JR. Adolescent obesity increases significantly in second and third generation U.S. immigrants: the National Longitudinal Study of Adolescent Health. J Nutr 1998;128(4):701–6.
89. Gordon-Larsen P, Harris KM, Ward DS, et al. Acculturation and overweight-related behaviors among Hispanic immigrants to the US: the National Longitudinal Study of Adolescent Health. Soc Sci Med 2003;57(11):2023–34.
90. Gomez SL, Kelsey JL, Glaser SL, et al. Immigration and acculturation in relation to health and health-related risk factors among specific Asian subgroups in a health maintenance organization. Am J Public Health 2004;94(11):1977–84.
91. August KJ, Sorkin DH. Racial/ethnic disparities in exercise and dietary behaviors of middle-aged and older adults. J Gen Intern Med 2011;26(3):245–50.
92. Barcenas CH, Wilkinson AV, Strom SS, et al. Birthplace, years of residence in the United States, and obesity among Mexican-American adults. Obesity (Silver Spring) 2007;15(4):1043–52.
93. Steyn K, Lombard C, Gwebushe N, et al. Implementation of national guidelines, incorporated within structured diabetes and hypertension records at primary level care in Cape Town, South Africa: a randomised controlled trial. Glob Health Action 2013;6:20796.
94. Ena J, Casan R, Lozano T, et al. Long-term improvements in insulin prescribing habits and glycaemic control in medical inpatients associated with the introduction of a standardized educational approach. Diabetes Res Clin Pract 2009; 85(2):159–65.

95. Ciccone MM, Aquilino A, Cortese F, et al. Feasibility and effectiveness of a disease and care management model in the primary health care system for patients with heart failure and diabetes (Project Leonardo). Vasc Health Risk Manag 2010;6:297–305.

96. Kuhne-Eversmann L, Fischer MR. Improving knowledge and changing behavior towards guideline based decisions in diabetes care: a controlled intervention study of a team-based learning approach for continuous professional development of physicians. BMC Res Notes 2013;6:14.

97. Ku GM, Kegels G. Effects of the first line diabetes care (FiLDCare) self-management education and support project on knowledge, attitudes, perceptions, self-management practices and glycaemic control: a quasi-experimental study conducted in the Northern Philippines. BMJ Open 2014;4(8):e005317.

98. Ku GM, Kegels G. Integrating chronic care with primary care activities: enriching healthcare staff knowledge and skills and improving glycemic control of a cohort of people with diabetes through the First Line Diabetes Care Project in the Philippines. Glob Health Action 2014;7:25286.

99. Collins-McNeil J, Edwards CL, Batch BC, et al. A culturally targeted self-management program for African Americans with type 2 diabetes mellitus. Can J Nurs Res 2012;44(4):126–41.

100. Williams E, Curtis A. Implementation of a diabetes management flow sheet in a long-term care setting. Can J Diabetes 2015;39(4):273–7.

101. Bhojani U, Kolsteren P, Criel B, et al. Intervening in the local health system to improve diabetes care: lessons from a health service experiment in a poor urban neighborhood in India. Glob Health Action 2015;8:28762.

102. Bailie R, Si D, Dowden M, et al. Improving organisational systems for diabetes care in Australian Indigenous communities. BMC Health Serv Res 2007;7:67.

103. Shehab A, Elnour A, Abdulle A. A clinical audit on diabetes care in patients with type 2 diabetes in Al-ain, United Arab Emirates. Open Cardiovasc Med J 2012; 6:126–32.

104. Gagliardino JJ, Etchegoyen G. A model educational program for people with type 2 diabetes: a cooperative Latin American implementation study (PED-NID-LA). Diabetes Care 2001;24(6):1001–7.

105. Al-Adsani A, Al-Faraj J, Al-Sultan F, et al. Evaluation of the impact of the Kuwait Diabetes Care Program on the quality of diabetes care. Med Princ Pract 2008; 17(1):14–9.

106. Rothe U, Muller G, Schwarz PE, et al. Evaluation of a diabetes management system based on practice guidelines, integrated care, and continuous quality management in a Federal State of Germany: a population-based approach to health care research. Diabetes Care 2008;31(5):863–8.

107. Hsu CC, Sandford BA. The Delphi technique: making sense of consensus. Pract Assess Res Develop 2007;12:1–8. Available at: http://pareonline.net/getvn.asp?v=12&n=10. Accessed October 12, 2015.

108. Nieto-Martínez R, Hamdy O, Marante D, et al. Transcultural diabetes nutrition algorithm (tDNA): Venezuelan application. Nutrients 2014;6(4):1333–63.

109. Mechanick JI, Marchetti AE, Apovian C, et al. Diabetes-specific nutrition algorithm: a transcultural program to optimize diabetes and prediabetes care. Curr Diab Rep 2012;12(2):180–94.

110. Su HY, Tsang MW, Huang SY, et al. Transculturalization of a diabetes-specific nutrition algorithm: Asian application. Curr Diab Rep 2012;12(2):213–9.

111. Joshi SR, Mohan V, Joshi SS, et al. Transcultural diabetes nutrition therapy algorithm: the Asian Indian application. Curr Diab Rep 2012;12:204–12.

112. Hussein Z, Hamdy O, Chin Chia Y, et al. Transcultural diabetes nutrition algorithm: a Malaysian application. Int J Endocrinol 2013;2013:679396.

113. Gougeon R, Sievenpiper JL, Jenkins D, et al. The transcultural diabetes nutrition algorithm: a Canadian perspective. Int J Endocrinol 2014;2014:151068.

114. Galvis AB, Hamdy O, Pulido ME, et al. Transcultural diabetes nutrition algorithm: the Mexican application. J Diabetes Metab 2014;5(9):1–10.

115. Moura F, Salles J, Hamdy O, et al. Transcultural diabetes nutrition algorithm: Brazilian application. Nutrients 2015;7(9):7358–80.

116. Hamdy O, Marchetti A, Hegazi RA, et al. The transcultural diabetes nutrition algorithm toolkit: survey and content validation in the United States, Mexico, and Taiwan. Diabetes Technol Ther 2014;16(6):378–84.

117. Fixsen D, Naoom S, Blase K, et al. Implementation research: a synthesis of the literature. Tampa (FL): National Implementation Research Network, University of South Florida; 2005.

118. American Psychological Association. Guidelines on multicultural education, training, research, practice, and organizational change for psychologists. Am Psychol 2003;58(5):377–402.

119. Bernal G, Jiménez-Chafey M, Domenech R. Cultural adaptation of treatments: a resource for considering culture in evidence-based practice. Prof Psychol Res Pract 2009;40(4):361.

120. Yoon KH, Lee JH, Kim JW, et al. Epidemic obesity and type 2 diabetes in Asia. Lancet 2006;368(9548):1681–8.

121. Garvey WT, Garber AJ, Mechanick JI, et al. American Association of Clinical Endocrinologists and American College of Endocrinology position statement on the 2014 advanced framework for a new diagnosis of obesity as a chronic disease. Endocr Pract 2014;20(9):977–89.

122. American Diabetes Association. Standards of medical care in Diabetes—2016. Diabetes Care 2016;39(Suppl 1):S1–112.

123. Pan A, Wang Y, Talaei M, et al. Relation of active, passive, and quitting smoking with incident type 2 diabetes: a systematic review and meta-analysis. Lancet Diabetes Endocrinol 2015;3(12):958–67.

124. Axelsson T, Jansson PA, Smith U, et al. Nicotine infusion acutely impairs insulin sensitivity in type 2 diabetic patients but not in healthy subjects. J Intern Med 2001;249(6):539–44.

125. Koppes LL, Dekker JM, Hendriks HF, et al. Moderate alcohol consumption lowers the risk of type 2 diabetes: a meta-analysis of prospective observational studies. Diabetes Care 2005;28(3):719–25.

126. Hivert MF, Vassy JL, Meigs JB. Susceptibility to type 2 diabetes mellitus—from genes to prevention. Nat Rev Endocrinol 2014;10(4):198–205.

127. Field MJ, Lohr KN. Institute of Medicine (US) Committee to Advise the Public Health Service on Clinical Practice Guidelines. Washington (DC): National Academies Press (US); 1990.

128. Bernal G, Bonilla J, Bellido C. Ecological validity and cultural sensitivity for outcome research: issues for the cultural adaptation and development of psychosocial treatments with Hispanics. J Abnorm Child Psychol 1995;23(1):67–82.

129. Gagliardi AR, Brouwers MC, Palda VA, et al. How can we improve guideline use? A conceptual framework of implementability. Implement Sci 2011;6:26.

130. Proctor E, Silmere H, Raghavan R, et al. Outcomes for implementation research: conceptual distinctions, measurement challenges, and research agenda. Adm Policy Ment Health 2011;38(2):65–76.

131. Gaglio B, Shoup JA, Glasgow RE. The RE-AIM framework: a systematic review of use over time. Am J Public Health 2013;103(6):e38–46.

132. Bernal G, Domenech-Rodriguez M. Cultural adaptations: tools for evidence-based practice with diverse populations. Washington, DC: American Psychological Association; 2012.

133. Pronk NP. Designing and evaluating health promotion programs: simple rules for a complex issue. Dis Manag Health Outcomes 2003;11(3):149–57.

134. Juni P, Altman DG, Egger M. Systematic reviews in health care: assessing the quality of controlled clinical trials. BMJ 2001;323(7303):42–6.

135. National Institute for Health and Care Excellence, editor. Developing NICE guidelines: the manual [Internet]. London: National Institute for Health and Care Excellence (NICE); 2015. Process and Methods Guides No. 20. NICE Process and Methods Guides.

136. Paulweber B, Valensi P, Lindstrom J, et al. A European evidence-based guideline for the prevention of type 2 diabetes. Horm Metab Res 2010;42(Suppl 1): S3–36.

137. Handelsman Y, Bloomgarden ZT, Grunberger G, et al. American Association of Clinical Endocrinologists and American College of Endocrinology—clinical practice guidelines for developing a diabetes mellitus comprehensive care plan—2015. Endocr Pract 2015;21(Suppl 1):1–87.

138. Ryden L, Grant PJ, Anker SD, et al. ESC guidelines on diabetes, pre-diabetes, and cardiovascular diseases developed in collaboration with the EASD: the task force on diabetes, pre-diabetes, and cardiovascular diseases of the European Society of Cardiology (ESC) and developed in collaboration with the European Association for the Study of Diabetes (EASD). Eur Heart J 2013;34(39):3035–87.

139. Cheng AY. Canadian Diabetes Association 2013 clinical practice guidelines for the prevention and management of diabetes in Canada. Introduction. Can J Diabetes 2013;37(Suppl 1):S1–3.

140. Elkan AC, Engvall IL, Cederholm T, et al. Rheumatoid cachexia, central obesity and malnutrition in patients with low-active rheumatoid arthritis: feasibility of anthropometry, mini nutritional assessment and body composition techniques. Eur J Nutr 2009;48(5):315–22.

141. Erselcan T, Candan F, Saruhan S, et al. Comparison of body composition analysis methods in clinical routine. Ann Nutr Metab 2000;44(5–6):243–8.

142. Eto C, Komiya S, Nakao T, et al. Validity of the body mass index and fat mass index as an indicator of obesity in children aged 3-5 year. J Physiol Anthropol Appl Human Sci 2004;23(1):25–30.

143. IDF. International Diabetes Federation (IDF). Consensus on type 2 diabetes prevention. 2007. Available at: http://www.idf.org/webdata/docs/IDF_prevention_consensus_DM.pdf. Accessed January 20, 2016.

144. Giorda C, Picariello R, Nada E, et al. The impact of adherence to screening guidelines and of diabetes clinics referral on morbidity and mortality in diabetes. PLoS One 2012;7(4):e33839.

145. Walsh JL, Harris BH, Roberts AW. Evaluation of a community diabetes initiative: integrating diabetes care. Prim Care Diabetes 2015;9(3):203–10.

146. Davies B, Edwards N, Ploeg J, et al. Insights about the process and impact of implementing nursing guidelines on delivery of care in hospitals and community settings. BMC Health Serv Res 2008;8:29.

147. Barcelo A, Cafiero E, de Boer M, et al. Using collaborative learning to improve diabetes care and outcomes: the VIDA project. Prim Care Diabetes 2010;4(3): 145–53.

148. O'Connor PJ, Crain AL, Rush WA, et al. Impact of an electronic medical record on diabetes quality of care. Ann Fam Med 2005;3(4):300–6.
149. Wallgren S, Berry-Caban CS, Bowers L. Impact of clinical pharmacist intervention on diabetes-related outcomes in a military treatment facility. Ann Pharmacother 2012;46(3):353–7.

Evolving to Personalized Medicine for Type 2 Diabetes

S. Sethu K. Reddy, MD, MBA, FRCPC, MACE

KEYWORDS

- Personalized • Precision • Diabetes • Big data • Genomics • Proteomics

KEY POINTS

- Type 2 diabetes is an expensive public health problem that threatens our society at many levels.
- Precision medicine applies not only to medical interventions but also to psychosocial measures, nutrition, and exercise that may also affect individuals differently.
- Using this highly personalized approach, one hopes to achieve better outcomes, more effectively.
- The striking evolution in generating "Big Data," Bio-marker Fingerprints, and the Internet of Things will force all clinicians to be familiar with the terminology and understand the clinical relevance.

To imagine potential future treatment options for type 2 diabetes (T2DM), one must understand past approaches to management. Therapies have been based on traditional herbal therapies to accidental discoveries and more recently based on understanding of the underlying pathophysiology of T2DM. Thus, there is predictable innovation, but we must also be ready to accept disruptive innovation as well. In this brief overview, potential treatments in the near horizon are discussed and also precision medicine approaches and novel disruptive techniques that the clinician needs to be familiar with.

TYPE 2 DIABETES MELLITUS

T2DM accounts for about 85% of the nearly 30 million[1] individuals with diabetes in the United States.[2] Hyperglycemia, the hallmark of diagnosis of diabetes, results after years to decades of dysfunctional physiology of insulin secretion and insulin action. The challenge has been akin to treating a patient with aortic

The author has no relevant conflicts of interest.
Endocrinology, Diabetes & Metabolism, F20, Cleveland Clinic, 9500 Euclid Avenue, Cleveland, OH 44195, USA
E-mail address: sethu.k.reddy@gmail.com

regurgitation and heart failure today instead of treating the patient 20 years earlier for aortic stenosis.

Current Treatments

There have been several excellent summaries of evidence-based approaches to using approved medications for T2DM (American Association of Clinical Endocrinologists and American Diabetes Association/European Association for the Study of Diabetes[3]). These statements have evolved to a shared vision of glycemic targets and the need for an individualized approach. The mantra, "the right medication for the right patient at the right time," is still a universal goal of all practitioners.

The management of hyperglycemia is limited by the occurrence of hypoglycemia. Treatment options can be considered as either hypoglycemic or nonhypoglycemic antihyperglycemic therapies. Because euglycemia is an impractical target, we are generally advised to aim for glycemic targets that are safe for the individual.

Customized Approaches to Diabetes Management

Even though the distinction between at least 2 types of diabetes was made centuries ago, the discovery of insulin in 1921 led to a therapy-based differentiation: IDDM, insulin-dependent diabetes mellitus, and NIDDM, non-insulin-dependent diabetes mellitus. In the former, insulin was absolutely critical for maintaining life, whereas, in the latter, lifestyle measures and oral agents may control the hyperglycemia for many years. Of course, the age of onset appeared different, and thus, IDDM was always synonymous with juvenile diabetes and NIDDM was often called adult-onset diabetes mellitus. This distinction led to a variety of clinical approaches.

In the 1980s, the nomenclature was updated to the labels of Type 1 Diabetes Mellitus and Type 2 Diabetes Mellitus, indicating a specific pathophysiology underlying the conditions. This etiologic classification led to active research into immunoregulatory approaches to Type 1 Diabetes Mellitus and clearer recruitment of subjects for clinical research (**Table 1**).

Although this nomenclature has served well for the last 30 years, it was apparent very early on that there are other types of diabetes that do not neatly fit into a predetermined category.

Table 1
Features of type 1 versus type 2 diabetes mellitus

Feature	Type 1	Type 2
Prevalence (%)	0.4	6.6
Annual incidence in United States	15,000	500,000
Ketosis prone	++++	+
Anti-islet cell antibody	+++	−
Anti-GAD antibody	++++	−
Prevalence of other autoimmune conditions	+++	−
Usual age of onset (y)	<30	>40
Prevalence of obesity	+	++++
Family history	+	++++
HLA linkage	DR3, DR4	−
DQ β-polymorphism	++	−

SECONDARY DIABETES MELLITUS AND DIABETES DUE TO PANCREATIC DESTRUCTION

An early consideration for an individualized approach to management was in treating diabetes from other causes than those of typical types 1 and 2 DM. Secondary DM[4] may present in individuals with the following conditions:

- Chronic pancreatitis
- Cystic fibrosis
- Hemochromatosis
- Pancreatectomy

Conditions associated with elevated counterregulatory hormones—pheochromo-cytoma, acromegaly, and Cushing syndrome—may also precipitate DM. Drugs may also cause hyperglycemia; these include glucocorticoids, thiazide diuretics, phenytoin (Dilantin), interferon-α, pentamidine (Pentam 300 or NebuPent), and diazoxide (Proglycem or Hyperstat I.V.) Anti-retroviral agents and high-dose statins have also been linked to the development of hyperglycemia.

Many of the secondary causes of DM have other associated comorbidities, such as malabsorption with chronic pancreatitis, cystic fibrosis, and with near-total pancreatectomy. In addition to insulin deficiency, patients may also have glucagon deficiency, which could result in brittle diabetes. Hemochromatosis should encourage the search for other manifestations, both endocrine and nonendocrine, of this systemic disorder. Of all the medication-induced causes of hyperglycemia, steroid-induced hyperglycemia is by far the most prevalent and the most challenging. The pathophysiology is neither type 1 nor classical T2DM. Abnormalities in insulin secretion as well as insulin action have been described. Clinically, patients on oral steroid regimens often present with relatively normal fasting glycemia but with profound postprandial hyperglycemia. Because of the severity of patients' primary condition, appropriately timed insulin therapy is often the best choice.

Certainly, these scenarios call for a patient-centric approach as opposed to a "cookie-cutter" approach for types 1 or 2 DM. An increasingly common occurrence is the development of T2DM among adolescents, who are reflexively treated as type 1 DM. Occasionally, a lean elderly individual may develop type 1 DM and be reflexively treated as T2DM.

COSTS OF DIABETES MELLITUS: MORBIDITY

As the prevalence of T2DM approaches 30 million individuals in the United States, the downstream costs of diabetes could be overwhelming.[5] The prognosis for an individual with T2DM may be affected by the following:

- Inherent background morbidity pattern of the nondiabetic in his or her population
- Competing risks
- Pattern of risk factors
- Quality and quantity of available health care
- Possible differences in cause of the patient's T2DM

More than 10 studies have documented an excess mortality in T2DM; several studies have estimated a 5- to 10-year loss in life expectancy in patients older than 40 years. DM is the leading cause of blindness in adults 25 to 74 years old in Europe and North America. Women appear to be predisposed to retinopathy, and blacks appear to be at more risk than whites. DM also is the leading cause of end-stage renal disease, which also has major implications for a patient's quality of life. DM, which also may have an adverse effect on productivity, leads to a greater use of health care resources. The direct and indirect costs of DM are extremely high. In the United States, it has been estimated that DM care costs more than $100 billion per year, with patients with DM requiring 2 to 3 times the cost of health care of individuals without DM.

A careful medical history must always be obtained to assess the risk of DM. It should include the use of the following medications that adversely affect glucose tolerance:

- Diazoxide
- Furosemide (Lasix)
- Thiazides
- Glucocorticoids
- Oral contraceptives
- Adrenaline
- Isoproterenol (Isuprel)
- Nicotinic acid
- High-dose statins
- Anti-retroviral therapy for human immunodeficiency virus (HIV)
- Phenytoin (Dilantin)
- Tacrolimus
- Cyclosporin

If necessary, these medications may need to be withdrawn (if possible).

Toward Precision Medicine

Advances in medicine, in particular, in oncology and developments in diagnostic technology in the fields of genomics,[6] proteomics, and metabolomics,[7] have led to an explosion of knowledge about disease cause and responsiveness to medications and natural history. This has led to the development of personalized medicine, or as more recently termed, precision medicine.[8]

Table 2 illustrates one potential concept of personalized medicine applied to the natural history of T2DM. On the x-axis, the various stages of diabetes are depicted.

Table 2
A wholistic view of the concept of personalized medicine as applied to diabetes mellitus

	Stages of Disease				
"FingerPrint"	Prevention	Prediabetes/ Metabolic Syndrome	Diagnosis	Ongoing Management	Complications of Diabetes
Genomic Proteomic Metabolomic	Predictor of condition, response to treatment, likelihood of adverse events to interventions, likelihood of complications and comorbidities				
Phenotypic	Clinical differentiation of T2DM into various subtypes; correlation with biomarkers				
	Personalized care delivery plans				
	Big data and clinical research and analytics				
	Self-care to coach, to peer-to-peer, to community				
Socioeconomic	Living situation, access to medical care and medications, access to community				
	Adherence; social safety net				
Epigenetic	Interaction of environment and genotype				
	Risk management/sharing				

On the y-axis are some potential means to "fingerprint" the patient with respect to the specific nature of one's diabetes. Rather than just the label of "type 2 diabetes," by using the techniques of genomics, proteomics, and metabolomics, one might determine the exact cause(s) of diabetes as well as the likelihood of developing long-term complications of diabetes. One might also be able to determine the chances of a drug being effective as well as the potential risk of drug-related adverse events.

The clinician could build on this type of data by assessing other important health variables, such as patient's clinical features, response to diet or exercise, and the presence of a support network. A comprehensive assessment of patient's social safety net, understanding his/her condition, is as important as the biological variables.

Finally, the field of epigenetics is still in its infancy, but the interaction between environment and genetic factors could be a major influence on disease progression.

Personalized medicine could use these approaches for any condition, including diabetes.

The US Government sponsored a key National Institutes of Health initiative in precision medicine that hopes to advance the oncology field initially, but certainly other chronic conditions, like diabetes and heart failure, are also in the scope.[9]

The other area in which there has been a paradigm shift in drug discovery is a novel nonpathophysiologic approach that holds much promise for truly customized, innovative therapies. The confluence of the ability to analyze vast health data sets[10] (Big Data) as well as a variety of social sources (the Internet of Things) promises to add another layer of context to biological factors.

The traditional approach has been to study a disease in depth, in both animal and clinical models, find a dysfunctional metabolic pathway, and then discover a targeted therapy to correct the defect. This approach takes decades to progress and is dependent on disease experts and follows a neat, logical path. It takes typically 15 years or more for a potential drug to be fully tested and then approved by the US Food and Drug Administration (FDA).

The new approach to drug discovery does not require disease expertise per se but requires access to vast sets of biological samples from both control and affected cohorts with concomitant clinical phenotypic data as well. This approach, if successful, can take years rather than decades and a therapeutic intervention for an unpredicted target may come to fruition more quickly.

In the remainder of this article, these 2 areas are reviewed, as related to diabetes.

Pharmacogenomics

Pharmacogenomics, the study of the relationship of genetic attributes to drug metabolism and drug effects, can help identify responders and tolerability.

- Drug exposure and clinical response variability
- Risk for adverse events
- Genotype-specific dosing
- Mechanisms of drug action
- Polymorphic drug target and disposition genes

Many medications are metabolized by the cytochrome P450 system in hepatic mitochondria. An assessment of the cytochrome P450 system of genetic variability may help predict potential chances for toxicity.

When such data are included in the label for a drug, one can theoretically screen an eligible patient for a particular genetic trait, which may predict response or potential for adverse events and thus exclusion from taking the medication. Thus, this information can help direct a clinical decision.

As an example, one should avoid sulfonylurea if a patient has glucose-6-phosphate dehydrogenase deficiency because this may lead to hemolytic anemia.

More recent examples are human monoclonal antibodies for proprotein convertase subtilisin-kexin type 9 inhibitors, which can reduce low-density lipoprotein (LDL)-cholesterol levels by up to 60% in those with LDL receptor mutations (familial hyper-cholesterolemia).[11] These patients do not respond to statin therapy. Therefore, one could envision genetic testing to confirm the genotype before initiating this expensive regimen.

Everyone is familiar with warfarin. Several genetic variants impact on warfarin dosing and the likelihood of bleeding side effects. The *CYP2C9* gene encodes one of the main enzymes responsible for metabolizing warfarin. If a certain *CYP2C9* allele is associated with reduced enzyme activity and lower clearance rates of warfarin, the clinician would start with a lower dose of warfarin.[12]

Most of the scenarios using pharmacogenomics involve oncology. In oncology, because the treatments are often both expensive and toxic, it is critical to avoid major side effects and to have a predictably favorable response to therapy.

With diabetes,[13] because medications are generally safer and work faster than those for cancer, a clinician is more likely to test the medication clinically to see if the patient responds, and so forth. This different philosophy has an impact on drug pricing. If a medication is proven to be very effective in a small, identifiable niche cohort, before FDA approval, then the medication is likely to be quite expensive. On the other hand, if the medication can be used in almost all patients with a condition, then the price is likely to be more modest. This type of scenario has an impact on when the manufacturer conducts pharmacogenomics studies in the life cycle of a drug.

Recent work from the Icahn School of Medicine at Mt. Sinai in New York[14] analyzed electronic medical records (EMRs) and genotype data for more than 11,000 patients. Patients were grouped into 3 distinct subtypes based on the EMR data (1: more likely to have nephropathy and retinopathy; 2: more likely to have cancer or cardiovascular disease; and 3: neurologic disease, allergies, or HIV). Subsequently, genomic single-nucleotide polymorphism analysis was performed, and there appeared to be cluster-specific genetic variants in hundreds of genes. More studies with more correlation of biomarkers with the clinical phenotypic markers are necessary to develop a useful subcategorization of T2DM.

Sulfonylureas (SFU) have been used in practice for more than 75 years, but in the recent past, an interesting scenario of diabetes in infants has been found to be responsive to SFU. In these particular cases, the potassium inwardly rectifying channel, subfamily J, member 11 (*KCJN11*), a site of action for SFU, was associated with T2DM.[15] Variation in this locus affected the response to sulfonylurea in 1268 patients[16] as measured by fasting glucose and HbA1c. It has been suggested that transcription factor 7-like 2 (*TCF7L2*) is also associated with variation in the insulin secretory response to GLP-115 and with change in HbA1c after the initiation of SFU.[17]

Genome Wide Association Studies (Caveat: P-Values do not Imply Causality)

In the last 20 years, more than 150 genetic variants have been statistically found to be linked to a higher chance of T2DM.[18] Although this is exciting news, it is premature to say that any one of them will be highly predictive of developing T2DM. Studying genetic association in groups of patients numbering in the thousands provides huge statistical power but may not necessarily point to clinically significant results.[19]

The first candidate gene reproducibly associated with T2DM was *PPARG*, encoding the nuclear receptor PPAR-γ.[20] The PPAR-γ receptor is a nuclear target for thiazolidinediones. This variant (transcript expressed in adipose tissue has an extra exon B and a substitution of a proline for alanine at position 12 of this protein, which is seen in about 15% of the European population) has been shown to be associated with increased adiponectin levels, increased insulin sensitivity, and reduced likelihood of developing T2DM.

It is difficult to make sense of the entire long list of all of the genetic variants associated with T2DM, but a key summative observation must be noted. Of the genetic variants with T2DM that have been described, more than 80% are related to insulin molecule or insulin secretion. Very few variants have been associated with insulin resistance.

A Hopeful Glimpse into the Future

What is a clinician to do? As the clinician is bombarded with another genetic association with a particular condition, almost on a weekly basis, a question to ask might be, is there any physiologic relevance to any of these findings?

It has been well known that different polymorphisms in the fat-mass and obesity-associated gene (FTO) have been strongly associated with traits related to obesity and metabolic syndrome. Claussnitzer and colleagues[21] from the Broad Institute, Boston, by using advances in genomic technology, were able to determine that a particular FTO variant influenced mitochondrial respiration and adipocyte browning. The investigators were thus able to link the genetic variant to a biological cause for adipocyte differentiation and the development of obesity.

Epigenetics

Without modifying the DNA sequence itself, methylation of DNA, posttranslational acetylation/de-acetylation of histones, or activation of microRNAs can lead to epigenetic changes that can affect the phenotype.

It is premature to describe any definitive data of causality to T2DM, but some have suggested that epigenetic mechanisms may impact glucotoxicity in islets and/or progression of diabetic complications.[22]

Epigenetics may play a role in what is called "metabolic memory" or the "legacy effect." Periods of good metabolic control and histone modification in endothelial cells may be associated with downstream protection from diabetic complications many decades later, as evidenced by the UKPDS (United Kingdom Prospective Diabetes Study) and DCCT (Diabetes Control and Complications Trial) studies.[23]

Future Drugs for Diabetes and Beyond

The traditional formula for drug discovery was discussed, but a tantalizing approach is to leverage systems biology[24] and enhanced information technology; data analytics involves clinicians, epidemiologists, statisticians, and pharmacologists proficient in computer-aided design.

Instead of many years of studying diabetes and identifying a viable target related to the pathophysiology of diabetes, the modern discovery team has no preconceived notion on where the answer may lie.

Step 1. Determine a genomic, proteomic, and/or metabolomic "fingerprint" of the condition of interest. One can generate a profile of control subjects as well as those with the condition and do a subtraction analysis. The difference in the patterns then would represent the pattern associated with diabetes. The condition may be associated with genes that are turned "on" as well as genes that are turned "off."

A similar approach could be applied to proteomic and metabolomics data as well.

Step 2. Performing a "social network" analysis of the data may also point to which of all these variables are key nodes (important).

Step 3. Because this is an open-ended query for key associated variables, there may be surprise targets that become evident.

Note that to engage in this type of discovery process, there is no prerequisite for deep pathophysiologic knowledge of diabetes.

Step 4. Exposing patients or cells to potential therapies and examining the resulting "fingerprint" genomic-proteomic-metabolomic profile to see if it matches or overlays with the disease "fingerprint." A good fit might indicate that that particular agent may be effective.

As one can imagine, this process would take far less time. There are already case studies of specific antibiotic therapy based on the characteristics of the pathogen. In the future, one can envision a precision medicine that is both safe and effective in a small, specific population. It is likely the costs for the development of such treatments would be exponentially less than the current cost of a typical development program (more than 1 billion dollars).

Beyond Biomarkers

Although determining the patient's genomic, proteomic, and metabolomics profile should lead to the best medicine for the right patient, psychosocial determinants may be equally important.[25]

Knowing the patient's social situation and the quality of his/her social safety net is critical. The individual's physical activity, mental status, shopping habits, and adherence to medication regimens are also important factors in achieving healthy outcomes.

We have come to realize that diabetes is not a quarterly condition that only shows up when the patient seeks medical attention; in an ideal world, the patient needs daily assistance/coaching/oversight. Although this is physically impossible to offer to all patients, refinements and advances in digital technology may be able to offer scalable solutions.

The Internet of Things is a reality.[26] As medical, biological, and social data are connected, one can derive more precise, contextual conclusions and recommendations.

SUMMARY

T2DM is an expensive public health problem that threatens our society at many levels. There are many therapeutic options in 2016, but we can perform even better.

Precision medicine will be increasingly part of the regular practice in the future. It behooves us to be aware of the need to subcategorize T2DM to subgroups that can direct the clinician to find the most effective and safe therapeutic regimen. Precision medicine applies not only to medical interventions but also to psychosocial measures, nutrition, and exercise that may also affect individuals differently.

Using this highly personalized approach, one hopes to achieve better outcomes, more effectively. There are also rapid changes occurring that necessitate all clinicians to be aware of systems biology and its potential of innovative drug discovery.

The striking evolution in generating "Big Data," bio-marker fingerprints, and the Internet of Things will force all clinicians to be familiar with the terminology and understand the clinical relevance. Increasingly, these topics are being reviewed by primary care journals, and although considered esoteric a few years ago, in 2016, all physicians should be familiar with the terminology and approaches to personalized medicine.

REFERENCES

1. Garber AJ, Abrahamson MJ, Barzilay JI, et al. American Association of Clinical Endocrinologists/American College of Endocrinology' comprehensive diabetes management algorithm 2015. Endocr Pract 2015;21:e1–10.

2. Centers for Disease Control and Prevention. National diabetes statistics report: estimates of diabetes and its burden in the United States, 2014. Atlanta: US Department of Health and Human Services; 2014.

3. Inzucchi SE, Bergenstal RM, Buse JB, et al. Management of hyperglycemia in type 2 diabetes, 2015: a patient-centered approach. Update to a position statement of the American Diabetes Association and the European Association for the Study of Diabetes. Diabetes Care 2015;38:140–9.

4. Reddy SSK, Zimmerman R. Diabetes mellitus: control and complications. In: Stoller JK, Michota F, Mandell B, editors. Chapter 42 intensive review of internal medicine. Wolters Kluwer; 2015. p. 500–16.

5. American Diabetes Association. Economic costs of diabetes in the US in 2012. Diabetes Care 2013;36:1033–46.

6. McCarthy MI. Genomic medicine at the heart of diabetes management. Diabetologia 2015;58:1725–9.

7. Walford GA, Porneala BC, Dauriz M, et al. Metabolite traits and genetic risk provide complementary information for the prediction of future type 2 diabetes. Diabetes Care 2014;37:2508–14.

8. Hamburg MA, Collins FS. The path to personalized medicine. N Engl J Med 2010; 363:301–4 [Erratum appears in N Engl J Med 2010;363:1092].

9. Collins FS. Exceptional opportunities in medical science: a view from the National Institutes of Health. JAMA 2015;313:131–2.

10. Billings LK, Florez JC. The genetics of type 2 diabetes: what have we learned from GWAS? Ann N Y Acad Sci 2010;1212:59–77.

11. Raal FJ, Honorpour N, Blom, et al. Inhibition of PCSK9 with evolocumab in homozygous familial hypercholesterolemia (TESLA part B): a randomized, double-blind, placebo-controlled trial. Lancet 2014;385(9965):341–50. Available at: http://www.thelancet.com.

12. Dean L. Warfarin therapy and the genotypes CYP2C9 and VKORC1. Bethesda (MD): National Center for Biotechnology Information (US); 2012. Medical Genetics Summaries [Internet]. Available at: http://www.ncbi.nlm.nih.gov/books/NBK84174/.

13. Moore AF, Florez JC. Genetic susceptibility to type 2 diabetes and implications for antidiabetic therapy. Annu Rev Med 2008;59:95–111.

14. Li L, Cheng WY, Glicksberg BS, et al. Identification of type 2 diabetes subgroups through topological analysis of patient similarity. Sci Transl Med 2015;7:311ra174.

15. Gloyn AL, Weedon MN, Owen KR, et al. Large-scale association studies of variants in genes encoding the pancreatic beta-cell KATP channel subunits Kir6.2 (KCNJ11) and SUR1 (ABCC8) confirm that the KCNJ11 E23K variant is associated with type 2 diabetes. Diabetes 2003;52(2):568–72.

16. Feng Y, Mao G, Ren X, et al. Ser1369Ala variant in sulfonylurea receptor gene ABCC8 is associated with antidiabetic efficacy of gliclazide in Chinese type 2 diabetic patients. Diabetes Care 2008;31(10):1939–44.

17. Schäfer SA, Tschritter O, Machicao F, et al. Impaired glucagon-like peptide-1-induced insulin secretion in carriers of transcription factor 7-like 2 (TCF7L2) gene polymorphisms. Diabetologia 2007;50(12):2443–50.

18. Prasad RB, Groop L. Genetics of type 2 diabetes-pitfalls and possibilities. Genes 2015;6:87–123.

19. Vella A. Pharmacogenetics for type 2 diabetes: practical considerations for study design. J Diabetes Sci Technol 2009;3(4):705–9.

20. Altshuler D, Hirschhorn JN, Klannemark M, et al. The common PPARgamma Pro12Ala polymorphism is associated with decreased risk of type 2 diabetes. Nat Genet 2000;26(1):76–80.

21. Claussnitzer M, Dankel SN, Kim KH, et al. *FTO* obesity variant circuitry and adipocyte browning in humans. N Engl J Med 2015;373:895–907.

22. Kato M, Natarajan R. Diabetic nephropathy—emerging epigenetic mechanisms. Nat Rev Nephrol 2014;10:517–30.

23. Brasacchio D, Okabe J, Tikellis C, et al. Hyperglycemia induces a dynamic co-operativity of histone methylase and demethylase enzymes associated with gene-activating epigenetic marks that coexist on the lysine tail. Diabetes 2009; 58:1229–36.

24. Zhu J, Zhang B, Schadt EE. A systems biology approach to drug discovery. Adv Genet 2008;60:603–35.

25. Hill J, Nielsen M, Fox MH. Understanding the social factors that contribute to diabetes: a means to informing health care and social policies for the chronically ill. Perm J 2013;17(2):67–72.

26. Jara AJ, Zamora MA, Skarmeta AFG. An internet of things-based personal device for diabetes therapy management in ambient assisted living (AAL). Pers Ubiquit Comput 2011;15:431–40.

Index

Note: Page numbers of article titles are in **boldface** type.

A

A1C, in diabetes, CGM impact on, 896–898
    decrease of, with metformin vs. other glucose-lowering drugs, 821–822
    inpatient diabetes management and, in noncritically ill patients, 876, 878–879
    insulin therapy and, 853, 858–864
    islet cell transplantation effect on, 925
    mobile medical applications and, 944, 960–961, 963
    nutrition and, 800, 806, 808
    population management and, 934, 936, 938
        global, 989
    post-bariatric surgery, 914–915
  in NASH, 771, 773
  in prediabetes, 751–752, 757
    treatment of, 758
  in T2DM, genotype data analysis of, 1016
  weight loss effect on, 907–908
ABPAT2 gene, in CGL, 786–787
Access to care, patient, in diabetes population management, 935
Accountable care organizations, for diabetes population management, 935–936
Accu-Chek Aviva Expert (Roche) mobile application, for diabetes management, 948, 951
    discussion on, 960–963
    overview of, 958
    study results on, 952, 956
Accu-Chek Connect (Roche) mobile application, for diabetes management, 948, 951
    discussion on, 960–963
    overview of, 958
Acculturation, in transcultural endocrinology, for T2DM, 969
Acquired generalized lipodystrophy (AGL), 784, 788, 790
  subtype classification of, 790
Acquired lipodystrophies, 784, 788, 790–792
  generalized, 784, 788, 790
  HAART-induced, 784, 790–791
  localized, 784, 791–792
  main types of, 784
  partial, 784, 790, 793
  treatment of, 791–794
Acquired partial lipodystrophy, 784, 790, 793
Acromegaly, diabetes related to, 1013
ADA. See *American Diabetes Association (ADA); American Dietetic Association (ADA).*
Adipocytokines, in lipodystrophies, 784
  in T2DM with obesity, 906–907
Adiponectin, in lipodystrophies, 784

Endocrinol Metab Clin N Am 45 (2016) 1021–1058
http://dx.doi.org/10.1016/S0889-8529(16)30115-3
0889-8529/16/$ – see front matter

endo.theclinics.com

C

UNITED STATES POSTAL SERVICE

Statement of Ownership, Management, and Circulation
(All Periodicals Publications Except Requester Publications)

1. Publication Title
ENDOCRINOLOGY AND METABOLISM CLINICS OF NORTH AMERICA

2. Publication Number
000 – 275

3. Filing Date
9/18/2016

4. Issue Frequency
MAR, JUN, SEP, DEC

5. Number of Issues Published Annually
4

6. Annual Subscription Price
$313.00

7. Complete Mailing Address of Known Office of Publication (Not printer) (Street, city, county, state, and ZIP+4®)
ELSEVIER INC.
360 PARK AVENUE SOUTH
NEW YORK, NY 10010-1710

Contact Person
STEPHEN R. BUSHING

Telephone (Include area code)
215-239-3688

8. Complete Mailing Address of Headquarters or General Business Office of Publisher (Not printer)
ELSEVIER INC.
360 PARK AVENUE SOUTH
NEW YORK, NY 10010-1710

9. Full Names and Complete Mailing Addresses of Publisher, Editor, and Managing Editor (Do not leave blank)

Publisher (Name and complete mailing address)
ADRIANNE BRIGIDO, ELSEVIER INC.
1600 JOHN F KENNEDY BLVD. SUITE 1800
PHILADELPHIA, PA 19103-2899

Editor (Name and complete mailing address)
LAUREN BOYLE, ELSEVIER INC.
1600 JOHN F KENNEDY BLVD. SUITE 1800
PHILADELPHIA, PA 19103-2899

Managing Editor (Name and complete mailing address)
PATRICK MANLEY, ELSEVIER INC.
1600 JOHN F KENNEDY BLVD. SUITE 1800
PHILADELPHIA, PA 19103-2899

10. Owner (Do not leave blank. If the publication is owned by a corporation, give the name and address of the corporation immediately followed by the names and addresses of all stockholders owning or holding 1 percent or more of the total amount of stock. If not owned by a corporation, give the names and addresses of the individual owners. If owned by a partnership or other unincorporated firm, give its name and address as well as those of each individual owner. If the publication is published by a nonprofit organization, give its name and address.)

Full Name	Complete Mailing Address
WHOLLY OWNED SUBSIDIARY OF REED/ELSEVIER, US HOLDINGS	1600 JOHN F KENNEDY BLVD. SUITE 1800 PHILADELPHIA, PA 19103-2899

11. Known Bondholders, Mortgagees, and Other Security Holders Owning or Holding 1 Percent or More of Total Amount of Bonds, Mortgages, or Other Securities. If none, check box ▶ ☐ None

Full Name	Complete Mailing Address
N/A	

12. Tax Status (For completion by nonprofit organizations authorized to mail at nonprofit rates) (Check one)
The purpose, function, and nonprofit status of this organization and the exempt status for federal income tax purposes:
☐ Has Not Changed During Preceding 12 Months
☐ Has Changed During Preceding 12 Months (Publisher must submit explanation of change with this statement)

13. Publication Title
ENDOCRINOLOGY AND METABOLISM CLINICS OF NORTH AMERICA

14. Issue Date for Circulation Data Below

PS Form **3526**, July 2014 [Page 1 of 4 (see instructions page 4)] PSN: 7530-01-000-9931 PRIVACY NOTICE: See our privacy policy on www.usps.com.

---

15. Extent and Nature of Circulation

		Average No. Copies Each Issue During Preceding 12 Months	No. Copies of Single Issue Published Nearest to Filing Date
a. Total Number of Copies (Net press run)			
b. Paid Circulation (By Mail and Outside the Mail)	(1) Mailed Outside-County Paid Subscriptions Stated on PS Form 3541 (Include paid distribution above nominal rate, advertiser's proof copies, and exchange copies)		
	(2) Mailed In-County Paid Subscriptions Stated on PS Form 3541 (Include paid distribution above nominal rate, advertiser's proof copies, and exchange copies)		
	(3) Paid Distribution Outside the Mails Including Sales Through Dealers and Carriers, Street Vendors, Counter Sales, and Other Paid Distribution Outside USPS®		
	(4) Paid Distribution by Other Classes of Mail Through the USPS (e.g., First-Class Mail®)		
c. Total Paid Distribution (Sum of 15b (1), (2), (3), and (4))	▶		
d. Free or Nominal Rate Distribution (By Mail and Outside the Mail)	(1) Free or Nominal Rate Outside-County Copies included on PS Form 3541		
	(2) Free or Nominal Rate In-County Copies Included on PS Form 3541		
	(3) Free or Nominal Rate Copies Mailed at Other Classes Through the USPS (e.g., First-Class Mail)		
	(4) Free or Nominal Rate Distribution Outside the Mail (Carriers or other means)		
e. Total Free or Nominal Rate Distribution (Sum of 15d (1), (2), (3) and (4))	▶		
f. Total Distribution (Sum of 15c and 15e)	▶		
g. Copies not Distributed (See Instructions to Publishers #4 (page #3))	▶		
h. Total (Sum of 15f and g)	▶		
i. Percent Paid (15c divided by 15f times 100)	▶		

* If you are claiming electronic copies, go to line 16 on page 3. If you are not claiming electronic copies, skip to line 17 on page 3.

16. Electronic Copy Circulation

	Average No. Copies Each Issue During Preceding 12 Months	No. Copies of Single Issue Published Nearest to Filing Date
a. Paid Electronic Copies	▶	
b. Total Paid Print Copies (Line 15c) + Paid Electronic Copies (Line 16a)	▶	
c. Total Print Distribution (Line 15f) + Paid Electronic Copies (Line 16a)	▶	
d. Percent Paid (Both Print & Electronic Copies) (16b divided by 16c × 100)	▶	

☐ I certify that 50% of all my distributed copies (electronic and print) are paid above a nominal price.

17. Publication of Statement of Ownership
☒ If the publication is a general publication, publication of this statement is required. Will be printed in the DECEMBER 2016 issue of this publication. ☐ Publication not required.

18. Signature and Title of Editor, Publisher, Business Manager, or Owner

STEPHEN R. BUSHING - INVENTORY DISTRIBUTION CONTROL MANAGER

[signature] Stephen R. Bushing

Date 9/18/2016

I certify that all information furnished on this form is true and complete. I understand that anyone who furnishes false or misleading information on this form or who omits material or information requested on the form may be subject to criminal sanctions (including fines and imprisonment) and/or civil sanctions (including civil penalties).

PS Form **3526**, July 2014 (Page 3 of 4) PRIVACY NOTICE: See our privacy policy on www.usps.com.

Moving?

Make sure your subscription moves with you!

To notify us of your new address, find your **Clinics Account Number** (located on your mailing label above your name), and contact customer service at:

Email: **journalscustomerservice-usa@elsevier.com**

800-654-2452 (subscribers in the U.S. & Canada)
314-447-8871 (subscribers outside of the U.S. & Canada)

Fax number: **314-447-8029**

Elsevier Health Sciences Division
Subscription Customer Service
3251 Riverport Lane
Maryland Heights, MO 63043

*To ensure uninterrupted delivery of your subscription, please notify us at least 4 weeks in advance of move.

Printed and bound by CPI Group (UK) Ltd, Croydon, CR0 4YY

08/05/2025

01864696-0004